PHARMACOLOGY EXAMS EXPERT CRACKER

PHARMACOLOGY EXAMS EXPERT CRACKER

PHARMACOLOGY EXAMS EXPERT CRACKER

Dr. Jagadish Prasad

Formerly Professor and Head
Department of Pharmacology
Osmania Medical College
Hyderabad-Telangana

PharmaMed Press

An imprint of BSP Books Pvt. Ltd.
4-4-309/316, Giriraj Lane,
Sultan Bazar, Hyderabad - 500 095.

Pharmacology Exams Expert Cracker
by Dr. Jagadish Prasad

Published by:

PharmaMed Press
An imprint of BSP Books Pvt. Ltd.
4-4-309/316, Giriraj Lane, Sultan Bazar, Hyderabad - 500 095.
Phone: 040-23445688; Fax: 91+40-23445611
e-mail: info@pharmamedpress.com
www.pharmamedpress.com/pharmamedpress.net

ISBN: 978-93-48734-90-7 (Hardback)

Preface

"Today one might be at door steps, tomorrow can reach greater heights and soon to reach great peaks. It is the great endeavour, patience, and committed work that makes all the difference to reach one's goal and find a place of distinction in the peer circles and recognition by the valued teachers"

Author

Pharmacology is a distinct discipline and offers core knowledge to broaden student programs in the provision of health care (medicine, pharmacy, nursing and related subjects) as well as research-oriented programs. Therefore, knowledge and information on core pharmacology topics, prescription medication, drug interactions, dosage adjustments, and correct dosage calculation for the medicine are essential for preventing and reducing medication errors, which is a key element to the patient. Moreover, Pharmacology is a demanding interdisciplinary subject requiring fairly good knowledge and skills from the entry level into the medical field and to a later stage of super speciality of any branch in medicine.

Conventionally Pharmacology is taught and followed through text books and other study material which offer a sound knowledge of the subject. However, it is also essential for one to get prepared on sound footing for the evaluation and assessments at the end of the study period and also during the study period. In this book an effort is made to meet the requirements of pharmacology students who are preparing for a forthcoming university examination with more confidence and commitment. The curriculum suggested by National medical commission and Pharmacy council of India are followed in the preparation of the book with more attention for written examination, MCQs, Viva voce, clinical case studies, prescription writing and correction of a given prescription. However, more additions are also made which include descriptive advanced topics in the form of review articles and recent advances in Pharmacology to provide an overall relevant and up-to-date information in the subject. All the topics covered in the book are clinically oriented to serve the best on hand information in all branches of pharmacology related courses.

- Jagadish Prasad

Acknowledgements

In the process of executing the work for this book, a well-planned and well thought out process was made with a balanced and accurate coverage of the subject with merits and which meets the requirements of the students. This enables the student to easily grasp the subject and to recollect and recall at the time of preparation for various internal as well for the final university examinations. Every effort is made to include and cover the entire subject of Pharmacology to the maximum possible extent in different categories present in the book.

In my effort to undertake the job I sincerely thank Mr. Anil Shah, Mr. Nikhil Shah and Mr. Naresh Davergave, Mrs. Rajitha of BSP Books Pvt. Ltd. who gave their consent to proceed with the work. I thank them for their nice gesture. I appreciate the inspiration, encouragement and cooperation extended by my wife Kameswari whose invaluable services at home facilitated me to get the work done most peacefully and successfully. I also have great pleasure and appreciation for the services rendered by my grandchildren Sishir, Suchir Shreyas and Shriya who helped me greatly in the data processing, compiling, editing and for giving a final shape to the book. I have great pleasure in complimenting my assistant Naveen Kumar whose services for the past many years helped me to complete my job through his periodical and regular meetings and through regular responses. I solemnly recollect my parents who were responsible for my upcoming and for the acquisition of my education and career.

- Jagadish Prasad

Aspiring Doctors

Aspiring doctors must not only excel academically but also embrace a set of values and practices that align with the country's healthcare ethos. Here are a few essential guidelines that all medical students in India should follow to ensure a successful and fulfilling career in the medical field.

1) **RESPECT FOR DIVERSITY AND CULTURAL SENSITIVITY:** India is a melting pot of various cultures, traditions, and languages. Medical students have the privilege of interacting with patients from various backgrounds, each with unique beliefs and practices. It is crucial to approach patient care with cultural sensitivity and an open mind.

   Understanding and respecting patients' cultural preferences can lead to better communication, trust, and ultimately, more effective medical care. Taking the time to learn about the customs and beliefs of different communities can significantly improve patient-doctor relationships and outcomes.

2) **ETHICAL PRACTICE AND PROFESSIONALISM:** Medical ethics and professionalism are the cornerstones of a successful medical career. Indian medical students must adhere to the ethical principles outlined in the Indian Medical Council (Professional Conduct, Etiquette, and Ethics) Regulations, 2002.

   These guidelines emphasize the importance of patient confidentiality, informed consent, and maintaining the highest standards of integrity. Upholding ethical values not only ensures the well-being of patients but also contributes to building a trustworthy reputation within the medical community.

3) **DEVELOP EFFECTIVE STUDY HABITS:** As a medical student, you will be bombarded with a vast amount of information. To succeed, it is crucial to develop effective study habits. Create a study schedule that allows for regular breaks and incorporates active learning techniques such as summarizing, flashcards, and teaching others.

   Additionally, prioritize understanding concepts rather than memorising facts. This will not only help you retain information better but also prepare you for clinical practice.

4) **HOLISTIC PATIENT CARE:** In a country where access to healthcare can be a challenge for many, medical professionals often find themselves treating not just physical ailments, but also addressing socio-economic factors.

   Indian medical students should be prepared to deliver holistic patient care by considering the patient's economic, social, and psychological background. This approach may require a more comprehensive diagnosis and treatment plan that considers all aspects of the patient's well-being.

5) **EMBRACE TECHNOLOGICAL ADVANCEMENTS:** The healthcare landscape in India is rapidly evolving with technological advancement. From electronic health records to telemedicine, embracing these innovations can streamline patient care and enhance medical practice.

   Medical students should stay updated on the latest technologies, as they have the potential to revolutionize healthcare delivery, especially in remote and underserved areas. Integrating technology into medical practice can lead to increased efficiency, accuracy, and accessibility of healthcare services.

6) **LIFELONG LEARNING AND ADAPTABILITY:** The field of medicine is characterized by constant advancements in research, treatments, and medical knowledge. Indian medical students should cultivate a mindset of lifelong learning to stay up to date with the latest medical developments.

   Pursuing continuing medical education, attending conferences, and engaging in research activities can help doctors-in-training refine their skills and expand their knowledge base. Adaptability to new medical techniques and practices is essential for providing the best possible care for patients.

Becoming a successful medical professional in India goes beyond academic achievements. It requires a deep-rooted commitment to cultural sensitivity, ethical practice, holistic care, technological integration, and continuous learning. As the healthcare system in India continues to evolve, medical students have a pivotal role in shaping its future. By following these few essential guidelines, aspiring doctors can not only excel in their careers but also contribute positively to the well-being of the nation's population. Remember, the journey may be tough, but the impact you will have on the lives of patients makes it all worthwhile.

Contents

Clinical Case Studies

Review Articles

Recent Advances

Answers to University Question Papers

Model Question Paper as per MCI Regulations-1

As per recent MCI guidelines the examination pattern at the end of 3rd semester would be like this

1) 2 Theory papers of 100 marks each = 2×100

Consisting of structured essays, short assay questions, short answer questions

a) Short assay questions 2×10 = 20

b) Short assay answers 6×5 = 30

c) Short answer questions 10×3 = 30

Total = 80

MCQs and Quizzes = 20

Total = 100

2) Practicals = 100

3) Viva = 20

4) Practicals and Viva 80+20 = 120

5) Internal assessment – Theory =40 + Practicals 20=60

6) Grand Total for assessment = 420 marks

There might be variations in the updated notifications from NMC

Model Question Papers

PAPER I

Total Marks 100

1) **Long Essay Questions** 2 x 10 = 20
   a) Mention the halogenated general anesthetics and mention the advantages and disadvantages of any two of them.
   b) Explain the bioavailability of drugs and the factors modifying the same

2) **Short Essay Questions** 6 x 5 = 30
   a) G-Protein couples' receptors.
   b) Cardio-selective Beta receptor blockers
   c) Selective serotonin reuptake inhibitors.
   d) Non-depolarizing skeletal muscle relaxants.
   e) Inhalational drugs used to treat bronchial asthma
   f) Mechanism of action of bupivacaine and its clinical uses

3) **Short Answer Questions** 10 x 3 = 30
   a) Explain therapeutic drug monitoring and give few examples
   b) Cholinesterase Inhibitors and their uses
   c) Drug addiction
   d) Dobutamine
   e) Tachyphylaxis
   f) Verapamil
   g) Phenylephrine
   h) Uses of H1 Receptor blockers
   i) Uses of Carbamazepine
   j) Tremadol

PAPER II

Total Marks 100

1) **Long Essay Questions** 2 x 10 = 20
   a) Classify Antidiabetic Drugs. Explain the mechanism of action of any two groups of the drugs and enumerate their adverse effects.
   b) Classify the drugs used for acid peptic disease and discuss the mechanism of action of any two major groups and their indications.

2) **Short Essay Questions** 6 x 5 = 30
   a) Explain the mechanism of action of high ceiling diuretics and their clinical indications.
   b) Explain the mechanism of action of oral anticoagulants and their clinical uses.
   c) Mention the drugs used to treat Herpes viral infections and their clinical uses.
   d) Mention the drugs used to treat acne vulgaris.
   e) Mention the selective estrogen receptor modulators and their clinical uses.
   f) Explain the antiarrhythmic action and clinical uses of lidocaine.

3) **Short Answer Questions** 10 x 3 = 30
   a) Levothyroxin
   b) Methocobalamine
   c) Enoxaparin
   d) Indications of Sodium Nitropruside
   e) Clinical uses of methotrexate
   f) Indications of Fluconazole
   g) Explain the rationale of combination of Sulfamethoxazole and Trimethorprim
   h) Clinical uses of Artemether
   i) Indications and adverse effects of INH
   j) Domperidone

Answers to Model Question Paper I

1. Long Essay Questions:

(a) How do you classify general anesthetics? Mention their mechanism of action and anesthetic properties and disadvantages with suitable examples.

Ans: General anesthetics are classified as

a) **Volatile inhalational anesthetics**

i. Gases: - Nitrous oxide

ii. Liquids: - Halothane, euflurone, isoflurane, desflurane and sevoflurane

b) **Non-volatile/ Non-inhalational anesthetics or IV anesthetics**:

Thiopental, Thiamylol, propofol, methohexital, ketamine, etomidate.

Mechanism of Action

General anesthetics enhance the activity of inhibitory neurons, increase the levels of inhibitory neurotransmitters, and lower the actions of excitatory neurons and the levels of excitatory neurotransmitters glutamate and aspartate.

At the molecular level general anesthetics act at the GABA receptor enhancing the inhibitory neurotransmission which is also mediated by glycine. They act on GABA cl^- ion channel which acts as a receptor or augmenting cl^-conductance gated by cl^-channel. General anesthetics depress spontaneous and evoked activity in many areas of central nervous system, involving the synaptic processes inhibiting synaptic transmission. In addition, there is hyperpolarization of the neurons through activation of K^+ channels which leads to decreased production of action potentials. Ketamine and nitrous oxide do not act through GABA receptor.

Site of Action

General anesthetics cause generalized inhibition of central nervous system, and act primarily in areas like reticular activating system, central cortex, the cuneate nucleus, the obfactory cortex, hippocampus and dorsal horn of the spinal cord. Inhaled general anesthetics primarily act on the spinal cord to produce immobility.

1. Anesthetic properties and disadvantages of Enflurane.

Anesthetic Properties	Disadvantages
1. Blood-gas partition coefficient is 1.8. **2.** MAC 1.68% in pure oxygen and 0.5% in 70% nitrous oxide+ 30% oxygen. **3.** Provides rapid induction and rapid recovery. **4.** Has an adequate analgesic and skeletal muscle relaxation property?	**1.** Causes fall of blood pressures and reduced cardiac output. **2.** Causes respiratory depression. **3.** In higher doses it can cause spike and wave pattern in EEG causing generalized muscle twitching and contra indicated in patients with a history of epilepsy. **4.** Can cause postoperative shivering. **5.** Can cause mild simultaneous of tracheobronchial secretions

2. Anesthetic properties and disadvantage of Nitrousoxide.

Anesthetic Properties	Disadvantages
1. Blood-gas partition coefficient is 0.47; **2.** MAC 1.68% **3.** Because of poor solubility, it passes very quickly from the inspired gas mixture and quickly attains alveolar concentration and induces equilibrium in all compartments quickly thereby producing rapid onset and rapid recovery.	**1.** It is more an analgesic than a potent anesthetic because of its MAC of more than 100%. It is a less potent general anesthetic. **2.** It can increase cerebral blood flow but not to the extent produced by liquid general anesthetics. **3.** Not a skeletal muscle relaxant and muscle relaxants should be adequately supplemented with general anesthetic agent and used simultaneously. **4.** It gets exchanged with N_2 in any air-containing cavity in the body and enters the cavity faster and increases the volume or pressure inside it.

(b) Explain the drug-related factors modifying the drug action.

There are many factors that influence the drug action which may be a decrease or an increase or that produce an altogether different action or can even produce adverse effects.

The factors affecting the drug action may be broadly termed as – Drug related and patient related.

Drug related factors modifying the drug action:

a) **Physical Properties**
   i. The poor solubility of procaine penicillin confers on it a longer duration of action compared to benzyl penicillin.
   ii. Thiopental sodium is highly lipid soluble and gets distributed in the body compartments quickly and rapidly enters brain to produce general anesthesia.

b) **Rate of Administration:** The drug effects also depend upon the rates at which the drug is administrated.
   i. Aminophyllin if given rapidly causes fall of blood pressure and respiratory distress and hence given over a period of 10 minutes.
   ii. Thiopental if given rapidly causes respiratory depression but if given too slowly causes laryngospasm and cough.

c) **Selective Distribution**
   i. Chloroquine is used in hepatic amebiasis mainly because it is selectively concentrated is the liver
   ii. Aminoglycoside cause nephrotoxicity and ototoxicity because they get accumulated in the kidneys and perilymph and endolymph of the inner ear.

d) **Biotransformation:** Acetylcholine is rapidly hyrolized by acetylcholinesterage and has a very shorter duration of action. But carbachol and bethanechol can resist enzymatic destruction and can have longer duration of action.

e) **Presence of Other Drugs:** The effects of an individual drug may be affected by the concomitlant administration of another drug. The actions of warfarin can be affected by drugs like sulfonamides, aspirin (increased action) and barbiturates (decreased action).

f) **First-pass Metabolism:** Drugs such as propranolol, morphine, lidocaine and glyceryltrinitrate undergo varying degress of first-pass metabolism resulting in decreased bioavailability.

g) **Additive and Enhanced Effects:** When a drug is combined with another drug and if both the drugs have similar pharmacological responses, the total response or net response of the two drugs is equal to the arithmetic sum of their individual responses. Thus, a combination of aspirin and paracetamol provides a more qualitative response for the relief of pain.

On the other hand, when the combination of two drugs having different mechanisms of action produces a greater than the arithmetic sum of the individual effects of the drugs, the net effect is termed as synergism. It is a quantitative effect. For example, enalapril in combination with a thiazide diuretic yields a greater antihypertensive effect.

h) **Diminution of Effect:** when the effects of a drug are blocked or reduced in the presence of another drug, the feature is known as antagonism. A drug having affinity and efficacy for a receptor, is called an agonist. On the other hand, if a drug is having only affinity without efficacy the feature is know as antagonism. Here the antagonist simply occupies the receptor site and blocks the actions of agonist at the same site. For example, ach actions are blocked by atropine and D-tubocurarine working at two different sites (Ach M and Ach N receptor sites respectively).

i) **Chemical Antagonism:** In this case, one drug chemically reacts with and neutralizes the other drug. For example, an antacid or alkali will nullify the corrosive action of an acid. Similarly, protamine annuls the anticoagulant action of heparin, the former has a strong electropositive charge which antagonizes the electronegative charge of the later to which its action is due.

j) **Physiological Antagonism:** Here the two drugs have opposite effects but they are mediated through different mechanism or receptor systems. For example, adrenaline causes a rise in blood pressure, but nitrates cause a fall: therefore, the two are antagonistic to each one. While adrenaline causes vasoconstriction acting through α-receptors, nitrates cause vasodilatation acting on the smooth muscle of the blood vessel.

2. Short Essay Questions:

a) **G-Protein Coupled Receptors:** They are transmembrane receptors, also called metabotropic receptors coupled to intracellular effective systems/ second messengers like cAMP, cGMP, Ca^+, IP_3 and DAG through G-Proteins (guanine nucleotide binding protein). Example of G-Protein coupled receptors include muscarinic acetylcholine(mAch), α_2, opioid, β – adrenergic, 5 – HT and histamine receptors and also receptors for several hormones, including glucagon. G – Proteins are of three types namely G_S, G_I, and G_q. $G_s$mediates the actions of adrenergic, histaminergic, and 5 – HT (serotonin) receptors, glucagon receptors and receptors of several other hormones. G_I mediates the actions of α_2, mAch and opioid receptors. $G_q$mediates the actions of mAch, 5-HT_{1c}, vasopressin type1 redeptors and angiotensin 11 receptors.

b) **Cardioselective Beta-blockers:** β_1 – blockers are also known as cardio-selective blockers as they exclusively block β1 receptor – by virtue of B1 receptor blockade located in the heart (SA nodal, AV nodal and Ventricular tissues). Examples include metoprolol, atenolol, esmolol, acebutolol, bisoprolol and nebiolol.

By virtue of their β_1–blockade on the myocardium, they reduce heart rate, force of contraction, and sympathetic activity such as seen during exercise. They have an antihypertensive action due to the reduction of heart rate, cardiac output, inhibition of release of renin from GJ apparatus, inhibition of presynaptic nor-adrenaline release. They also elicit antiarrhythmic effect predominantly because of their action on phase-4 depolarization of cardiac action potential.

They are clinically useful to treat hypertension, angina prophylaxis (chronic stable angina) and early phase of acute myocardial infarction, supraventricular arrhythmias, and chronic congestive heart failure. Their use is associated with decreased morbidity and mortality post MI. Treatment with β_o-blockers reduces the risk of stroke, coronary artery disease and congestive heart failure.

c) **Selective Serotonin Reuptake Inhibitors:** Citalopram, venlafaxine, duloxetine, escitalopram, fluoxetine, paroxetine, sertraline, and fluvoxamine are the selective serotonin reuptake inhibitors. They act by preventing the reuptake of 5-HT into the tryptaminergic nerve terminal thereby increasing the 5-HT levels. They are used as antidepressants is anxiety disorders (velnafaxine, duloxetine) and used to treat panic, generalized anxiety disorder, phobia and obsessive-compulsive disorder. They are also effective to treat posttraumatic stress disorder.

d) **Non-depolarizing Muscle Relaxants:** D – tubocurarine, atracurium, cisatracurium, mivacurium, doxacurium, metocurium are the non-depolarizing skeletal muscle relaxants that are in clinical use. They act on the $\mathbf{N_m}$ type of cholinergic receptors and block the actions of Ach and prevent the muscle contraction. As the action is a total blockade of the end plate potential, a type of faccid paralysis occurs in comparison to depolarizing agents which produce initial spasticity followed by flaccidity.

They are used as adjuvant to general anesthesia, in intensive care units to facilitate mechanical ventilation, or endotracheal intubation and in acute respiratory distress syndrome to assist normal or assisted ventilation; Neostigmine is the antagonist for non-depolarizing skeletal muscle relaxants.

e) **Inhalational drugs used to treat bronchial asthma:** Terbutaline, metaproterenol, salbutamol, fenoterol, formoterol, and salmeterol are used by inhalation, and act as β_2 agonists to cause relaxation of bronchial smooth muscle. They are used to treat acute and chronic bronchial asthma. Ipratropium is a $\mathbf{M_3}$ receptor antagonist used to treat acute episodes of bronchial asthma. Budesonide, fluticasone, beclomethasone, flunisolide, mometasone are the cortiostemids used to treat acute episodes of chronic bronchial asthma. Steroids do not have any bronchodilatory effects. They suppress the airway inflammation which is responsible for bronchoconstriction. This is brought about by suppression of inflammatory mediators, including cytokines, chemokines adhesion molecules, leukotreins, prostaglandins. Both ipratropium and $\beta_2$agonists cause bronchodilation releiving the symptoms.

f) **Mechanism of action of bupivacaine:** Bupivacaine is a local anesthetic and acts by blocking the voltage-gated Na+ channels which contain the receptor site for the agents located at its cytoplasmic (inner portion) thereby preventing the permeability of or flux of Na+ into the excitable membrane. It blocks the generation of action potentials in the nerve cells by increasing the threshold for electrical excitation.

It is used to provide spinal, epidural, regional, local, and infiltration anesthesia. Its onset of action is slow but has a longer duration of action of nearby 2 to 9 hours. Bupivacaine is more cardiotoxic than other local anesthetics as its duration of the cardiac action potentials is longer than that of the rest of local anesthetics. This is because of its slow diassaociation from the binding sites.

3. Short Answer Questions:

a) **Explain therapeutic drug monitoring and give few examples:** when a drug is administered it is likely to give not only the desired pharmacological and clinical responses but also the undesirable adverse effects. These adverse effects may be mild, moderate, and severe depending upon the dose given, the patient's response and duration of action of the drug.

Therapeutic drug monitoring is a process by which it becomes necessary sometimes to monitor the drug response with the corresponding dose given and the incidence of adverse effects it produces. The monitoring is necessary for a drug that is being administered over extended periods and those with narrow margin of safety. Therapeutic drug monitoring facilitates mainly to know plasma levels of the drug and the corresponding therapeutic response, adverse effects observed and adjust the dose accordingly. The drugs which require therapeutic dry monitoring include lithium, digoxin, antimalignancy drugs and anticonvulsants.

b) **Cholinesterase inhibitors and their uses:** These drugs act by inhibiting acetylcholinesterase thereby increasing the actions of endogenous acetylcholine levels and inducing cholinomimetic effects. Edrophonium, neostigmine, physostigmine, demecarium are the reversible cholinesterase inhibitors. Organophosphorus compounds like ecothiophate, diisopropyl flurophosphate, parathion is some of examples of irreversible cholinesterase inhibitors. They are used mainly to treat myasthenia gravis, glaucoma, atropine poisoning, paralyticus ileus and atony of the urinary bladder.

c) **Drug addiction:** when a drug or non-therapeutic agent is used for extended periods it is likely to produce a state of tolerance which is a feature of reduced pharmacological response and that may lead to an increase in dose or over consumption to get the same response. Initially there would be physical dependance followed by psychic dependence as in the case of non-prescriptional and non-therapeutic agents like alcohol, opioids, LSD, phencyclidine, anabolic steroids. Addiction is the term used to include the development of either physical or psychic dependence or both.

d) **Dobutamine:** It is a direct acting inotropic drug; the action being mediated through cardiac β_1– receptors increasing cardiac contractility and cardiac output. Dobutamine is mainly used in cardiac decompensation that occurs after cardiac surgery or in patients with congestive heart failure or myocardial infarction. It increases cardiac output without any significant effect on heart rate or blood pressure.

e) **Tachyphylaxis:** It is a term used to denote acute tolerance observed usually in experimental procedures. It develops very quickly with successive doses with reduced pharmacological responses, and it cannot be overcome immediately by increasing the dose. Indirectly acting sympathomimetic drugs such as ephedrine, tyramine and amphetamine are the examples which show tachyphylaxis. The phenomenon of tachyphylaxis is due to exhaustion of the stores of sympathetic amines or may be due to metabolic degradation of the agent by the corresponding enzymes.

f) **Verapamil:** It is a calcium channel blocker and acts by blocking the voltage gated calcium channels in the blood vessels and heart. It causes relaxation of the vascular smooth muscle followed by vasodilation, decreased cardiac contractility producing negative inotropic and chronotropic effects. It is mainly used in hypertension, variant or prinzmetal angina, exertional angina, and cardiac arrhythmias.

g) **Phenylephrine:** It is α_1– receptor agonist. It is not a catecholamine and hence not inactivated by COMT and has much longer duration of action. It is mainly used as vasopressor to raise the blood pressure in conditions of hypotension, and along with local anesthetics to produce local vasoconstriction and slow its absorption and to provide longer duration of action. It is also used as a mydriatic drug (10% solution) without any effect on intraocular pressure. It is also used as nasal decongestant.

h) **Use of H_1 receptor blockers:** H_1 blockers are mainly used in allergic conditions like urticaria, dermatosis, conjunctivitis, seasonal rhinitis and common cold to relieve sneezing, rhinorrhea, itching of the eyes, nose, and throat. They are often combined with nasal decongestants like pseudoephedrine, phenylephrine; and with acetaminophen (paracetamol) for better relief of symptoms.

i) **Uses of carbamazepine:** It is an antiepileptic drug. It acts by blocking Na^+ channels and limits repetitive firing of action potentials evoked by sustained depolarizations in the cortical areas. It abolishes maximum electroshock – induced convulsions. It has no GABA like action. It is mainly used in generalized tonic – clonic contractions, simple and partial complex seizures (Temporal lobe epilepsy), trigeminal and glossopharyngeal neuralgia, pain disorders like multiple sclerosis, and postherpetic neuralgia.

j) **Tremadol:** It is a synthetic codeine analog with a weak opioid receptor agonist activity. It is mainly effective in relieving mild-to-moderate pain such as labor pain, pain due to injuries, toothache, neurological pain, and many other not so severe types of pain. It is not effective to relieve pain of musculoskeletal origin. It is not effective to relieve pain due to malignancy. It is available in combination of paracetamol for a better therapeutic effect. It is available as immediate release and sustained release dosage forms, while the immediate release preparation is useful for acute pain and the the sustained preparation is useful for chronic pain.

Answers to Model Question Paper II

1. Long Essay Questions:

(a) What are Aminoglycosides? Give examples and mention their clinical uses and adverse effects.

Ans: Aminoglycosides are the antibiotics effective against many Gram-negative organisms such as E. coli, salmonella, shigella, enterobacter, citrobacter, klebsiella, morganella, pseudomonas and mycobacterium tuberculosis. They also have efficacy against enterococci and streptococci in combination with betalactams and vancomycin to produce synergistic effect. Aminoglycosides consist of streptomycin, gentamicin, tobramycin, amikacin, netilmicin and kanamycin.

The common properties of aminoglycosides include:

- They contain amino sugars linked to a hexose through a glycosidic bridge.
- They are effective against Gram negative infections with the exception of amikacin which has remarkable activity against methicillin – resistant S. aureus (MRSA).
- They are administered mainly parenterally (IM/IV).
- They are usually given in once daily doses and also as twice daily doses.
- The exhibit concentration dependent bactericidal activity with an increase of action with corresponding increase of the dose of the drug.
- They possess post antibiotic effect and they continue to kill the bacteria even after their plasma levels fall below the minimum inhibitory concentration (MIC).
- They cause ototoxicity and nephrotoxicity with slight variability among the compounds.
- All of them are useful in fulminating conditions like bacterial endocarditis, urinary tract infections, septicemias and pulmonary tuberculosis (Streptomycin, Kanamycin and amikacin).

Clinical uses of Aminoglycosides

1) Streptomycin is useful in bacterial endocarditis caused by enterococci, D streptococci, viridans sfreptococi in combination with penicillin or vancomycin. It is used to treat mycobacterium tuberculosis in combination with other anti TB drugs like pyrazinamide, INH, rifampicin, ethambutol). It is also effective to treat plague, tularemia, and brucellosis.
2) Gentamicin is the most preferred drug to treat serious, life – threatening Gram – negative infections such as septicemia, systemic bacteremia, infected burns, osteomyelitis, pneumonia and peritonitis caused by P aeruginosa, enterobacter, klebsiella, serratia, proteus and acinobacter. It is usually combined with extended spectrum penicillin or a cephalosporin which provides a synergistic effect.

   The other uses of gentamiain include urinary tract infections, bacterial endocarditis caused by enterococci, streptococci, strepococcus pneumoniae; nosocomial pneumonia and sepsis. Topically it can be used for infected burns, wounds or skin infections and external ocular infections (eye drops).
3) Tobramycin is used mainly for infections caused by P. aeruginosa
4) Amikacin has the same uses as gentamicin and tobramycin and particularly if the bacterial strains are not sensitive and resistant to the earlier drugs.

Adverse effects of Aminoglycosides:

All aminoglycosides produce potential dangerous reversible and irreversible adverse effects such as ototoxicity, nephrotoxicity and neuromuscular effects. Ototoxicity produced by aminoglycoside is irreversible (both cochlear and vestibular dysfunction). Nephrotoxicity is manifested as increased excretion of brush border enzymes, proteinuria, and appearance of casts in the urine, and decrease of GFR. Neomycin is the most nephrotoxic because of its high accumulation in the renal cortex and streptomycin is beast nephrotoxic.

(b) Classify Antithyroid Drugs. Explain the mechanism of action of the principal group, and their uses.

Ans: Antithyroid drugs can be classified as

1) Thioamides – Propylthiouracil, methimazole, carbimazole
2) Anion inhibitors – Potassium perchlorate, thiocyanate, pertechnetate
3) Iodine and iodates – Lugol's iodine, potassium iodide
4) Iodinated contrast media – Diatrizoate, iohexol
5) Radioactive iodine – ^{131}i

Mechanism of Action Thioamides: They decrease thyroid hormone production. They interfere with peroxidase –catalyzed reactions and prevent the iodination of tyrosine to form mono and diiodotyrosin residues, coupling of iodotyrosine residues to form T4 and T3 and prevent the conversion of T4 to T3 (Propylthiouracil) peripherally by inhibiting 5' – deiodinase. Due to this additional property, propylthiouracil is often used to provide rapid relief from severe thyrotoxicosis. Thioamides also inhibit thyroid release. Propylthiouracil provides rapid reversal of symptoms compared to methimazole and has a short half-life of 1.5hr compared to 6 hrs with methimazole. Propylthiouracil is also the drug of choice during 1st trimester of pregnancy and also the drug of choice during the recovery phase of thyrotoxic crisis.

Uses of Antithyroid Drugs

1) Thioamides are used in the management of hyperthyroidism and thyrotoxic crisis and in the preparation of patients for surgical subtotal thyroidectomy.
2) Anion inhibitors act as competitive inhibitors of thyroid transport mechanism and prevent the uptake of iodide by the gland. They are effective in treating iodine – induced hyperthyroidism which may occur in patients treated with antiarrhythmic compound amiodarone.
3) Lugol's iodine inhibits the uptake and incorporation of iodine into the thyroid gland and inhibits TSH control over the thyroid gland and decreases the levels of T4 and T3. It also inhibits the release of thyroid hormones. Lugol's iodine is used in combination with propylthiouracil in the management of thyrotoxic crisis to rapidly inhibit thyroid secretion. Most commonly it is used in the preoperative preparation of patients about to go for thyroid surgery to decrease the vascularity and turgescence of the thyroid gland.
4) Iodinated contrast media are used in the treatment of hyperthyroidism as they rapidly inhibit the peripheral conversion of T4 to T3.
5) Radiolabeled iodine (^{131}I) is used in the treatment of hyperthyroidism while other isotopes of radioactive iodine are used for thyroid ablation by emitting β – particle emission.
6) B – adrenergic blockers (propranolol) are used to control the sympathetic effects associated with hyperthyroidism, particularly cardiovascular sympathetic effects (increased here rate, blood pressure). It is also used in thyrotoxic crisis for the similar effects.

(c) Write about the following.

a. Mechanism of action of clomifene and its adverse effects.

Ans: clomifene is an ovulation inducing agent and has partial agonist and antagonist actions. It binds to the estrogen receptors (ERα and ERβ) because of its antagonistic action and blocks the negative feedback inhibition of release pituitary gonadotropins (FSH, LH) by estrogen and facilitates their release. The FSH and LH release during midcycle facilitates ovulation. Women who are infertile suffer from polycystic ovary syndrome (poly follicular syndrome) which is characterized by amenorrhea, anovulation, dysfunctional uterine bleeding (DUB), and infertility. Hence clomifene is used in the treatment of ovulatory dysfunction.

The adverse effects of clomifene include hot flushes similar to those seen in menopausal syndrome. It can cause enlargement of ovaries, increased incidence of multiple births, ovarian cysts, and GI side effects like nausea and vomiting.

b. Mechanism of action of methotrexate, its uses and important adverse effects.

Ans: Methotrexate is an antimetabolite and inhibits the enzyme dihydrofolate reductase thereby preventing the conversion of dihydrofolate to tetrahydrofolate (antifolate action). This blocks regeneration of tetrahydrofolate and prevents synthesis of purines and pyrimidines which in effect results in interfering with the formation of DNA, RNA, and key cellular proteins. Formation of methotrexate polyglutamate derivatives is essential for its antitumor activity.

Methotrexate is used in the treatment of childhood leukemias with reasonable periods of remissions. It is also effective for choriocarcinoma, hydatiform mole, breast cancer, and solid tumors such as osteogenic sarcoma, psoriasis and rheumatoid arthritis.

The adverse effects of methotrexate include anorexia, nausea, vomiting, progressive weight loss, bloody diarrhea, and leucopenia. It causes maximum damage to bone marrow and GI mucosa. **Leucovorin** (5-fromyl derivative folic acid) is indicated to diminish toxicity and counteract the effects of impaired methotrexate elimination or inadvertent overdosage of methotrexate.

c. Clinical uses of corticosteroids

Ans: Corticosteroids (glucocorticoids) can be used for hormonal and non- hormonal uses.

Hormonal indications mainly are related to replacement therapy, and the non-hormonal uses are by virtue of their antiinflammatory and immunosuppressant actions.

Hormonal uses include acute adrenal insufficiency (Addison's disease), chronic adrenal insufficiency, congenital adrenal hyperplasia, Cushing syndrome secondary to an ACTH secretary pituitary adenoma after surgical removal of the tumor.

Non- hormonal uses include

1) Rheumatic fever and rheumatic arthritis.
2) As adjuvant with other drugs to treat psoriatic arthritis, ankylosing spondylitis, post traumatic osteoarthritis, acute and subacute bursitis, synovitis, osteoarthritis (OA), tenosynovitis and acute gout and chronic rheumatoid arthritis.
3) Renal diseases (nephrotic syndrome).
4) Allergic conditions like angioneurotic edema, hay fever, serum sickness, urticaria (including for topical use), contact dermatitis, drug reactions, including anaphylactic shock.
5) Bronchial asthma, both for acute and chronic episodes.
6) Dermatological conditions like psoriasis eczema, atopic dermatitis seborrheic dermatitis, acne vulgaris, and acne rosacea and in bacterial infections along with topical antibiotics.
7) GI diseases like inflammatory bowel syndrome.
8) Immuno suppression after organ transplantation, tissue grafting and several graft rejections.

9) Autoimmune diseases like Guillain – Barre syndrome, multiple sclerosis, myasthenia gravis, systemic lupus erythematosus, autoimmune hemolytic anemia, polymyositis, autoimmune uveitis, scleroderma and Sjogren syndrome.
10) Cerebral edema due to space occupying lesions.
11) Ocular diseases like allergic conjunctivitis, keratitis and Kerato conjunctivitis.

(d) Drugs for Nosocomial Infections.

Ans: Nosocomial infections are hospital acquired infections during the process of receiving health care that were not present during the time of admission. They can be acquired by the patients, hospital staff (doctors, nursing sisters, and paramedical staff) and can occur anywhere (area) in the hospital from person to person, or by the use of invasive procedures, surgery, indwelling catheters, prosthetic devices, all of which are infected with microorganisms. They are more likely to occur in closed areas such as ICUs, surgical theatres and isolated hospital wards. The most common forms of nosocomial infections include pneumonia, skin and soft tissue infections, GI infections, blood stream infections, and urinary tract infections. Both Gram positive and Gram-negative bacteria can be the source of infection apart from opportunistic fungal and viral infections in immunocompromised patients.

Treatment is usually started with ceftriaxone 1 – 2g IM/IV twice daily or levofloxacin 750mg (PO) once daily or moxifloxacin 400mg (PO)once daily all being empirical drugs to begin with keeping in view that the pathogens for the infections might be or proven to be streptococcus pneumoniae, H. influenzae, methicillin – sensitive staphylococcus aureus. The other important drug for use is vancomycin 15-20mg/kg IV 8th hourly, or linezolid 600mg/orally, 12th hrly for 10 -14 days or Ertapenem 1g once daily IV/IM for 14 days to cover Gram negative infections caused by E. coli, Klebsiella pneumoniae, enterobactor, proteus and serratia. Similarly, antiviral and antifungals may also be added in immunocompromised patients.

(e) Fibrinolytic Drugs.

Ans: Fibrinolytics (fibrinolytic agents) are the agents used to facilitate lysis of already formed clots and thereby restore the patency of the obstructed blood vessel. Fibrinolytic drugs are life saving in acute thrombotic disordered like MI, pulmonary embolism, deep vein thrombosis and cerebrovascular thrombotic stroke. The following drugs are used as fibrinolytic agents.

1) Streptokinase though exerts most striking and potentially beneficial effects in fresh thrombi,

   its action is limited by two factors. It is capable of producing antigenic reactions and likely to cause anaphylactic reaction if reused when it was given once earlier. It is relatively nonspecific and can result in systemic fibrinolysis causing bleeding episodes.

2) Urokinase

   It lacks antigenecity unlike streptokinase. It directly vonverts plasminogen to active plasmin which in turn leads to the breakdown of fibrin mesh structure in the clot. It is mainly used for restoration of blood flow in peripheral blood vessels, occluded catheters used in dialysis, and also for other embolic disorders such as MI, stroke, pulmonary embolism and deep vein thrombosis.

3) Tissue plasminogen activators like alteplase, reteplase, tenectiplase and anistreplase are the most preferred agents used in acute MI and cerebrovascular stroke. They are the recombinant derivatives of naturally occurring tissue plasminogen activator and have the same indications as the rest of the fibrinolytic drugs.

   All the fibrinolytic drugs act by converting of the inactive zymogen, plasminogen to the active protease plasmin. Plasmin is a relatively nonspecific protease that digests fibrin to fibrin degradation products with dissolution of the clot.

(f) Prophylactic use of antibiotics with examples.

Ans: Antibiotics are not only effective in acute bacterial infections but also serve as prophylactic agents for the prevention of a possible infection by microorganisms (chemoprophylaxis).

a. Rifampin is administered to prevent meningococcal meningitis in people who are in close contact with an infected person.

b. Prevention of gonorrhea and syphilis soon after contact with an infected person.

c. Chemoprophylaxis is recommended in patients with valvular lesions of the heart who are likely to be predisposed to endocarditis, and those undergoing dental, surgical or other procedures which are likely to produce bacteremia. Similarly, patients with valvular heart disease undergoing tonsillectomy are recommend chemoprophylaxis

d. Travellers visiting endemic areas of malaria can be protected by prior administration of sulfadoxine and pyrimethamine or mefloquine.

e. Chemoprophylaxis can prevent cardiac valvular disease at a later age in patients with childhood rheumatic arthritis. Long – acting penicillin like benzathine penicillin is given for the purpose.

f. Prior administration of a broad-spectrum antibiotic can prevent wound infection or any other abdominal/thoracic infection is a person to undergo surgery.

Model Question Papers

PAPER III

1. Long Essay Questions:

1. **Classify non – insulin antidiabetic drugs. Explain the mechanism of action of any two groups and enumerate their adverse effects.**

Ans:

a) Insulin secretagogues
   i) Sulfonylureas – glibenclamide, glimepiride, gliclazide, glipizide
   ii) Non – sulfonylurea derivatives – Nateglinide Repaglinide
b) Biguanides – Metformin
c) Thiazolidinediones – Rosiglitazone, Pioglitazone
d) α – glucosidase inhibitors – Acarabose, Volgibose, Miglitol
e) GLP – 1 analogue – Exenatide, liraglutide, semaglutide
f) Dipeptidyl peptidase inhibitors – Sitagliptin, saxagliptine, alogliptin
g) Sodium – glucose Co – transporter – 2 (SGLT – 2) inhibitor – Dapagliflozin empagliflozin canagliflozin
h) Amylinomimetics – Pramlintide
i) Bile acide Sequestrants – Colesevelam
j) Dopamine agonists – Bromocriptine

a) Insulin secretagogues

i) Sulfonylurea's derivatives: Glibenclamide, glimepiride, gliclazide, glipizide is the second-generation sulfonylurea derivative. Chlorpropamide and tolbutamide belong to the first – generation drugs of the same class. Because of undue hypoglycemia and other unsuitable administrative procedures, caused by first generation drugs, the second-generation group of drugs is the most commonly prescribed oral antidiabetic drugs.

Mechanism of Action: Sulfonylurea drugs act by liberating insulin from the pancreatic β – cells. This is brought about by binding of sulfonylureas to a 140 KD sulfonylurea receptor (SUR1) which is an integral part of the ATP – sensitive potassium channel (KATP) that is present on the β – cell membrane surface. Closure of the KATP channel prevents the outflow of potassium with an increase in the intracellular K^+ levels that triggers the opening of voltage gated Ca^+ channels (inward flux of Ca+) leading to depolarization of the cell membrane followed by degranulation and release of insulin. Sulfonylureas may further facilitate increased insulin levels by reducing hepatic clearance of the hormone.

Adverse effects: The most common adverse effect associated with sulfonylureas administration is hypoglycemia which may be substantiated by inadequate calorie intake. The chances of hypoglycemia are higher in the elderly with hepatic or renal impairment. Chlorpropamide by virtue of its long half – life is more likely to produce hypoglycemia. In the second-generation sulfonylurea preparations, glibenclamide has a more chance for the development of hypoglycemia.

The other important adverse effects, sulfonylureas include weight gain which is undesirable in persons who are already obese. There is a possibility of drug interactions with sulfonamides, clofibrate, and salicylates which displace sulfonylureas from plasma binding sites and increase their plasma levels. Chlorpropamide is likely to develop alcohol – induced flush similar to that produced by disulfiram. Chlorpropamide has ADH – potentiating effects, the actions of which make it useful in mild forms of central diabetes mellitus.

Nonsulfonylurea derivatives

Repaglinide (structurally related to glybenclamide (glyburide) and Nateglinide act by binding to sulfonylurea receptor (SUR1) which is an integral part of ATP-sensitive potassium channel present on the β-cell membrane similar to sulfonylurea derivatives. They inhibit K+ outflux, depolarizing the β-cell membrane liberating insulin release through ca+ influx.

Both the drugs cause a brief rapid pulse of insulin when given before meal and reduce the postprandial rise in blood glucose levels. They can be used as monotherapy or in combination with biguanides (metformin) to reduce postprandial glucose levels and should be given just before meals.

ii) **GLP – 1 agonists:** Incretins are hormones that work to increase insulin secretion. There are two main incretins in the body, namely GLP – 1 (glucagon – like peptide – 1) and GIP (glucose – dependent insulotropic peptide, also known as gastric inhibitory peptide). Both of them are secreted by the endocrine cells (L – type cells) that are located in the epithelium of the small intestine. Incretins are carried through the circulation to the target tissue, the pancreatic β – cell. Incretin stimulation of β – cells cause them to secrete more insulin in response to the same amount of blood glucose.

Mechanism of action: GLP – 1 agonists (exenatide, liraglutide, dulaglutide, albiglutide, lixisenaside, semaglutide) act through GLP – 1 receptors expressed in pancreatic β- cells. Binding of agonists to GLP – 1 receptor activates cAMP – PKA pathway that results in increase of insulin secretion followed by exocytosis. GLP – 1 agonists also increase pancreatic β – cell function, cause decrease of glucagon, reduced glucose production in the liver by reducing hepatic gluconeogenesis and an increase of glucose uptake in the skeletal muscle and adipose tissue.

Adverse effects: GLP – 1 agonists may produce nausea, diarrhea, hypoglycemia and vomiting. Less common side effects include headache, constipation, dyspepsia, fatigue.

2. **Classify the drugs for acid peptic disease and discuss the mechanism of action of any two major groups and their indications.**

Ans: Drugs for acid – peptic disease can be classified as

a) Acid – neutralizing agents (antacids) – Aluminum hydroxide, magnesium hydroxide, magnesium tricylicate.
b) H_2 receptor antagonists – Ranitidine, famotidine, nizatidine.
c) Proton pump inhibitors – Omeprazole, rabiprazole, lansoprazole, pantoprazole, esomeprazole.
d) Anticholinergic drugs – Pirenzepine, glycopyrolate, mepenzolate.
e) Prostaglandin analogues – Misoprostal.
f) Mucosal protective agents – Sucralfate, colloidal bismuth compounds.
g) Drugs for H – pylori infection - Metronidazole, amoxacillin, clarithromycin.

1) **H_2 receptor antagonists:** They inhibit the acid production by reversibly competing with histamine for binding to H_2 receptor on the basolateral membrane of parietal cells. They also suppress basal acid secretion and suppress the acid secretion due to feeding, gastrin, hypoglycemia or vagal stimulation.

   These agents are particularly useful in suppressing nocturnal acid secretions which reflect mainly basal parietal cell activity. These agents promote ulcer healing because of their predominant effect on the nocturnal basal secretion. H_2 antagonists are available both for oral and parenteral use.

   Therapeutic uses: H_2 receptor antagonists are useful to treat all types of acid peptic disorders and they are as effective as proton pump inhibitors in providing ulcer healing when given in adequate doses and for adequate duration. Thus, they are indicated in healing of gastric and duodenal ulcers, to treat uncomplicated GERD and to prevent the occurrence of stress – induced ulcers, including prevention of bleeding from stress related gastritis, and for treating drug – induced ulcers. They are most effective for duodenal ulcers than for gastric ulcers.

2) **Proton pump inhibitors (PPIs)** (Omeprazole, lansoprazole, pantoprazole, rabeprazole, esomiprazole).

   Mechanism of Action: PPIs are inactive prodrugs which are activated in the acid medium in the parietal cell canaliculi. Oral preparations of these drugs are enteric coated to prevent premature activation. In the local acidic pH of the canaliculi, these become active and protonated to form the sulfonamide cations, which then react with a cysteine residue on the H^+/K^+/ATPase (Proton pump) to form a covalent disulfide bond. This binding inhibits the activity of the proton pump irreversibly, leading to prolonged and nearly complete suppression of acid secretion.

   Therapeutic uses

   (1) PPIs are used to treat active duodenal ulcers, H-Pylori associated ulcers in combination with antibiotics like amoxacillin, clarithromycin, and metronidazole; hemorrhagic ulcers and steroids induced ulcers. They provide more rapid relief of epigastric pain and heart burn and more rapid and effective gastric ulcer and esophageal ulcer healing than H_2 blockers.

   (2) They are the drugs of choice to treat Zolinger– Ellison syndrome

   (3) They are the first drugs of choice to treat gastroesophageal reflux disease (GERD). They ae useful to treat erosive and nonerosive reflux disease (erosive esophagitis, Barretts esophagitis, esophageal strictures and esophageal adenocarcinoma).

   (4) PPIs ae useful to reduce the risk for upper GI bleeding.

   (5) PPIs are extremely useful in treating pathological hypersecretory conditions like gastrinomas which are inoperable or metastatic in nature. By giving PPIs, the development of peptic ulceration, erosive esophagitis, and malabsorption can be prevented.

   (6) PPIs are useful in NSAID induced gastric and duodenal ulcers.

2. Short Essay Questions:

1. Explain the mechanism of action of high ceiling diuretics and their clinical indications.

Ans: High ceiling diuretics are also known as loop diuretics. They have high ceiling effect as far as natriuresis and diuresis are concerned in comparison to other groups of drugs in the category. High ceiling means the maximum capacity or the highest natriuresis when compared to the effect produced by other groups of diuretics.

High – ceiling diuretics have a predominant effect on thick ascending loop of Henle inhibiting reabsorption of Nacl. Frusemide, ethacrinic acide, bumetanide, torsemide are the available loop diuretics for clinical use. At the thick ascending limb of Loop of Henle, they inhibit NKCC2 (Sodium potassium chloride cotranporter-2) in the apical (luminal) membrane of the loop epithelial cells and reduce the reabsorption of Nacl up to 25% of filtered load of Na+. They also cause a loss of Mg^+ and Ca^+ by inhibiting positive luminal potential.

Clinical uses

1) Loop diuretics are used to treat edematous states such as pulmonary edema, edema due to congestive heart failure, hepatic cirrhosis, nephrotic syndrome and hypertension.
2) They also cause a decrease of serum Ca^+ levels by increasing Ca^+ elimination and can be used in hypercalcemic states such as hyperthyroidism or parathyroid malignancy associated hypercalcemia.
3) They are also used to counteract hyperkalemia caused by potassium – retaining diuretic or ACE inhibitors.
4) They can be used to induce forced diuresis to facilitate rapid removal of toxic drugs when taken in excessive doses.

2. Explain the mechanism of action of oral anticoagulants and their clinical uses.

Ans: Oral anticoagulants can be broadly classified as Vitamin K antagonists and factor Xa and thrombin (FIIa) inhibitors. Vitamin K inhibitors like warfarin, acenocoumarol, dicoumarol and anisindione act as antagonists of vitamin K which is essential for the synthesis of coagulation factors II, VII, IX and X and the anticoagulant proteins C and S (coagulation regulatory factors).

Factor Xa (FXa) inhibitors like rivaroxaban, apixaban, edoxaban, betriaxaban prevent the formation of thrombin from prohrombin and thereby inhibit the conversion of fibrinogen to fibrin clot.

Factor IIa (FIIa) like dabigatran is a direct thrombin inhibitor.

Clinical uses of oral anticoagulants: Oral anticoagulants are used to treat conditions like venous thromboembolism, including deep venous thrombosis and pulmonary embolism. They are also used to prevent thrombus formation in conditions like atrial fibrillation, mechanical and prosthetic devices implants, in conditions like prosthetic cardiac valve replacement and thereby to prevent stroke, peripheral venous thromboembolism.

3. Mention the drugs used to treat Herpes viral infections and their clinical uses.

Ans: The drugs used to treat Herpes viral infections include idoxuridine, acyclovir, valacyclovir, famciclovir, docosanol, penciclovir.

Clinical uses of drugs for Herpes infections: Acyclovir and other drugs of this class are used to treat herpes simplex and varicella zoster infections. Herpes simplex virus – 1 causes herpes labialis (Cold sores) or herpes esophagitis; herpes simplex – 2 causes genital herpes, Varicella Zoster causes chicken pox and shingles. Acyclovir is also effective against Epsten – Barr viral infection which causes infectious mononucleosis, and cytomegalovirus infection which produces pneumonia, gastroenteritis, retinitis, encephalitis and mononucleosis in immuno compromised patients. Acyclovir is also used to treat herpes encephalitis and neonatal herpes simplex infections. Acyclovir is available for oral use as well as for topical use for genital herpes.

4. Mention the drugs used to treat acne vuglaris.

Ans: Acne vulgaris is a skin disorder seen in adolescents and is caused by Cubibacterium acnes and consists of lesions of comedones (small flesh – colored, white or dark bumps on the face, forehead, and chin) and inflammatory papules, pustules and nodules.

Drugs used to treat acne vulgaris

1) Topical antibiotics like clindamycin (1% gel); erythromycin (4% lotion); metronidazole (0.75%) cream; azelaic acid (20% cream and 15% gel); benzyl peroxide (2.5% gel)

2) Systemic antibiotics like erythromycin, tetracyclines, sarecycline (tetracycline derivative)
3) Topical retinoids like retinol, tretinoin, isotretinoin, acitretin, Tazarotene, bexarotene, adapalene.
4) Systemic retinoids like isotretinoin.

5. Mention the selective estrogen receptor modulators and their clinical uses.

Ans: Selective estrogen receptor modulators (SERMs) are the drugs that modulate the actions (differentiation of actions) of estrogen acting at different target sites. Thus, tamoxifene, the first SERM to be developed blocks the estrogen receptors (ER_{α}, ER_{β}) in the breast and causes regression of breast tumor growth in women with ER – Positive tumors. Tamoxifene produces estrogen effects (acts as agonist) on bone and plasma lipids and facilitate bone turnover and an increase of bone mineral density. However, tamoxifene demonstrates partial agonist activity in the uterus which explains the endometrial hyperplasia and the possible endometrial malignancy with its use.

Raloxifene is the second generation SERM has significant agonist activity of estrogen on bone mineral metabolism and hence useful to treat osteoporosis in post menopausal women and also for risk reduction of invasive breast cancer in post menopausal women. It has anti – estrogen action on the uterus and does not cause uterine hyperplacia. The third generation of SERMS includes ormeloxifene, toremifene, lasoxifene, arzoxifene and bazedoxifene and all of them are approved for the treatment of osteoporosis.

Clinical uses of SERMs

1) Breast cancer: Tomoxifene is used primarily in estrogen-positive breast tumor in women after the patients have completed their primary treatment with surgery and radiation and those with non-invasive breast tumor (ductal carcinoma in situ) and as prophylactic drug for invasive breast tumor. It is efficacious in younger women and is particularly recommended if there is a family history of invasive breast cancer.
2) Osteoporsis: Raloxifene and the third generation of SERMs are used to treat osteoporosis in post menopausal women. They reduce bone resorption and facilitate bone formation acting on osteoclastic and osteoblastic cells respectively.
3) Abnormal uterine bleeding (AUB) and contraception: Ormeloxifene is used for AUB and contraception.
4) Prevention of atherosclerosis – By virtue of their positive lipid lowering effects, they can be used for prevention of atherosclerosis and cardiovascular events.

6. Explain the antiarrhythmic action and clinical uses of lidocaine.

Ans: Lidocaine blocks both activated and inactivated Na^+ channels and causes minimal phase-0 depression, decrease automaticity in Purkinje fibers, decrease the abnormal and triggered activity thus abolishing early and delayed after-depolarizations in Pukinje fibers. It also causes depression of slope of phase 4 depolarization and increase of excitability threshold in punkinje fibre. Refractory period is prolonged and reentry arrhythmias are abolished.

Uses: it is mainly used for rapid control of ventricular arrhythmias due to myocardial infarction, and those caused by inhalational general anesthetics.

3. Short Answer Questions:

1. **Levothyroxine:** It is used to treat hypothyroidism. It serves as replacement therapy if the natural production of thyroxine is inadequate or if there is total absence of the hormone after thyroid surgery. It is also used in pregnancy associated hypothyroidism wherein serum thyroxin – binding globulin levels are increased resulting in decrease of serum free thyroid hormone secretions (FT4). Hence requirements of the

hormone are increased during pregnancy. This is particularly important because total brain development of the fetus depends on maternal thyroid dose. Levothyroxine is also useful to treat myxedema coma.

2. **Methocobalamine:** It is used to treat megaloblastic anemia associated with Vitamin B12 deficiency or folate deficiency or both. B12 deficiency tends to cause neurogenic syndrome while folate deficiency is related to hematological changes. Methocobalamine is the active form of vitamin B12 and can be given both orally and parenterally. The oral dose is 500 – 1000mcg/ day and the parenteral dose is 500mcg IV/IM in 3 times a week. Improvement of neurological symptoms like paresthesias, burning sensations in the hand and feet, unsteadiness of gait, personality changes improve within a period of 3 months after initiation of therapy while the hematological changes may take a longer time for recovery.

3. **Enoxaparin:** It is a low – molecular weight heparin and exhibits more predictable anticoagulant activity than unfractionated heparin. Its bioavailability is more due to lesser plasma and endothelial binding. It has longer half – life and allows less frequent administration and has lesser antigenic reactions. Its action on osteoclasts is also less with lesser bone loss. It can be used safely during pregnancy.

   The chances of thrombocytopenia are also less and also lesser platelet aggregation when compared to unfractionated heparin. It is given in 30 – 40 mg once daily dose by subcutaneous route for prophylaxis of venous thromboembolism, deep vein thrombosis, pulmonary embolism, and acute coronary syndrome, percutaneous coronary intervention (PCI) for stent placement and in conditions of acute MI. It is given in patients who are bed ridden for longer periods due to any reason for prevention of any thromboembolic events.

4. **Indications of sodium Nitroprusside:** It is a vasodilator used in acute decompensated cardiac failure. It is given IV as infusion and has an onset of action of 30 seconds. It reduces both the preload and afterload thereby reduces cardiac workload and oxygen consumption and thus increases cardiac output. This is usually combined with loop diuretics like frusemide to off load the extracellular fluid volume to reduce the work load on the heart. It is also used to lower the blood pressure in hypertensive emergencies wherein it lowers the blood pressure rapidly.

5. **Clinical uses of methotrexate:** It is an antifolate. It inhibits the enzyme dihydrofolate reductase which catalizes the reduction of dihydrofolate to tetrahydrofolate and thus blocks the regeneration of tetrahydrofolate and prevents synthesis of purines and pyrimidines which in effect prevent the formation of DNA or RNA and key cellular proteins. Formation of methotrexate polyglutamate is essential for the antitumor activity.

   It is used mainly in childhood leukemias, choriocarcinoma, hydatiform mole, breast cancer and solid tumors such as osteogenic sarcoma in higher doses. It is also used in rheumatoid arthritis and psoriasis and psoriatic arthritis, squamous cell carcinoma of lungs, epidermoid cancers, and cutaneous T – Cell lymphoma.

   It produces anorexia, nausea, and vomiting affecting GI mucosa. It causes maximum damage to bone marrow and causes leucopenia, thrombocytopenia, and even agranulocytosis. **Leucovorin** (5- formyl derivative of folic acid) is given to reduce its toxicity and to counteract its adverse effects and to facilitate its elimination due to inadvertent over dosage.

6. **Indications of fluconazole:** Fluconzole is hydrophilic triazole and can be used both orally and intravenously for different fungal infections. Fluconzole is especially useful for cryptococcal and coccidiodial meningitis because of its high penetration into CSF. It is also useful to treat oropharyngeal candidiasis, esophagial candidiasis, for the prevention of systemic fungal infections in bone marrow transplant recipient and AIDS patients. It is also useful in vaginal candidiasis.

7. **Explain the rationale of combination of sulfamethoxazole and trimethoprim.**

Ans: Timethoprim/ pyrimethamine have antibacterial and antimalarial actions and it is because of their high affinity for dihydrofolate reductase. It binds the enzyme competitively and inhibits it in bacteria and mammalian cells. Thus, trimethoprim inhibits the conversion of dihydrofolate to tetrahydrofolate (THF) and blocks the formation of thymidines, purines, methionine and glycine in bacteria leading to their rapid lysis. Sulfonamides (sulfamethoxazole and others) are structural analogs of PABA and competetively inhibit it, preventing the utilization of PABA by bacteria for folic acid synthesis.

When sulfamethoxazole and trimethoprim are given in a fixed dose ration of 5:1 equivalent to 800mg and 160mg respectively, they reach peak plasma levels (40mcg/ml and 2mcg/ml in that order). Thus, the combination of the two drugs causes sequential blockade of essential synthetic processes for the formation of folinic acid required for its vonversion to RNA and DNA in the bacteria. It provides a synergistic action and the combination is known as **cotrimoxazole.** Individually both the drugs are bacteriostatic but in combination produce bactericidal effect. The half-lives of trimethoprim and sylfamethoxazole are approximately 11 and 10 hours respectively. Cotrimaxazole is used in many bacterial infections like urinary tract infections, respiratory infections like chronic bronchitis, and upper respriratory tract infections, otitis media, acute maxillary sinusitis, Shigellosis, salmanosis, pneumocystis jiroveci infection (pneumonia in immunocompromised patients) and for gram negative infections in neutropenic patients.

8. **Clinical uses of Artemether**

Ans: Artemether is a derivative of dihydroartemicinin. It can be given orally, parenterally and rectally also. It is used in **multidrug – resistant P. falciparum malaria** infection. It is used in combination with lumifantrine and given for severe acute cases of drug – resistant P. falciparum malaria. When used alone it is given orally on a 7-day course with 4mg/kg/day for 3 days, followed by 1.6mg/kg/day for 4 days. But when nused in combination with lumifatrine it is given in a dose of 120 mg along with artemether dose of 20 mg.

9. **Indications and adverse effects of INH:** Isonicotinic acid hydrazine – **isoniazid (INH)** is the principal first line drug in the treatment of tuberculosis and given in combination with rifampicin, pyrazinamide and ethambutol during intensive 2 months therapy in a dose of 300 mg/day and in a dose of 600 – 900mg two times a week in the continuous 4 months treatment. Adverse effects of INH include hepatotoxicity, peripheral neuropathy, hypersensitivity reactions like rash, fever, jaundice. Hepatotoxicity usually occurs in patients with existing liver dysfucntion, and with the simultaneous use with other hepatotoxic toxic drugs like pyrazinamide or rifampicin and is chronic alcoholics. Peripheral neuropathy occurs in the absence of pyridoxine and also due to slow acetylation of the enzymatic (N – acetylation) metabolism of the drug.

10. **Domperidone:** It is a prokinetic drug and has antiemetic action. It blocks predominantly D2 receptors without any major effect on other receptors. Unlike metoclopramide, it does not cross blood – brain barrier and consequently is less prone to produce central side effects. It is indicated in delayed gastric emptying of functional origin with GERD and/ or dyspepsia, control of nausea and vomiting of central and local origin, as an antiemetic in patients receiving cytotoxic drugs and radiation chemotherapy. It is also used to facilitate radiological examination of upper GI tract and in acute attacks of migrane. It is also indicated in diabetic patients with gastroperesis.

Answers to Question Paper given by Kaloji Narayana Rao University, Warangal – April/May 2022

1. Classify Antiepileptic drugs. Write the mechanism of action, therapeutic uses and adverse effects of sodium valproate.

Ans: Antiepileptic drugs can be classified as follows

1) **Hydantoin derivatives** – Phenytoin, phosphenytoin, mesantoin, ethotoin
2) **Barbiturates** – Phenobarbitone, mephobarbitone, thiopentone
3) **Succinimides** – Ethosuximide, methosuximide
4) **Benzodiazepines** – Diazepam, clonazepam, clobazam, clorazepate, lorazepam
5) **Iminostilbenes** – carbamazepine, oxcarbazepine
6) **Oxazolidinediones** - Trimethadiane, paramethadione
7) **Carboxylic acid derivatives (partial GABA agonists)** – valproic acid
8) **GABA agonists and GABA promoters** – Gabapentine, pregabalin, vigabatrine, tiagabine.
9) **Sulfonamide derivatives** – Zonisamide
10) **Miscellaneous** –Topiramate, lamotrigine, levetiracetam, retigabine, lacosamide, rufinamide.

Mechanism of action of sodium valproate (valproic acid)

- It abolishes both pentylenetetrazol, and maximum electroshock induced convulsions
- It blocks sustained, high – frequency, rapid, repetitive neuronal firing in the cortical areas. This action is brought about by blockade of Na+ channels similar to Phenytoin and carbamazepine.
- It blocks NMDA receptor – mediated excitatory responses.
- It blocks low threshold Ca2+ currents ('T' currents) similar to ethosuximide
- It also exhibits GABA like action by an increase of GABA levels by different mechanisms, such as increased synthesis, inhibition of GABA reuptake, or inhibition of GABA degradation.

Therapeutic uses of valproic acid

1) Valproic acid is very effective against **absence seizures** particularly when the patient also suffers from generalized tonic – clonic seizures simultaneously
2) Myoclonic seizures.
3) Primary generalized tonic – clonic seizures
4) Complex partial seizures as monotherapy or in combination therapy that occur either in isolation or in association with other types of seizures.
5) Prophylaxis for migraine, but not for an acute attack.
6) Manic episodes associated with bipolar disorder.

Adverse effects of valproic acid: Valproic acid causes GI effects like nausea, vomiting, anorexia; CNS effects like sedation, ataxia and tremors and is most likely to cause hepatotoxicity. It is also likely to cause insulin resistance, anovulatory cycles, and spinabifida. It is contraindicated in patients of hepatic disorders.

2. **Classify Beta blockers. Write the mechanism of action, therapeutic uses and adverse effects of propranolol. What are the advantages of cardioselective beta blockers?**

Ans: Beta blockers can be classified on the basis of their development.

1. **First generation** – Propranolol, Nadolol, Pindolol, Timolol, levobutanol, Penbutolol, sotalol, carteolol.
2. **Second generation** – **(β1 selective)** – Acebutolol, atenolol, metoprolol, bisoprolol, esmolol
3. **Third generation -**
   a. **With α – receptor blocking action** – Carvedilol, labetalol, bucindolol, medroxalol
   b. **β1 selective** – Betoxalol, celiprolol (with partial Beta-2 selectivity), nebivolol

Mechanism of action of propranolol

β – Blockers depending on their receptor selectivity completely block the receptor activity preventing the actions of catecholamines. Propranolol is a non – selective β blocker. It blocks both the β1 and β2 receptors present in different effector sites in the body

β1 receptor are present on cardiac myocytes, including the SA and AV nodes. When there is activation of these receptors, there is an increase in cyclic AMP, which leads to increased intracellular calcium which in turn leads to contractility of cardiac muscle fibres. When propranolol is given, this contractile force of heart is decreased followed by decreased cardiac workload which further causes a decrease of oxygen demand and myocardial remodelling. Similarly, propranolol decreases heart rate and cardiac output. Propranolol also blocks β**2** receptors present in the bronchial smooth muscles, the effect of which is not noticed in normal individuals. However, in patients of bronchial asthma and COPD, it results in severe bronchoconstriction.

Therapeutic uses of propranolol

Propranolol, similar with other β-blockers has wide variety of clinical uses that include hypertension, ischemic heart disease (IHD) (in early phase of acute myocardial infarction), prophylactic use for angina pectoris,(selective β1 receptor blockers are the drugs of choice in the IHD and prophylactic use for angina), cardiac arrhythmias, congestive heart failure (more preferentially carvedilol, bisoprolol, metoprolol), prophylaxis of migraine (propranolol is the drug of choice), alcohol withdrawal, thyrotoxicosis (for controlling the sympathomimetic effects associated with hyperthyroidism), situational anxiety states, for reduction of portal venous pressure, pheochromocytoma, and Marphan syndrome to effect a slow progression of aortic dilation.

Adverse effects of Propranolol

Common adverse effects of propranolol include bradycardia, cold extremities and aggravation of pre-existing peripheral artery disease, and withdrawal effects if the drug is stopped suddenly (rebound sympatomimetic activity). Propanolol can also cause bronchoconstriction and increase of airway resistance. Propranolol can cause hypoglycemia if the person is also taking antidiabetic drugs simultaneously.

Advantage of cardioselective β – blockers

Cardio selective β1 blockers like atenolol, metoprolol, bisoprolol, nebivolol have specific action on cardiac β1 receptors and thus have more selective and more effective action in the treatment of hypertension (antihypertensive activity), cardiac arrhythmias (antiarrhythmic action – supraventricular arrhythmias), ischemic heart disease, prophylaxis for angina pectoris, and congestive heart failure (bisoprolol and metoprolol). However, they are likely to cause bradycardia, decreased exercise capacity, hypotension, and AV-nodal block. They do not cause any bronchoconstrictin and hence can be used safely in patients of bronchial asthma and COPD. However, they should be used with more causion to avoid potential risk. The advantage with their use is that they do not cause hypoglycemia when combined with antidaibetic drugs and also, they do not cause any peripheral vasoconstriction and hence do not cause Raynauod's disese or any other peripheral vascular disorder.

3. Write a short note on the following.

1) Define receptors, Explain ion channel receptors

Ans: Receptors are specific cell targets for the drug action. They are macromolecular components of the cell, which are regulatory proteins and for which the drug molecules (signalling molecule or ligand) show affinity and efficacy to varying degrees. The interaction between them results in the changes in the biological systems leading to the development of pharmacological actions. The receptors may be located on the cell surface or inside the cell (intracellular receptors). For each type of hormone (thyroid hormone, insulin, sex hormones, ovarian hormones), neurotransmitter (AD, NAD, DA, Ach, GABA, NMDA), growth factor or autacoids (Histamine, serotonin, prostaglandins), there is at least one specific receptor along with their subtypes commonly.

Ion receptors (Ligand gated ion channels)

They are also known as inotropic receptors and present on the surface of the cell. These ligand gated channels contain a ligand – binding site (receptor). The ligands that act through these channels include Ach, GABA, glutamate, glycine and 5 – HT (Serotonin) and the corresponding binding sites (receptor) are nicotinic acetylcholine – (nAch); 5 – HT1,5-HT2, and subtypes, glycine receptors, GABAA, GABAB, and glutamate receptors. In some channels the conductance of ligand is regulated by changes in the voltage across the plasma membrane. These channels are called Voltage gated ion channels that include Na+, Cl^-, Ca+,. These channels participate in neuronal transmission, cardiac conduction, and skeletal muscle contraction. G-protein coupled receptors are known as metabotropic receptors (adrenergic, histaminergic, serotonergic (5-HT), receptors for glucogon and other hormones.

2) Mention five prostaglandins with specific therapeutic uses.

Ans:

1. **PGE2 and PGF2α** – (**Dinoprostone, Carboprost**), Medical and therapeutic abortion (**Medical termination of pregnancy**).
2. **PGE1 (Alprostadil) – Erectile dysfunction.**
3. **PGE1 (Misoprostol) – NSAID induced gastric ulcers, protection against NSAID – induced GI adverse effects.**
4. **PGF2α (Bimatoprost, Latanoprost)** – **glaucoma** by facilitating better drainage of aqeous humor and reducing intraocular pressure.
5. **PGI2 (Epoprostenol, iloprost) – Pulmonary hypertension effecting pulmonary vasodilation**.

3) Explain teratogenic agents with examples.

A teratogenic or mutagenic drug is one which causes characteristic fetal abnormalities or malformations if taken during the first trimester of pregnancy (period of organogenesis). Teratogenic effects produced by drugs may be the result of interference with the passage of oxygen or nutrients to the foetus through the placenta. Teratogenicity can also occur due to direct meternal and foetal toxicity of the drug.

Some drugs such as thalidomide, cytotoxic drugs (methotrexate), antithyroid drugs (Propylthiouracil), aromatic retinoids like isotretinoin (used for acne vulgaris, acne rosaseae) directly act on the fetus and produce several foetal abnormalities; other drugs that can cause fetal damage include alcohol (fetal alcohol syndrome), tetracyclines can cause yellow-gray-brown discoloration of teeth,hypoplasia of enamel and deposition in the bones in the infancy and later), Quinolones (abnormalities like arthralgia, and joint swelling in infants), ACE inhibitors (pregnancy fetopathy), Phenytoin(foetal hydantoin syndrome), and smoking during pregnancy can produce potential teratogenic effects, and alcohol consumption during pregnancy can cause fetal alcohol syndrome characterized by craniofacial abnormalities, central nervous system dysfunction, pre and postnatal stunting of growth, hearing defects and speech disorders.

Answers to Question Paper given by King George Medical University, Lucknow

1) Classify Antimalarial Drugs. Describe the mechanism of action, uses and adverse effects and contraindications of chloroquine.

Ans: Antimalarial drugs can be classified based on chemical structure

1) 4 – aminoquinolines – chloroquine, amodioquine
2) 8 – aminoquinolines – Primaquine
3) 4 – Quinoline methanol – Mefloquine
4) Cinchona alkaloids – Quinine, quinidine
5) Antimetabolites – proguanil, chlorproguanil, sulfadoxine, pyrimethamine (folate antagonists)
6) Sequiterpene lactone endoperoxides – Artemisinins
7) Antibiotics – Doxycycline, clindamycin, azithromycin
8) Hydroxynaphthoquinone - Atovaquone

Mechanism of action of chloroquine: Erythrocytic forms of the parasite thrive on the hemoglobin of the host erythrocytes in their food vacuoles and produce highly reactive byproducts like ferroprotoporphyrin, also known as **heme** and free radicals. Chloroquine is a weak base that in its neutral form freely diffuses into the food vacuole of the parasite and gets protonated (ionized) with a rise of internal PH. The protonated chloroquine binds to the toxic heme and prevents its polymirization to hemozoin (nontoxic product). Prevention of detoxification of heme (conversion toxic heme to non – toxic hemozoin) results in oxidative damage to the parasite due to the build-up of toxic heme, thereby causing lysis of the parasite.

Uses of chloroquine:

1) Chloroquine is used in the treatment of acute attack of malaria caused by P. Vivax and P. malaria. It is also effective against falciparum malaria, but resistance to its action on the parasite is common. Its action is on the erythrocyte forms of the parasites, and has no effect on the hypnozoites.
2) Chloroquine is also effective as suppressive chemoprophylactic agent of falciparum infection in endemic areas. In combination with proguanil it is used to eradicate P. Vivax and P. Ovale malaria
3) Other uses of chloroquine include its indication for amoebic abscess of the liver and chronic recurrent progressive rheumatoid arthritis, systemic lupus erythematosus and lepra reaction

Adverse effects of chloroquine: The adverse effects are usually dose related and reversible. They include nausea, vomiting, headache, anorexia, blurred vision, dizziness and fatigue. In prolonged usage permanent retinal damage (optic neuritis) can occur. The other adverse effects of chloroquine include bleaching of hair, widening of QRS interval and 'T' wave abnormalities.

Contraindications and precautions for use of chloroquine: Chloroquine is contraindicated in the presence of retinal or visual field changes. It is also contraindicated in patients with psoriasis and porphyria where it may aggravate the condition. Chloroquine should be used with caution in patients with liver disease or neurologic or hematologic disorder.

2) Enumerate low molecular weight heparins. Describe with clinical relevance their differences with ultra fractionated heparin

Ans: Enoxaparin, dalteparin, and tinzaparin, nadroparin are the low molecular weight heparins **(LMWH).** They act by inhibition of the final common pathway of coagulation cascade. The final common pathway is the conversion of fibrinogen into fibrin by the activity of thrombin. LMWH inhibit coagulation by activating antithrombin III. Antithrombin III binds to and inhibits factor Xa thereby preventing the conversion of prothrombin to thrombin. This leads to inhibition of conversion of fibrinogen into fibrin for the formation of the clot.

Clinical Relevance of differences of LMWHs and ultra fractionated heparin:

1) The inability of ultra fractionated heparin (Heparin) to inactivate surface – bound thrombin and factor Xa is of limited efficacy in unstable angina, high – risk coronary angioplasty, and coronary thrombolysis. This has led to the development of low molecular weight heparins (LMWHs) which have more activity of Antithrombin III and also have activity against factor Xa thereby increasing its efficacy.

2) Advantages of LMWHs include

- More predictable anticoagulant activity
- Improved safety profile over unfractionated heparin
- More bioavailability due to lesser plasma and endothelial binding
- Longer half-lives
- Less frequent administration and lesser antigenic reactions
- Less activation of osteoclasts and less bone loss (osteopenia) as a result of less binding to osteoclasts
- Safe for use during pregnancy because the incidence of thrombocytopenia is less than 2% with LMWHs, which do not cross the placental barrier.
- Not inactivated by factor IV unlike heparin (UFH)
- Increased platelet aggregation does not occur unlike that is seen with UFH use.

Clinical uses of LMWHs

- prophylaxis and treatment of deep vein thrombosis and pulmonary embolism in medium and high – risk groups (persons undergoing surgical, orthopedic, and medical procedures)
- Pulmonary embolism (PE) due to other causes
- Venous thromboembolism in pregnancy
- Peripheral artery embolism
- Treatment of embolization associated with atrial fibrillation or prosthetic valve replacement
- Prophylaxis of postoperative deep vein thrombosis (DVT)
- For prevention of possible DVT and PE in patients who are bedridden for longer periods
- Renal dialysis, blood transfusions
- Unstable angina or non – ST segment elevation or non – Q wave MI

3) What is menopausal hormone therapy (MHT) Mention the indications and describe the advantages and disadvantages of MHT.

Ans: Menopause by definition is the final menstrual period in a women's reproductive life. Menopause is diagnosed after 12 months of amenorrhea and is characterized by a myriad symptom. Hormonal changes and clinical symptoms occur over a period leading up to and immediately following menopause. This period is frequently termed as **climacteric** or **perimenopause** and symptoms begin years before the menopause and usually in the form of delayed and irregular menstrual cycles and mild to moderate clinical features as that occur during the period of regular menopausal stage. The symptoms can be hastened because of oophorectomy, hysterectomy, autoimmune disorder, use of chemotherapy and radiation therapy.

The classical features of menopause include hot flushes, night sweats, insomnia, weight gain, floating mood changes, irregular menstruations, depression, anxiety states, headache, feelings of tiredness, vaginal dryness, reduced sex drive, dyspareunia, build – up of fat around waist, weight gain and charges skin colour.

Menopausal hormone therapy (**MHT**) is indicated in menopausal women when the expected benefits of treatment are anticipated to be greater than any possible adverse effects. MHT includes the use of conjugated equine estrogens, bazedoxifene (selective estrogen receptor modulator – SERM) and tibolone (an estrogen preparation having estrogenic, progestational and androgenic effect). MHT is the most effective treatment for vasomotor symptoms associated along with menopause related complaints such as joint and muscle pains, mood changes, sleep disturbances, CV risk, genitourinary complains, irregular menstrual cycles, and bone changes (osteoporosis). Vasomotor symptoms include hot flashes and nocturnal sweats.

Disadvantages of MHT: MHT can cause GI symptoms like anorexia, nausea, vomiting, increase of gall bladder stones, cholestatic jaundice. The cardiovascular effects include thrombophlebitis, thromboembolism producing deep vein thrombosis (DVT), increased risk of CV disease, uterine hyperplasia and uterine bleeding, and salt and water retention. MHT is contraindicated in women with underlying CV disease, history of earlier episodes of thromboembolism, hypercholesterolemia, stroke, and gall bladder disease and breast cancer.

4) **Mention the limitation of benzylpenicillin (Penicillin – G). Describe with suitable examples how the other penicillins are useful to overcome these limitations.**

Ans: Limitations of Benzyl Penicillin (Penicillin - G) include its short half – life of 20 – 30 minutes and frequent administrations, ingestion of food may delay oral absorption with an oral bioavailability of 30%, inactivation by β – lactamase enzyme, unstable in acid medium, hypersensitivity reactions and the need for administration by IM/IV routes for therapeutic effect. These short comings of Penicillin- G are overcome by the following mechanisms.

1) **Penicillin V** (potassium phenoxymethyl penicillin) – It is more stable in the acid medium and well absorbed from the gastrointestinal tract.
2) **Procaine Penicillin** – G – It is the suspension of penicillin - G in aqueous medium and is a long-acting penicillin and needs to be given by IM route only once daily. A dose of 3 lakh units produces plasma levels of 0.9 μg/ml within 1 – 3hr which falls to 0.1μg/ml at the end of 24hrs, further to 0.03 μg/ml at 48hrs.
3) **Benzathine Penicillin** – It is a suspension of Penicillin G - It is a suspension of Penicillin G in aqueous medium and made poorly soluble by the addition of ammonium (0.02%) and is long-acting penicillin that provides longer duration of action. Available in 6 lakh units given once in a month. A dose of 1.2 million units produces plasma levels of 0.09 μg/mL on the first, 0.02 μg/mL on the 14th and 0.002 μg/mL on the 32nd day after administration.
4) **Penicillinase resistant penicillins** – (**cloxacillin, dicloxacillin, methicillin, nafacillin, and oxacillin**) – These penicillins are resistant to the inactivation by β – lactamases produced by the sensitive organisms. They have a narrow spectrum of activity compared to natural penicillins (Penicillin G, Penicillin V). Their antimicrobial efficacy is aimed directly against penicillinase producing strains of Gram – Positive Cocci, particularly staphylococci.
5) **Combination penicillin G with Probenecid** – Higher and sustained plasma levels of Penicillin can be obtained when it is administered with Probenecid that blocks renal tubular secretion of Penicillin.

5) Enumerate five biological agents for rheumatoid arthritis (RA). Briefly describe mechanism of action and administration of each.

Ans: Biologic disease – modifying antirheumatic drugs (bDMARDs) include TNFα inhibitors, tocilizumab, and IL – 1 inhibitor like anakinra.

Mechanisms of action of bDMARDs

1) **TNFαinhibitors (Adalimumab, Infliximab, etanercept)** Cytokines play an important role in immune response and rheumatoid arthritis (RA). Two important cytokines involved in RA are TNFα and IL1. The cellular function effects of TNFα are mediated through membrane bound receptors TNFR1 and TNFR2. Macrophages, mast cells, and activated TH cells secrete TNFα. TNFα increases phagocytic activity of macrophages. TNFα has also pyrogenic effect. It is implicated in the pathology of several autoimmune diseases like RA. TNFα inhibitors are shown to have beneficial effects in these conditions.
2) **IL6 inhibitors**: **Tocilizumab and sarilumab** are antagonists of IL6 receptor, IL-6 being a pivotal cytokine involved in the pathogenesis of RA. These agents have shown efficacy when combined with methotrexate or as monotherapy.
3) **IL1 inhibitors**: **Anakinra** is a recombinant human IL – 1 receptor antagonist and used as the second preferred drug to treat RA and less efficacious than other DMARDs.

Administration:

1. Adalimumab is administered in doses of 40mg subcutaneously on alternate weeks because of its long half – life of 10 – 20 days.
2. Infliximab – It is given as IV infusion in 5mg/kg single dose.
3. Etanercept – It is given in doses of 25mg twice weekly subcutaneously once in 3 – 4 days.
4. Tocilizumab – It is given IV in a dose of 4mg/kg as a 60-minute single drip infusion once every 4 weeks, which can be increased to 8 mg/kg given every 4 weeks as a 60- minute single drip.
5. Anakinra – It is given subcutaneously in a daily dose of 100mg

6) Classify antihypertensive drugs. Write mechanism of action, uses, adverse effects, and contraindications of calcium channel blockers.

Ans: Antihypertensive drugs can be classified as

1) Centrally acting – clonidine, α – methyldopa, guanfacine, moxonidine.
2) Adrenergic neuron blockers – guanethidine, guanadrel, bretylium
3) Ganglion blockers – Trimetaphan, mecamylamine, pempidine
4) Adrenergic receptor blockers – α – blockers – prazocin and its derivatives; β – blockers- Metoprolol, Nebivolol, bisoprolol
5) Calcium channel blockers - Nifedipine, verapamil, diltiazem, amlodipin, cilnidipine, lacidipine
6) ACE inhibitors – Enalapril, lisinopril, ramipril
7) AT1 receptor blockers –Losartan, Valsartan, telmisartan
8) Vasodilators – Arteriodilators – Hydralazine, minoxidil, dizoxide.
9) Arteriovenodilators- Sodium nitroprusside
10) Diuretics – Thiazide derivatives, Indapamide, hydrochlorothiazide, loop diuretics – frusemide; Potassium sparing diuretics – Eplerenone, Fenerenone
11) Renin antagonists – Aliskerin

Calcium channel blockers: Calcium channel blockers have predominant action on voltage gated Ca^{2+} channels and block the entry of Ca^{2+}, thereby causing relaxation of the vascular smooth muscle. Their action is most effective on depolarized cell membranes. They can act either on L type of Ca^{2+} channel or 'T' type Ca^{2+} channel. The calcium channel has two receptor binding sites, one for dihydropyridines such as nifedipine and its group and the other for verapamil and diltiazem.

Uses of calcium channel blockers: Calcium channel blockers are used in the treatment of hypertension, variant/Prinzmetal angina, exertional angina, cardiac arrhythmias, hypertrophic cardiomyopathy, peripheral vascular disorders, subarachnoid haemorrhage, renal failure, preterm labour, prophylaxis of migraine, and vestibular disturbances.

Adverse effects of Calcium channel blockers: Bradycardia, hypotension, cardiac depression, AV nodal block and heart failure can occur when they are used in excess doses. Dihydropyridines can cause reflex tachycardia and fluid retention. The other adverse effects include fatigue, flushing, constipation, gingivitis, gingival hyperplasia.

Contraindications of calcium channel blockers: Non – dihydropyridines (diltiazem, verapamil, bepridil) are contraindicated in those with heart failure with reduced ejection fraction, second or third – degree AV block, and sick sinus syndrome.

7) **On the basis of mechanism of action, classify drugs effective in the treatment of cardiac failure. Describe the current status of digoxin and its interaction with drugs with potassium levels.**

Ans: Classification of drugs for congestive heart failure based on the mechanism of action

a) **Positive inotropic drugs**
   i. Cardiac glycosides – Digoxin, Ouabain
   ii. Phosphodiesterase inhibitors – Amrinone, milrinone, vesnarinone, enoximone
   iii. Sympathomimetics – Dopamine, dobutamine

b) **Drugs affecting cardiac hemodynamic function**
   i. Angiotensin converting enzyme inhibitors (ACE inhibitors) – Ramipril, lisinopril
   ii. AT1 receptor blockers – Telmisartan, losartan, valsartan

c) **Drugs affecting cardiac – dynamics**: β-blockers- Carvedilol, Metoprolol, Bisoprolol, Nebiolol

d) **Drugs affecting renal function** – Diuretics

e) **Vasodilators** – Sodium nitroprusside, nitro-glycerine (arteriovenodilators) and hydralazine, minoxidil, diazoxide (arteriodilatoras)

f) **SGLT -2 inhibitors** – Dapagliflozin, empagliflozin, sotaglifilozin

g) **Aldosterone antagonists -** Spiranolactone, eplerenone, finerenone

h) **Newer agents –** Neprilysin and angiotensin receptor antagonists-sacubitril/valsartan

i) **Inodilators-** Levosimendon, ivabradin

Didoxin is a positive inotropic drug used earlier for the treatment of congestive heart failure. But of late it is not the first line of treatment or drug of choice for this condition, the reason being its narrow margin of safety and narrow therapeutic index. However, digoxin can be considered as a reserve drug when symptoms of the disease are not adequately controlled with ACE inhibitors and diuretics. In chronic congestive failure associated with cardiomyopathy, combination therapy with ACE inhibitors, digoxin, and positive inotropic drugs can reduce the morbidity greatly and mortality to a lesser extent.

Interaction of digoxin with drugs with potassium levels

Digoxin toxicity is caused by an excess of calcium or a deficiency of potassium (hypokalemia). Excess calcium increases to cardiac excitability and also the hypokalemia can cause the blockade of Na^+-K^+ - ATP ase pump which results in delayed outflux of Na^+, followed by accumulation of intracellular Ca+ which results in delayed after depolarizations (DADs), ventricular arrhythmias manifested as prolonged PR intervals, shortening of QT interval, inverted 'T' wave and ST segment depression. Loop diuretics which reduce potassium levels potentially Increase digitalis toxicity. Close monitoring of renal function and potassium levels are very important in appropriate use of digoxin. Hyperkalemia diminishes digoxin's effectiveness.

8) Describe with examples the additional mechanism of second generation H1 blockers. Describe their disadvantages over first generation H1 blockers. Mention two H1 blockers used for topical application.

Ans: 2nd generation **H1** blockers include loratadine, desloratadine, levocabastine, fexofenadine, ebastine, rupatadine, azelastine, cetirizine, levocetirizine, olapatadadine, alcaftadine

Additional Mechanisms of action:

1) They are hydrophilic polar compounds, do not cross the blood: brain barrier and hence do not cause sedation and drowsiness.
2) They are selective peripheral H1receptor blockers.
3) They have long half lives and hence given once daily.
4) They do not cause adverse autonomic effects (anticholinergic effects) unlike first generation H_1 blockers.
5) They do not cause cardiac irregularities.

Disadvantages of 2nd generation H1 blockers: In general, second generation H1 blockers are supposed not to cause drowsiness and sedation. However, drowsiness and moderate sedation can be produced by the use of them. They can also cause fatigue and lessened alertness. Astemazole, fexofenadine, ebastine can cause ventricular tachycardia.

Second generation H1 blockers used for topical uses: Azalastine 0.05% and olopatadine 0.1% are used as eye drops to treat allergic conjunctivitis and other superficial allergic condition of the eye. Alcaftadine 0.25%, can also be used for allergic conjunctivitis.

Question Paper given by Kerala University of Health Sciences - February 2022 Paper I Pharmacology

1. **MR. X, a 65 year – old teacher has severe retrosternal chest pain radiating to shoulder and left arm. He was profusely sweating and his E.C.G revealed ST elevation and a diagnosis of Acute Myocardial infarction (AMI) was made**
   a. **Write the management of AMI with rationale for use of each drug.**
   b. **Enumerate the drugs to be prescribed at the time of discharge.**
   c. **Mention the lifestyle modifications to be advised to the patient.**

Ans: Acute myocardial infarction (AMI) is an emergency clinical condition which should be diagnosed at the earliest by the clinical presentation of the case with the aid of requisite diagnostic tests. On admission to the hospital the said patient should be continuously monitored by ECG and laboratory readings of serum cardiac markers (troponin T – cTnT and cTnI tropnin C) taken to confirm the diagnosis. The immediate supportive measures include cardiopulmonary resuscitation and maintaining balance between oxygen supply and demand to prevent further ischemia. The other measures that follow include monitoring oxygen saturation by pulse oximetry, continuous oxygen supplementation in patients who are breathless and hypoxic (oxygen saturation < 90%) and electric cardioversion if there are ventricular arrhythmias.

Drug therapy

1) Analgesics – They reduce the pain thereby decreasing sympathetic stress with a reduced preload. They ensure comfort to the patient, reduce pulmonary arterial pressure, and provide sedative and anxiolytic effect necessary for patients who experience chest discomfort due to MI. Diamorphine 2.5 - 5mg given IV and repeated as necessary is the drug of choice.
2) Drugs for immediate benefit include sublingual nitroglycerine three doses each of 4 mg at 5 minutes intervals. Buccal absorption of a tablet of aspirin containing 160 – 325 mg is helpful for rapid inhibition of COX_1 in platelets and inhibition of TXA_2 preventing further platelet aggregation.
3) Antithrombotic agents – These agents prevent the formation of thrombus associated with MI, pulmonary embolism, and stroke. The drugs that are used commonly for this purpose include unfractioned heparin, low molecular weight heparins (enoxaparin), fondaparinux, and bivaluridin.
4) Thrombolytic agents – These agents immediately lyse thrombus, prevent recurrent thrombus formation, and facilitate rapid restoration of coronary artery patency and arrest hemodynamic disturbances. They are effective if given within 3 – 6 hours of onset symptoms. The agents that are used for this purpose are alteplase, reteplase, tenecteplase, anistreplase and streptokinase.
5) Vasodilators: They oppose coronary artery spasm, augment coronary blood flow, and reduce cardiac work decreasing preload and afterload. Nitroglycerine is the drug choice given IV is doses of 5 – 10 mcg/min and the dose are titrated by reducing the same by 10% periodically till the systolic blood pressure does not fall below 90mm.
6) β – blockers: They inhibit chronotropic and ionotropic responses to β – adrenergic activation and reduce blood pressure and cardiac contractility which decreases myocardial oxygen demands within 8 hours of onset of symptoms. They reduce the risk of reinfarction apart from decreasing the associated

pain arising out of increased myocardial O_2 demand. The drug of choice is metoprolol given IV in a dose of 5mg and the same is repeated twice later.

7) Follow up medications:
   a. Antiplatelet drugs like low doses of aspirin 75 – 80mg and clopidogrel 75mg/ day given orally.
   b. Cardioselective β – blockers – metoprolol 25 – 50mg/day
   c. Cholesterol lowering drugs like atorvastatin 2
   d. 0 – 40mg/day, rosuvastatin 10mg/day; pitavastatin 2mg/day. Either of them given regularly prevents the formation of fresh/new thrombi in coronary arteries when given along with antiplatelet drugs.
   e. ACE inhibitors like ramipril 2.5mg – 5mg/day may be needed to prevent the possible post – MI CV events particularly cardiac remodelling
8) Lifestyle charges needed by the patient include lesser intake of cholesterol containing foods like diary products, regular physical activity, anxiety free state, cessation of smoking in case the patient is a smoker, containment of alcohol intake if the person is an alcoholic and maintaining a healthy body weight/Body mass index of 20kg/m^2.

2. Classify opioid analgesics. Write the pharmacological effects, therapeutic uses, adverse effects and contraindication of morphine

Ans: Opioid analgesics can be classified as

Phenanthrenes – Natural – morphine, codeine Semisynthetic – Diacetylmorphine, dihydrocodone, hydrocodone, hydromorphone, oxycodone, oxymorphone.

1) **Piperidine derivatives** - Phenylpiperidines – Meperidine, difenoxilate, loperamide
2) **Anilidopiperidines** - Fentanyl, alfentanyl, sufentanyl, remifentanyl
3) **Phenyl heptylamines** – methadone, propoxyphene, dextro - propoxyphene
4) **Benzomorphans** – Pentazocin, phenazocin
5) **Morphinans** – Levorphanol, butorphanol
6) **Opioid antagonists** – Nalmefene, naltrexone, naloxone.

Pharmacological effects of morphine

1) Analgesia – Morphine and other opioids produce analgesia, drowsiness, changes in mood and mental clouding. Pain threshold is increased and sharp piercing pain becomes less intense and more tolerable, while dull aching pain disappears. Apart from the analgesic effect, morphine also reduces the affective component of pain that is accompanied by a state of wellbeing. Morphine also reduces the anxiety states, particularly when given as preanesthetic medication.
2) Sedation – Morphine produces drowsiness and mental clouding without producing amnesia. Phenanthrenes produce a more sedative effect then other groups of opioids.
3) Euphoric effect – Morphine produces a sense of well being or euphoria and freedom from anxiety and distress, and there is a sense of contentment. This is an essential component of its analgesic effect because the agitation and anxiety associated with painful illness or injury are thereby relieved. This is also an essential component for its effects of dependence and addiction.
4) Respiration: Morphine and other opioids depress respiration by acting on the brainstem respiratory centers – medulla oblongatae. Respiratory rate, respiratory minute volume and tidal exchange are depressed in a dose – dependent manner.

5) Antitussive effect: Morphine and related opioids codeine, pholcodine, dextromethorphan suppresses cough reflex by acting on the medullary cough center and used in dry unproductive cough.

6) Nauseant and emetic effects: Morphine – like drugs stimulate CTZ and produce nausea and vomiting which occurs even in normal therapeutic doses.

7) Miosis: Morphine produces constriction of the pupils due to stimulation of oculomotor nucleus (parasympathomimetic effect). Tolerance to the miotic actions of morphine does not develop.

8) Truncal rigidity: Morphine – like drugs increase the tone of the trunkal muscles and produce rigidity. This action is more prominent in high lipid – soluble opioids like fentanyl, sufentanil and alfentanil.

9) Effects on gastrointestinal system: Opioids decrease the mobility and increase the tone of the smooth muscle of the GI tract. Amplitude of propulsive contractions is markedly decreased in the large intestine and delays the passage of fecal mass and allows increased absorption of water which leads to constipation.

10) Neuroendocrine effects: Morphine acts on the hypothalamus and inhibits the release of gonadotropic releasing hormone (GnRH), Corticotropin releasing hormone (CRH), FSH, LH, ACTH thus decreasing their circulating concentrations. Prolactin levels increase due to removal of inhibition of its release by dopamine.

11) Effects on biliary tract: Opioids constrict the biliary smooth muscle which may result in biliary colic. The sphincter Oddi also gets contracted that leads to reflux of biliary and pancreatic secretions.

12) Effects on cardiovascular spem: This is well maintained in normal therapeutic dose. But when CVS function is not adequate, the release of histamine and depression on central vasomotor center may cause peripheral vasodilation resulting in a fall of blood pressure. Pentazocine causes tachycardia due to antimuscarinic effects.

13) Histamine release: Opioids produce flushing of the face, warming of the skin, sweating, and itching and bronchoconstriction due to liberation of histamine.

Therapeutic uses:

1) Analgesic action: Opioids are mainly used to provide analgesia and relief of anxiety and sedation in acute myocardial infarction. Opioids are also used to relieve postoperative pain, pain due to trauma and pain due to malignancy. Morphine also acts as a good analgesic for relief of pain due to renal and biliary colic in combination with atropine.

2) Pre – anesthetic medication: Morphine is given preanesthetically to relieve anxiety and produce quieting and sedative effect.

3) Adjuvant to general anesthesia: Morphine can be given as adjuvant to general anesthesia to reduce the requirements of the general anesthetic agent and used during the perioperative period.

4) Epidural and intrathecal analgesia: Morphine can be given by epidural and intrathecal routes to relieve chronic pain due to malignancy.

5) Acute pulmonary edema: Morphine provides relief from dyspnea due to pulmonary edema associated with left ventricular failure.

Contraindications of morphine: Morphine is contraindicated in head injury, in patients with atrial flutter and supraventricular tachycardia, hypotensive states, acute abdominal state, convulsions, hypoxia or reduced respiratory reserve, elderly debilitated patients, patients with renal or hepatic dysfunction, Addison’s disease, prostatic hypertrophy or urethral stricture, and use in children.

Answers to the Question Paper given in March 2022 Tamil Nadu MGR University of Health Sciences - Paper I

1. **60 years old is known HT and DM for the past 20 years has been admitted with c/o compressive swelling in the face and abdomen and legs for the past three months.**

   a) What is your diagnosis?

   b) Classify diuretics

   c) Describe the mechanism of action, uses and adverse effects of high ceiling diuretics

   d) Justify the rationality in combining high ceiling diuretics with ACE inhibitors

Ans: a) It is a case of chronic congestive heart failure secondary to hypertension with associated comorbidity of diabetes mellitus as per the presentation of symptoms of the patient.

b) Diuretics are classified as

1. Osmotic diuretics	–	Mannitol
2. Carbonic anhydrase inhibitors	–	Acetazolamide, Methazolamide, Dichlorphenamide
3. Thiazide diuretics	–	Hydrochlorothiazide, bendroflumethiazide, Chlorthalidone, indapamide, polythiazide.
4. Loop diuretics	–	Ethacrynic acid, furosemide, bumetanide, torsemide
5. Potassium sparing diuretics	–	Spironolactone, amiloride, triamterene, eplerenone, fenerenone

c) High ceiling diuretics or loop diuretics like frusemide act at the thick ascending limb of loop of Henle inhibiting reabsorption of the Nacl.

They inhibit NKCC2 transporter in the apical (luminal) membrane of loop epithelial cells thereby reducing reabsorption of Nacl (upto 25% of the filtered sodium). Loop diuretics also cause an increase of Mg^{+} and Ca^{2+} excretion by inhibiting positive luminal potential.

Uses of highceiling diueretics

- Loop diuretics are indicated in edematous conditions like pulmonary edema, edema due to congestive heart failure, hepatic cirrhosis, nephritic syndrome, and in the treatment of hypertension.
- Hypercalcemic conditions as they facilitate excretion of calcium as in the conditions like hyperparathyroidism, or parathyroid malignancy associated hypercalcemia.
- Hyperkalemia caused by potassium retaining diuretics or use of ACE inhibitors or due to renalinsufficiency causing increased potassium levels.
- To induce forced diuresis to facilitate rapid removal of toxic drugs if taken in excess doses.

Adverse effects of loop diuretics

Loop diuretics are very potent in their action and can cause volume and electrolyte depletion, leading to hyponatremia, hypokalemia, and hypotension which can further lead to reduced GFR, circulatory collapse. Excessicve potassium loss can induce arrhythmias particularly in those persons receiving digoxin.

Intially fluid and electrolyte loss causes dryness of mouth, thirst, weakness, drowsiness, muscle spasms, muscle fatigue, and nausea.

Loopm diuretics can cause ototoxicity, hyperuricemia, and hyperglycemia, increased plasma LDL-C levels and decreased HDL-C levels

d) ACE inhibitors like lisinopril are combined with high ceiling diuretics so as to potentiate more Na^+ and water loss (diuretic effect) and better and effective control of congestive heart failure. This results in off loading of fluid from the circulation thereby reducing the cardiac workload, improve contractility and force of contraction and thus improve the symptoms associated with CHF. The combination is also useful in the eventual reduction and control of hypertension associated with CHF. Another important benefit of the combination is to control the serum potassium levels in the therapeutic range. This is the result of an increase of K^+ levels (retention of K^+) seen with ACE inhibitors countered by the loss of K+ associated with loop diuretics. This prevents development of arrhythmias also.

2. A 65-year-old male on antipsychotic medications came with c/o of difficulty in walking, resting tremors and difficulty in swallowing.

a) What is the diagnosis?

b) How will you treat this patient?

c) Describe the mechanism of action, importance of combination therapy and adverse effects of Levodopa.

Ans: a) This is a case of Parkinsonism the symptoms of which also include muscular rigidity and postural instability apart from resting tremors and bradykinesia. As the patient is already on antipsychotic drugs therapy and the features described are more due to adverse effects caused by them, a probable diagnosis of drug induced Parkinsonism can be made out.

b) The drug induced Parkinsonism caused by the use of antipsychotic drugs like Phenothiazines, butyrophenones and metoclopramide and reserpine (all dopamine antagonists) can be treated with anticholinergic drugs like Benztropine, biperidin, procyclidine and trihexyphenidyl. Levodopa is not of use in the drug induced Parkinsonism and which may aggravate the mental disorders.

c) Levodopa is the initial drug to be prescribed for a case of classical Parkinsonism but not for drug induced Parkinsonism.

Dopamine by itself cannot cross the blood-brain barrier and hence its precursor levodopa needs to be given. However, when given orally 90% of levodopa is decarboxylated to dopamine peripherally and very little crosses the blood-brain barrier to enter the dopaminergic system. This peripheral conversion of levodopa to dopamine is responsible for many of its adverse effects. The peripheral conversion of levodopa to dopamine can be inhibited by dopa decarboxylase inhibitors carbidopa or benserazide, threby increasing the levels of levodopa, followed by its entry into the CNS.

The adverse effects that can be caused by levodopa include dyskinesia, behavioral effects, CVS responses like cardiac irregularities such as tachycardia and ventricular extrasystoles the incidence of which is very much limited when it is combined with carbidopa. Levodopa can also cause of GI side effects like anorexia, nausea and vomiting which are not seen when it is combined with carbidopa and also taken in divided doses. Most importantly, levodopa can cause fluctuations in the drug response after the end of successful treatment for 3-5 years. The simplest form of fluctuation is end-of-dose or wearing off reaction that will occur with re-emergence of parkinsonian symptoms.

I. Write short notes on:

1. Mechanism of action and clinical uses of statins.

Ans: Statins like levostatin, atorvastatin, fluvastatin, rosuvastatin act by inhibiting an enzyme HMG-COA reductase. Statins exert their major effect of reduction of LDL cholesterol by competitively inhibiting HMG-COA reductase, thereby preventing the conversion of HMG-COA to mevalonic acid and its further conversion to cholesterol.

Statins are used to treat primary and secondary hyperlipidemia and cause a dose dependant lowering of LDL cholesterol levels. They prevent the onset of atherosclerotic coronary vascular disease by lowering LDL-C levels and thus prevent many cardiovascular events like ischemic heart disease, MI and anginal episode in patients who have recovered from MI.

2. Pharmacovigilance: It is a type of continued monitoring of untoward effects and other safety related aspects of drugs that are already marketed and currently being used in general populations. In general, Pharmacovigilance refers to voluntary or spontaneous reporting systems which allow health care professionals and regulatory authorities to take suitable action and decisions for withdrawal of the drugs from general use when the drug is not safe for consumption. It involves detection, assessment, understanding and prevention of both short and long-term adverse drug effects.

3. Therapeutic effects of atypical antipsychotics.

Ans: Atypical antipsychotic drugs are 2nd generation antipsychotics drugs that include Clozapine, loxapine, olanzapine, risperidone, qetiapine, molindone, and ziprasidone act by blocking D_2 and 5-HT_2A receptors in the dopaminergic pathways of the brain-mesolimbic and mesocortical pathways. Atypical antipsychotics by virtue of their affinity for both D_2 and 5-HT_2A receptors alleviate both positive and negative symptoms of schizophrenia. They are safer and more efficacious. Apart from schizophrenia, they are also useful in acute mania, bipolar disorder, schizoaffective disorder, severe agitation, major depressive disorder along with antidepressants, Tourette syndrome, and obsessive-compulsive disorder and childhood autism (Clozapine is the drug of choice for the last two indications)

4. Brief phase II biotransformation reactions with suitable examples.

Ans: Phase II biotransformation reactions include **glucuronide, acetylation, glutathione, glycine, sulfate and methylation conjugation reactions**. The drugs which undergo phase I biotransformation initially also undergo phase II reactions subsequently by which the resultant drug product becomes highly ionized and rapidly eliminated.

i. Glucuronide conjugation – Morphine, Acetaminophen, Diazepam, Chloramphenicol.

ii. Acetylation – Sulphonamides, INH, dapsone, clonazepam

iii. Glutathione – Ethacrynic acid

iv. Glycine – Salicylic and Benzoic acids

v. Sulfate – Estrone, methyldopa

vi. Methylation – Dopamine, epinephrine

5. Therapeutic uses of adrenergic drugs.

Ans: Adrenergic drugs are used in a variety of clinical conditions that include mydriasis(phenylephrine), bronchial asthma(β_2 agonists), vasoconstrictor effect (adrenaline) to arrest local bleeding like epistaxis oral, facial,and nasopharyngeal bleeding; to prolong the duration of action of local anaesthetics (adrenaline, noradrenaline and phenylephrine); cardiogenic shock (adrenaline and isoprenaline), anaphylactic shock (adrenaline); hypotensive states that include orthostatic hypotension(ephedrine, midodrine, mephenteramine); for the arrest of premature labor (ritodrine and isoetharine); stress incontinence (ephedrine), attention-deficit hyperactivity disorder (dextroamphetamine); glaucoma (apraclonidine, brimonidine) and also as CNS stimulants (narcolepsy, modafinil is the drug of choice),and as anorectic drugs to suppress appetite and used in obesity (dextramphetamine).

6. Drugs used in prophylaxis of migraine.

Ans: Triptans like sumatriptan, zolmitriptan, rizatriptan, almotriptan, and naratriptan are the main drugs used for prophylaxis of migraine. The other drugs that can be used for the similar purpose include topiramate, sodium valproate, Beta blockers (propranolol, timolol), methysergide, calcitonin gene-related peptide (CGRP) receptor antagonists like Erenumab; tricyclic antidepressants like amitryptiline; calcium channel blockers, selective serotonin reuptake inhibitors (fluoxetine, paroxetine) and NSAIDS.

7. Role of leukotriene antagonists used in bronchial asthma.

Ans: Leukotrienes (LT_{B4}, LT_{C4}, LT_{D4}) produce potent contraction of the bronchial smooth muscle causing bronchospasm and respiratory difficulty seen in patients of bronchial asthma. They are also responsible for airway hyperreactivity, mucous secretion, mucosal oedema, which are all seen in episodes of bronchial asthma.

(a) Leukotriene synthesis inhibitor like zileuton is a potent and selective inhibitor of 5-lipoxygenase activity and thereby inhibits formation of leukotrienes (LT_{B4}, LT_{A4}).

(b) Leukotriene receptor antagonists like montelukast, zafirlukast act by binding to LT_{C4}, LT_{D4} and LT_{E4} which are strong bronchoconstrictors and thereby relieve bronchospasm seen in bronchial asthma.

8. Brief the drugs used in hypertensive emergencies.

Ans: Hypertensive emergency is high rise in blood pressure levels which may cause life-threatening signs and symptoms that result in potential damage to organ systems that in turn result in stroke, MI, ocular damage (changes in vision), bleeding from nose and other areas. These are apart from the very common immediate signs and symptoms that include headache, dizziness, and altered mental status, shortness of breath, decreased urine output, vomiting and chest discomfort. The blood pressure readings may exceed 180/100 mm Hg.

Hypertensive emergency is usually due to sudden withdrawal of antiadrenergic drugs like clonidine, β-blockers, sudden state of rage, anxiety, grief and similar conditions of unexpected emotional states.

The treatment of hypertensive emergency consults of administering labetalol, clevidipine, nicardipine, nitroglycerine, sodium nitroprusside, diazoxide, fenoldopam, hydralazine (in eclampsia and pre-eclampsia). All of them act by different mechanisms with the end result being lowering the elevated blood pressure levels as early as possible. It is always mandatory to monitor the doses of the drug in use so as to see that they do not cause abrupt fall of BP which may cause irreparable damage to the organ systems.

9. Heparin versus warfarin.

Ans: Heparin and warfarin are both anticoagulants which act by different mechanisms, given by different routes and indicated for different clinical conditions.

Heparin acts by binding to plasma protease inhibitor antithrombin III, which is an endogenous anticoagulant that inactivates thrombin, in addition to inactivating thrombin, antithrombin also inactivates coagulation factors IXa, Xa, XIIa, and IIa which leads to inhibition of conversion of fibrinogen to fibrin with the ultimate result of inhibition of both intrinsic and extrinsic coagulation pathways thus preventing coagulation. Heparin is indicated in a number of clinical conditions that include deep vein thrombosis (DVT), pulmonary embolism (PE), atrial fibrillation (AF) and for prevention of excess coagulation during surgery such as cardiac surgery, dialysis procedures, prevention of thrombosis due to chronic immobilization, as adjuvant in the treatment of unstable angina or non – ST segment elevation or non-Q wave MI.

Warfarin is an oral anticoagulant that acts as antagonist of vitamin K which is essential for the synthesis of coagulation factors II, VII, IX and X and the anticoagulant proteins C and S (coagulation regulatory factors). Warfarin is administered as continuation anticoagulation therapy after initiation with more rapid acting agents like heparin or synthetic heparin derivatives like fondaparinux. Warfarin is given for the prevention of thrombosis (DVT) and pulmonary embolism (further episodes). It is also indicated for prevention of thrombosis in stroke, during the process or during lifetime after cardiac valve replacement and atrial fibrillation.

10. Complication of spinal anesthesia.

Ans: The complications that could occur due to spinal anesthesia include neurotoxicity in the form back pain, pain in the buttocks, posterior thighs and in the groin. The cardiovascular adverse effects include hypotension. The effects on CNS include perioral and tongue numbness, visual and auditory disturbances, restlessness, sleepiness and light-headedness. Local anaesthetics can also produce allergic reactions, drug interaction with sulfonamides (procaine, benzocaine, tetracaine), and local sepsis if sterilization precautions not taken.

Answers to Question Paper given by March 2022 Tamil Nadu MGR University of Health Sciences

PAPER II

Long Essay Questions:

1. **a) Classify drugs used in peptic ulcer**

   b) Discuss the mechanism of action, uses and adverse effects of proton pump inhibitors

   c) Add a note on Anti-H-pylori drug regimens

Ans:

a) Classification of drugs used in peptic ulcer include the following:

1. Acid – Neutralizing agents (Antacids) – Aluminium hydroxide, Magnesium hydroxide, Magnesium trisilicate.
2. Gastric acid lowering agents:
   i. H2 receptor antagonists – Ranitidine, famotidine, nizatidine
   ii. Proton pump inhibitors – Omeprazole, lansoprazole, pantoprazole, rabeprazole, esomeprazole
   iii. Anticholinergic agents – Pirenzepine, glycopyrrolate, mepenzolate
   iv. Prostaglandin analogs (PGE_1 analog) – Misoprostol
3. Mucoprotective agents – Sucralfate, colloidal bismuth compounds
4. Drugs for eradication of H. Pylori – Metronidazole, amoxacillin, clarithromycin

b) Mechanism of action, uses and adverse effects of proton pump inhibitors.

Proton pump inhibitors are inactive prodrugs that require activation in the acid environment in the parietal cell canaliculi. Oral preparations of these drugs are enteric coated to prevent premature activation. They are concentrated in the secretory canaculus of the parietal cell where the local pH is less than 1.0. In this acid pH, the drugs become protonated to form the active sulfonamide cations, which then react with a cysteine residue on the H^+/K^+/ATP ase to form a covalent disulfide bond. Covalent binding of the drug inhibits the activity of the proton pump irreversibly leading to prolonged and nearly complete suppression of acid secretion.

Uses of PPIs: Proton pump inhibitors are used in peptic ulcer disease, gastroesophageal reflux disease (GERD), pathological hyper secretory conditions like gastrinomas which are inoperable, Zollinger – Ellison syndrome, H. Pylori infection in combination with antibiotics like amoxicillin, clarithromycin, NSAID – induced gastroduodenal ulcers, stress ulcers, reduction of risk for upper GI bleeding, add on therapy for patients on antiplatelet therapy with high risk of GI bleed, and prior to or following on endoscopy associated with an acute or high risk bleeding.

Adverse effects of PPIs: PPIs are usually well tolerated and the possible adverse effects include hypomagnesemia, possibility of intestinal infections with clostridium difficile, osteoporosis on long term use, a minor reduction of B_{12} absorption, hypergastrinemia, and minor GI adverse effects like nausea, abdominal pain and diarrhea can occur occasionally.

c) **Add a note on Anti – H. Pylori regimens**

For the eradication of H. Pylori infection, preventing acute ulceration and promoting healing of the ulcer, triple therapy is usually instituted in a combination regimen. It consists of one proton pump inhibitor, and two antibiotics. The proton pump inhibitor is given twice daily (Omeprazole 20mg twice daily), Clarithromycin 500mg twice daily and metronidazole/amoxicillin 500mg twice daily. Alternatively giving four drugs is also of therapeutic benefit. It consists of bismuth subsalicylate (two tablets of 262mg), tetracycline (500mg 4 times/day), omeprazole 20mg twice daily and metronidazole 250 mg 4 times a day. Any regimen is given for a period of 7 to 14 days.

2. **a) Classify antimalarial drugs**

   b) Describe the mechanism of action, uses and adverse effects of chloroquine

   c) Write briefly on Artemisinin based combination therapy

Ans:

a) **Antimalarial drugs can be classified as follows:(According to chemical groupings)**

i. 4 – aminoquinolines – Chloroquine, amodiaquine
ii. 8 –aminoquinolines – Primaquine
iii. 4 – Quinoline methanol – Mefloquine
iv. Cinchona alkaloids – Quinine, Quinidine
v. Antimetabolites – Proguanil, chlorproguanil, sulfadoxine, pyrimethamine
vi. Sequiterpene lactone endoperoxides – Artemisinins
vii. Antibiotics – Doxycycline, clindamycin, azithromycin
viii. Phenanthrene methanol – Halofantrine
ix. Hydroxy naphthoquinone – Atovaquone

b) **Mechanism of action, uses and adverse effects of chloroquine**

Erythrocytic forms of the malarial parasites thrive on the hemoglobin of the host erythrocytes in their acidic food vacuoles and produce highly reactive by products like ferroprotoporphyrin, also known as heme and free radicals. Chloroquine is a weak base that in its neutral form freely diffuses into the food vacuoles of the parasite and gets protonated with a rise in pH. The accumulated protonated chloroquine binds with the toxic heme and prevents its polymerization to nontoxic hemozoin. Prevention of polymerization / detoxification of heme results in oxidative damage in the parasite due to the accumulation of toxic heme, thereby damaging the parasite.

Chloroquine is used in acute clinical attack of malaria caused by P. Vivax, P. Malarial, P. Ovale and susceptible strains of P. Falciparum. It is also used as a suppressive chemoprophylactic agent in endemic areas of falciparum malaria. The other uses of chloroquine include amebic abscess of the liver and chronic recurrent progressive rheumatoid arthritis. Its other uses include systemic lumps erythematosus and lepra reaction.

Adverse effects of chloroquine include headache, nausea, vomiting, anorexia, blurred vision, dizziness and fatigue. The use of chloroquine in high doses can cause serious and permanent retinal damage (optic neuritis). The other adverse effects of chloroquine include bleaching of hair, widening of QRS interval and T wave abnormalities.

Artemisinin based combination therapy

Artemisinins (Artemisinin, artemether, artesunate) have shorter half lives requiring followup treatment with mefloquine or combination therapy with lumefantrine. The combination therapy is useful for severe acute cases of drug – resistant P. falciparum malaria.

II. Write short notes on

1. Role of bisphosphonates in osteoporosis

Bisphosphonates bind to hydroxyapatite crystals in the bone and inhibit osteoclast mediated bone resorption. They increase the density of the bone and decrease the incidence of fractures. The commonly used bisphosphonates include alendronate, etidronate, pamidronate, risedronate, and ibandronate. For maximum gut absorption, all oral bisphosphonates should be taken on empty stomach or two hours after food with plenty of water in a sitting or upright posture to avoid esophageal regurgitation.

2. Therapeutic uses and adverse effects of cisplatin

Cisplatin is an alkylating agent that kills tumor cells in all stages of the cell cycle by binding to DNA and preventing its replication by forming intra as well as inter-strand cross links. It is used to treat non-small-cell and small-cell lung cancers, esophageal and gastric cancers, head and neck and genitourinary cancers, particularly testicular, ovarian and bladder cancers. It is used also as a second-line drug for the treatment of colorectal cancer following treatment with the combination of 5-flurouracil and leucovorin.

3. Mechanism of action and uses of ciprofloxacin

Ciprofloxacin is a fluoroquinolone derivative. It elicits bactericidal action by inhibiting DNA gyrase (topoisomerase II) and topoisomerase IV which are required for the bacterial DNA replication, transcription, repair and recombination. Quinolone inhibition of bacterial topoisomerase is very rapid, which explains the concept of rapid killing with ciprofloxacin along with other quinolones.

Uses of ciprofloxacin include genitourinary infections (Urinary tract infections including those complicated due to renal stones, secondary to catheter use, obstructive uropathies), Prostatitis, respiratory tract infections (bacterial sinusitis, acute bronchitis, community acquired pneumonia, atypical pneumonia and nosocomial pneumonia); sexually transmitted infections (uncomplicated neisseria gonococcal urethritis, cervicitis, urethritis caused by H. Ducrei or chlamydia trachomatis; pelvic inflammatory disease in combination with cefoxitin, gastrointestinal infections (traveller's diarrhea), typhoid fever, bone, joint, and soft tissue infections. It is the most potent fluoroquinolone agent against pseudomonal infections.

4. Discuss alkylating agents used as anti cancer drugs

Alkylating drugs (mechlorethamine, cyclophosphamide, busulfan, chlorambucil, carmustine, lomustine, cisplatin and others) are highly reactive molecules and transfer their alkyl groups to important cellular components of DNA or RNA at an electron rich site making them nonfunctional. In general, they react with sulfydryl, amino, hydroxyl, carboxyl groups. Mechlorethamine is used in the treatment of Hodgkin's disease, lymphomas, chronic myelogenic leukemia, chronic lymphoblastic leukemia. Cyclophosphamide is used in malignant lymphomas, Hodgkin's disease, lymphocytic leukemia, Burkitt's lymphoma, multiple myeloma, adenocarcinoma of ovaries, carcinoma breast, and retinoblastoma. Carmustine, lomustine are used for the treatment of brain tumors like glioblastoma and metastatic brain tumours and Hodgkin's lymphoma.

Cisplatin and oxaliplatin are used in various types of malignancies that include ovarian, testicular, breast, colorectal cancers apart from small-cell lung cancer and head and neck cancers.

5. **Beta lactamase inhibitors**

   Clavulanic acid, sulbactam, tazobactam, avibactam are β-lactamase inhibitors that are able to inhibit the actions of many beta lactamases which are responsible for the inactivation of Beta lactam antibiotics. They are particularly useful against plasmid-encoded β-lactamases produced by staphylococci, H. influenzae, N. gonorrhoeae, Shigella, E. coli, Klebsiella pneumoniae.

   Clavulanic acid is combined with amoxicillin to enhance its antimicrobial action in a fixed dose of 250mg, 500mg and 875mg of amoxicillin and 125mg of clavulanic acid.

   Sulbactam is combined with ampicillin in equal proportions and given IM/IV. Tazobactam is combined with piperacillin in a fixed combination of 3g of piperacillin and 250mg of tazobactam and given parenterally every 6 hr in pseudomonal infections.

6. **Drugs for psoriasis**

   Psoriasis is a complex, chronic, multifactorial inflammatory disease of the skin that involves hyperproliferation of keratinocytes in the epidermis, with an increase of epidermal cell turnover rate. It is characterized by thickened patches of inflamed red skin covered with thick, silvery scales. It can occur in elbows, knees, scalp, feet, palms and nape of the neck.

   The drugs that can be used are topical corticosteroids (clobetasol, fludroxycortide, fludrocortolone, fluticasone), TNF-α inhibitors (infliximab, adalimumab given subcutaneously), immunosuppressive agents (alefacept, efalizumab, risankizumab given subcutaneously) and retinoids (acitretin, tazarotene given orally) and antiproliferative agents (methotrexate, cyclosporine, azathioprine given orally).

7. **Mechanism of action and adverse effects of Amphotericin B**

   Amphotericin B is fungicidal and binds to ergosterol in the fungal cell membrane thereby placing the membrane in less a fluid, more crystalline state and forming pores. The formation of pores allows the leakage of intracellular ions K^+, Mg^+ and macromolecules eventually leading to cell death.

   Adverse effects of amphotericin-B include hypersensitivity allergic reactions – fever, chills, headache, malaise, nausea and hypotension. It can also cause renal toxicity – decrease of GFR, renal tubular acidosis, potassium loss, hypomagnesemia and azotemia and normochromic, normocytic anemia.

8. **Mechanism of action, uses and adverse effects of Cyclosporine**

   Cyclosporin A is an immunosuppressant that supresses T-cell mediated immune responses that are associated with transplant rejection and autoimmune diseases. It inhibits antigen-triggered signal transduction in T lymphocytes preventing the release and function of many lymphokines including IL-2, IL-3 and TNFα

   Cyclosporine-A is used for prophylaxis against immune responses of organ transplantation of the kidneys, liver, heart and other allogenic transplants and used in combination with glucocorticoids.

   The adverse effects of cyclosporin-A include hypertension, cardiac failure, nephrotoxicity, hepatic dysfunction, headache, tremors, confusion, dizziness, insomnia, vertigo, impaired concentration, neuropathy, alopecia, bullous eruptions, hypertrichosis, urticaria, cataract, gynecomastia and several GI adverse effects.

9. **Selective estrogen receptor modulators**

   A selective estrogen receptor modulator interacts with estrogen receptors functioning as an agonist in some tissues and as antagonist in other tissues. Because of their high tissue selectivity, they produce the desired estrogenic effects (bone and plasma lipids) without possible stimulatory effects on the breast. There is variation in their selectivity. For example, Tamoxifene causes regression of breast tumor growth in women with estrogen receptor (ER) positive tumors, while at the same it shows partial agonist activity in the uterus which explains the endometrial hyperplasia and possible endometrial malignancy with its use. It has an estrogen like effect on bone metabolism in postmenopausal women and is associated with preservation of bone mineral density in lumbar spine and femoral bones preventing pathological fractures. Raloxifene has estrogen agonist actions on the bone, lipids and breast without any effects on the uterus. It is used to treat osteoporosis, breast tumor in postmenopausal women. Lasoxifene, bazedoxifene, toremifene are the other SERMs which have both agonist and antagonist actions on estrogen receptors and thus used to treat breast cancer and osteoporosis.

10. Multidrug resistant TB

The mutated forms of TB microbes are extremely resistant to at-least two of the most powerful anti TB drugs – INH and rifampicin. People infected with TB that is resistant to first line drugs will transfer this resistant form of TB to the people they infect. Multidrug resistant TB (MDR-TB) is due to resistance to INH and rifampicin. Extremely drug resistant (XDR-TB) is the one in which patients become resistant to many drugs at-least three of the six classes of second-line drugs (aminoglycosides, polypeptides, fluoroquinolones, thiamide, cycloserine and PAS). The treatment regimen of MDR-TB consists of 4 or 5 group of drugs which include streptomycin or kanamycin, fluroquinolone, ethambutol pyrazinamide and linezolid. The treatment is given for six months under direct observed therapy (DOT). Bedaquiline and delamanid are the other drugs used in combination with other anti TB drugs to treat MDR-TB.

Answers to the University Question Paper given by West Bengal University of Health Sciences – May 2022

1. **A 45-year-old male visits to a physician with complaint of insomnia due to stress in the office. He was prescribed one Benzodiazepine as hypnotic**
   a. **Enumerate two benzodiazepines used as hypnotic drugs**
   b. **Discuss mechanism of action and therapeutic uses of benzodiazepines as hypnotics**
   c. **Compare and contrast: Benzodiazepine and Barbiturates**

Ans:

a) Estazolam_with a half – life of 10 – 24 hrs has very quick onset of action. Flunitazepam is another benzodiazepine drug that also has quick onset of action and the dose of each drug is 1mg/day. However, the most commonly prescribed drugs for insomnia include alprazolam, clonazepam, and lorazepam followed by diazepam.

b) Benzodiazepines bind to molecular components (α and γ sub units) of GABA receptor present in the neuronal membranes in the CNS and facilitate the opening of cl^- channel indirectly (GABA ergic action). GABA is the major inhibitory neurotransmitter in the CNS and benzodiazepines potentiate the GABA ergic inhibition at different levels of CNS.

Uses of benzodiazepines

- To treat anxiety disorders including generalized anxiety disorder and panic disorder and institutional anxiety disorder. They are used to treat phobias, various psychological disorders associated with organic medical conditions like MI, hypertension and all types of chronic illnesses.
- They are useful to treat sleep disorders (insomnia) associated with organic diseases, age-related factors, and surgical procedures.
- They are also used in convulsive and spastic disorders. Diazepam is one of the choices to treat status epilepticus. They are also useful to treat absence seizures (clonazepam and clobazam), myoclonic seizures, central spastic disorders (multiple sclerosis and paraplegia), restless leg syndrome, and chorea and intension myoclonus.
- Preanesthetic medication to reduce anxiety, provide sedation and produce amnesia. They reduce anesthetic requirements. They provide safe and effective sedation for mechanical ventilation following cardiac surgery. They are also useful to provide anxiolytic, sedative and amnestic effects in a wide range of stressful diagnostic procedures such as bronchoscopy, laryngoscopy, endoscopy and orthopaedic procedures.
- Midazolam is the most preferred drug for induction and maintenance of general anesthesia.
- Benzodiazepines are also useful to treat alcohol withdrawal symptoms.
- They are also useful to control hyperexcitability of CNS produced by drugs like phencyclidine and toxic doses of atropine and other CNS stimulants.
- In combination with NSAIDS, they can be used to treat pain disorders.

Compare and Contrast Benzodiazepines and barbiturate:

		Barbiturates	Benzodiazepine
1)	CNS effects	Sedative, hypnotic actions; anticonvulsant action, antianxiety action, no skeletal muscle relaxant action	Sedative, hypnotic actions, anticonvulsant actions, antianxiety action, skeletal muscle relaxant action
2)	Type of CNS action	Non – specific, narrow margin of safety	Specific target action, wide margin of safety
3)	Respiratory function	Dose dependent respiratory depression	No respiratory depressant effects
4)	Uses	Sedative, hypnotic, anticonvulsant, induction of anesthesia, preanesthetic medication, hyperbilirubinemia and kernicterus	Sedative, hypnotic, anticonvulsant, anxiety states, preanesthetic medication, induction and maintenance of anesthesia, alcohol withdrawal, hyperexcitability of CNS
5)	Antidote	No specific antidose	Flumazenil

2. **A 23-year-old male arrives at emergency with difficulty breathing, with a history of recurrent episodes of seasonal breathlessness, relieved on inhalational medication. Now, the patient is diagnosed as a case bronchial asthma**

   a. **Classify the drug used in bronchial asthma**

   b. **How will you manage a case of acute bronchial asthma?**

   c. **How do inhalational drugs act better in bronchial asthma?**

Ans:

a) Classification of drugs for asthma

1) Sympathomimetics (β_2 agonists) – Salbutamol, terbutaline, salmeterol, metaproterenol, formoterol, fenoterol, Bitolterol, pirbuterol.
2) Anticholinergic agents – Ipratropium, tiotropium, oxitropium.
3) Glucocorticoids – Hydrocortisone, budesonide, beclomethasone, fluticasone, mometasone, triamcinolone.
4) Leukotriene synthesis inhibitors – zileuton.
5) Leukotriene receptor antagonists – Zafirleukast, monteleukast.
6) Anti – IgE monoclonal antibodies – omalizumab.
7) Drugs acting on the mast cells (mast cell stabilizers) – Cromolyn sodium, nedocromil

b) Status asthmatics is an acute exacerbation of a chronic case of bronchial asthma. It is a medical emergency that needs immediate attention and need hospitalization.

Status asthmaticus can be managed by the following measures

a) Oxygen saturation below 92% that need O_2 administration
b) Albuterol/ salbutamol – 0.5ml of 0.5% solution (2.5mg) in 2.5ml of normal saline as nebulization given intermittently or four puffs (0.36 mg) of metered dose inhaler with spacer given every 20 minutes for 3 doses
c) Adrenaline – 0.3mL of 1:1000 solution given subcutaneously every 20 minutes for 3 doses. It has to be used with caution in patients older than 40 years and contraindicated in patients older than

40 years and also contraindicated in patients of CVS disorders like hypertension, arrhythmias and CHF.

d) Corticosteroids – Methylprednisolone – 60 – 125 mg **or** hydrocortisone 100mg gaven IV every 6 hrs.

e) Anticholinergics – Ipratropium 0.5 mg by nebulization hourly **or** 4 – 8 puffs (0.08 mg/puff) with spacer every 20 minutes 3 doses.

f) Aminophylline – 5mg/kg/IV over 20 minutes (slowly), being the last preferred drug.

c) Inhalational drugs directly reach to their sites of action and clinical response sets in within few minutes. This mode of administration decreases the dose required for the desired effect compared to oral route as it bypasses the first dose metabolism. The reduced systemic bioavailability also minimizes the side effects. Inhalational drugs used in asthma (β_2 agonists, corticosteroids, anticholinergics) are given through a nebulizer machine, metered – dose inhaler administered through spacer, and drug powder inhalers. Aerosol drug particles of the size 2.5 μ are best suited for local deposition, and particles of the size of 10 μ do not pass through the alvelar cell membrane and particles of the size 1-2 μ remain suspended and may be exhaled.

3)

a) Write a note on prophylactic treatment of malaria. Outline mechanism of action and four adverse effects of chloroquine

b) Classify oral contraceptives. Describe the clinical uses oral contraceptives

c) Clinical uses and adverse effects of aminoglycosides

a) Chemoprophylaxis (prophylactic treatment) of malaria is the strategy that uses medications before, during and after the exposure period to prevent or suppress symptoms caused by malarial parasites. Chemoprophylaxis is advised and to be given for a person who is likely to enter endemic areas of malaria where the incidence of malaria is highly prevalent. The aim of prophylaxis is to prevent or suppress symptoms caused by blood – stage of parasites (RBC sehizonts)

Drugs used for chemoprophylaxis of malaria include chloroquine, mefloquine, atovaquone, and proguanil/primaquin combination; doxycycline and primaquine combination for terminal prophylaxis of P. falciparum malaria. The prophylactic treatment is started one to two weeks before a person enters the endemic areas, continued during his stay there and 2 to 4 weeks after he leaves the endemic area.

b) Oral contraceptives can be classified as

1. Estrogen and progesterone combination pills
2. Progesterone only contraceptive pills
    1. Estrogen and progesterone combination pills consist of an estrogen preparation (ethynyl estradiol) and progestin (norethindrone, norgestrel, norgestimate, levonorgestrel)
    2. Progesterone only pills contain only progesterone (mini pills) norethindrone, norgestral
    3. Progestin – only emergency/ post coital pill consists of levonorgestrel.

Clinical uses of oral contraceptives

1) Contraception is the main clinical use of oral contraceptives

2) Oral contraceptives have also found to have benefitial effects like reduced incidence of ovarian and endometrial cancer risk, reduced risk of colorectal cancer, reduced abnormal uterine bleeding,

decreased perimenopausal vasomotor symptoms, favourable bone mineral density profile, decreased anemia, improvement in acne and hypergonadism, reduced incidence of ectopic pregnancy, decreased incidence of pre-menstrual symptoms.

c) Clinical uses of Aminoglycosides

1) Streptomycin is useful in bacterial endocarditis caused by enterococci, D streptococci, viridans streptococi in combination with penicillin or vancomycin. It is used to treat mycobacterium tuberculosis in combination with other anti TB drugs like pyrazinamide, INH, rifampicin, ethambutol). It is also effective to treat plague, tularemia brucellosis.

2) Gentamicin is the most preferred drug to treat serious, life – threatening Gram – negative infections such as septicemia, systemic bacteremia, infected burns, osteomyelitis, pneumonia and peritonitis caused by P aeruginosa, Enterobacter, Klebsiella, Serratia, Proteus and Acinobacter. It is usually combined with extended spectrum penicillin or a cephalosporin which provides a synergistic effect.

   The other uses of gentamiain include urinary tract infections, bacterial endocarditis, nosocomial pneumonia and sepsis. Topically it can be used for infected burns, wounds or skin infections and external ocular infections (as eye drops)

3) Tobramycin is used mainly for infections caused by P.aeruginosa

4) Amikacin has the same uses as gentamicin and tobramycin particularly if the bacterial strains are not sensitive and resistant to the infections of eye, skin and ear.

Adverse effects of aminoglycosides

All aminoglycosides produce potentially dangerous reversible and irreversible adverse effects such as ototoxicity, nephrotoxicity, and neuromuscular effects. Adverse effects are both time-and – concentration dependent and usually do not occur till a threshold concentration is reached and once reached it may result in critical situation. Usually, predictive level for toxicity is 2mcg/mL. Ototoxicity produced by aminoglycosides is irreversible and usually manifested as vestibular and auditory dysfunction as the drug gets accumulated in the perilymph and endolymph over a period and proportional to the plasma concentration of the drug. Nephrotoxicity is reversible and the intial manifestation of renal toxicity is an increase of excretion of brush border enzymes, followed by a decrese in renal concentration ability, protinuria, and appearance of casts in the urine, which then followed by reduced GFR and a reise of serum creatinine levels. Neuromuscular toxicity is manifested as decresed skeletal muscle contractions and respiratory difficulty, the effects being reversible.

3. Write short notes on the following

a. Pharmacotherapy of diabetic ketoacidosis

b. Rifampicin (Mechanism of action, therapeutic uses and ADR)

Ans:

a. Diabetic ketoacidosis is an acute clinical emergency associated with diabetis mellitus which is poorly controlled due to inadequate or improper use of antidiabetic drugs. Biochemically hyperglycemia, hyperketonemia, and metabolic acidosis are the manifestations. The severity of ketoacidosis can be assessed by clinical manifestations and by measuring plasma bicarbonate levels, with severe acidosis resulting if the bicarbonate levels are less than 12mmol/lit. The clinical features of diabetic ketoacidosis include polyurea, thirst, weight loss, weakness, nausea, vomiting, leg cramps, blurred vision, dehydration, hypotension, tachycardia, hypothermia, confusion, drowsiness, coma and a characteristic smell of actone in breath.

Diabetic ketosis can best be managed by the administration of fluid replacement and administration of short acting soluble insulin, potassium replacement, and administration of antibiotics to control any associatyed bacterial infection.

1) Short acting soluble insulins are given intravenously at regular intervals. Insulin (lispro, aspart) is given as bolus IV in a dose of 0.3 U/kg, followed by 0.1U/kg/hr as IV infusion till a blood glucose level reaches 200-250 mg/dL. The insulin infusion is reduced later to a dose of 0.05U/Kg given 4th hourly till all the feeatues of DKA subside.
2) Fluid replacement – Intially, 1liter of 0.9% Nacl is given as infusion over a period of 30 minutes, followed by 0.5liter of the same solution after half an hour. This can be continued at hourly intervals before 5% glucose is given after 2½ hours.
3) Potassium replacement is done if the serum potassium levels are 3.5 – 5.5 mmols/L, 20mmols of KCL/L is infused for a period of nearly 2hrs after the patient is admitted with ketoacidosis.
4) 300ml of 1.26% sodium bicarbonate is given in patients who are severely acidotic (PH<7.0)

b. Rifampicin is an antituberculosis drug used in combination with pyrazinamide, INH and Ethambutol. Rifampicin is a bactrecidal drug that inhibits DNA dependent RNA polymerase of mycobacteria thereby inhibiting RNA synthesis. It is effective in both intracellular and extracellular microorganisms.

Therapeutic uses of rifampicin

The main indication of rifampicin is in the treatment of mycobacterium tuberculosis and given in combination with other drugs. The other important indications of rifampicin is its use for the treatment of leprosy. It is also useful or indicated for prophylaxis of meningococcal and H. Influenza meningitis in the carrier state. It also serves as a second – line drug for the treatment of skin and bone infections caused by staphylococci (osteomyelitis, cellulitis and wound infections)

Adverse reactions of rifampicin include hepatotoxicity which does not occur with normal hepatic function. However, in conditions of hepatic dysfunction, alcoholism, hepatotoxicity is considerably increased. Rifampicin can also have drug interactions with HIV protease inhibitors, digoxin, quinidine, disopyramide, oral contraceptives, ketoconazole, metoprolol and oral anticoagulants whose action is reduced due to enhanced metabolizing enzyme action.

4. Explain the following statements

a. Corticosteroid use over long term can be harmful

b. Tricyclic antidepressants are not preferred in elderly male subjects

c. Injection of thiopentone sodium is not used as maintenance agent in general anesthesia.

d. Ergometrine should not be used for induction of labor

e. Leucovorin rescue is mandatory in methotrexate therapy

Ans:

a. Long term use of glucocorticoids can cause the following conditions

1. Protein catabolism, gluconeogenesis that led to hyperglycemia and insulin resistance
2. Myopathy and muscle wasting
3. Retention of water and electrolytes (Na^+ retension) and loss of potassium leading to edema and hypokalemia, alkalosis, and hypertension.
4. Hypogonadism associated with decreased testosterone levels. In women anovulation, oligomenorrhea or dysfunctional uterine bleeding can occur.

5. Growth retardation in children
6. GI system may be affected causing gastric irritation and peptic ulcer
7. Subcapsular cataracts may occur
8. Osteoporosis, spontaneous fractures can occur
9. Several behavioural changes and neuropsychiatric disorders can also occur.

b. Anticholinergic antidepressants (tricyclic antidepressants) like amitryptiline, clomipramine, amoxapine, nortryptiline, desipramine, protryptiline, maprolitine can worsen the dementia, diabetis, and Parkinson's disease which are more common in elderly. Such drugs can cause postural hypotension and cardiac conduction abnormalities

c. Thiopentone is a short-acting barbiturate used mainly for induction of general anesthesia to be maintained by regular general anaesthetics like enflurane, sevoflurane, desflurane and isoflurane usually, and halothane occasionally. Thiopentone is having a very short duration of action and its action declines within 1-2 minutes after reaching peak blood levels. Hence it is not useful for the maintenance of general anesthesia which is required to last 1 to 1½ hours.

d. Ergometrine is used to control the postpartum hemorrhage as its action reaches to peak levels at the term of pregnancy. It causes rhythmic contractions of the uterus followed by relaxation in smaller doses and produces powerful and sustained contractions in higher doses. Its actions are most useful for the expulsion of the placenta after childbirth. It has an initial half-life of 10 minutes only and its action declines later. It cannot produce sustained contractions of the uterus which is required for initiation and maintenance of labor in conditions like delayed maturity, uterine inertia, premature rupture of membranes and preeclampsia.

e. Methotrexate is folate antagonist and can cause folate deficiency while it is being used in malignant conditions. Methtrexate toxicity due to overdosage is manifested as nausea, vomiting, diarrhea, stomatitis, mucositis, esophagitis, elevated hepatic enzymes, rash, renal failure, myelosupression, acute lung injury, hypotension, tachycardia, and neurologic dysfunction. The toxic features are due to accumulation of polyglutamated toxic product in the cells. It prevents the utilization of folic acid for the synthesis of purines, pyrimidines, and RNA and DNA synthesis. Hence folate deficiency occurs during methotrexate therapy. Leucovorin is 5-formyl derivative of folic acid and given as rescue therapy during methotrexate toxicity due to overdoasage. This is not needed for the conversion of dihydrofolate to tetrahydrofolate for utilization of DNA synthesis. It is a directly available folate preparation. It is started immediately before the toxic features appear (before the toxic polyglutamated product accumulates in the cells). It can be given orally, IM, and by IV routes. In methotrexate toxicity it is given IV in doses of $10 mg/m^2$ every six hours for a total of 10 doses after which it can be given orally in doses of 10 mg 3 times a day.

Answers to the Questions given by Odisha University of Health Sciences

1. **A patient was taking drug 'A' (Plasma half-life 12 hours) 500mg twice daily for his disease**
   a) **What is steady state plasma concentration of a drug and at what time drug 'A' will achieve it? Justify your answer**
   b) **Differentiate between zero order and first order kinetics**
   c) **Define the different types of drug half-lives and mention the clinical significance of plasma half-life**

Ans: a) Steady state concentration is defined as the time during which the concentration of the drug remains stable or consistent when it is given repeatedly or continuously (IV infusion) at regular intervels. The steady- state concentration of a drug depends upon its elimination half-life ($t_{½}$) and is achieved when the rate of the drug (units of a drug given at fixed intervals) entering the systemic circulation equals the rate the elimination (units of the drug eliminated at fixed intervals). This is also referred to as the plateau concentration of the drug in the plasma.

In the case of drug, A, if its first half-life is12 hours, the following sequence explain the steady state concentration

Dose given (mg)	Amount of the drug present in the body (mg)	Amount of the drug eliminated (mg)	Number of half-lives required
500	500	250	1
500	750 (500+250)	375	2
500	875 (500+375)	437.5	3
500	937.5 (500+437.5)	468.5	4
500	968.5 (500+468.5)	484.5	5
500	984.7 (500+484.5)	492	6
500	992 (500+492)	496	7

Hence 7 half-lives are required to achieve the steady state level of the drug A and 3½ hours is required to reach the level

Ans: (b) First order kinetics:

All the four parameters of kinetics (absorption, distribution, metabolism and excretion) are directly proportional to the drug concentration in the body. The movement of drug across the cell membrane is proportional to its concentrations; it is more in higher concentrations and less in lower concentrations. In the first order kinetics, a known fraction or percentage of the drug is eliminated at regular intervals, which is known as elimination half-life of the drug **($t_{½}$).** The rate of elimination and plasma concentrations are directly proportional. Majority of drugs follow first order kinetics.

Zero order kinetics: In the usual situations, the rate of elimination of a drug is directly proportional to its plasma concentrations. This process continues as long as the metabolizing enzymes are fully functional and non-saturated. But when enzyme system become saturated and reaches peak, further metabolism is not possible and it remains the same in spite of increase of dose. Here, certain amount of the drug is eliminated and the rate of elimination is not proportional to the plasma concentrations. Drugs which show zero order kinetics are alcohol and Phenytoin.

Ans: **(c)** There are three types of half-lives of a drug

1. Biological effective half life is the time in which the pharmacological effect of the drug and its active metabolites fall by one half or 50%
2. Elimination half life is the one in which the total amount of the drug in the body, after equilibrium of plasma with other compartments falls by one half or 50%
3. Plasma half life is the one where in the time taken for the plasma concentration to fall by 50% of its peak value.

Clinical significance of half life:

1. Half-life gives a gross idea about the pharmacokinetic and pharmacodynamic properties of a drug.
2. To predict the duration of a drug in the body
3. To formulate a dosage schedule- Amount of the drug to be given and to know the frequency of its administration. Drugs with long half-life can be given at lesser intervals and drugs with shorter half-life need to be given repeatedly.
4. To manage a case of overdosage of a drug.
5. To determine the time to achieve steady state concentration of the drug.

2. a) Classify parasympathomimetic drugs and discuss their clinical uses.

b) Discuss various types of drug antagonisms with examples

c) Give a note on the limitations of opioids as analgesics

d) What do you mean by microsomal enzyme induction? Give examples of such inducers. Discuss its clinical significance.

Ans: **(a)** Parasympathomimetic drugs can be classified as

1. Direct acting
   - Choline esters: Acetylcholine, Bethanechol, Carbachol, Methacholine
   - Cholinomimetic alkaloids: Muscarine, Nicotine, Pilocarpine, Physostigmine
2. Indirect acting (Cholinesterase inhibitors)
   - Reversible: Physostigmine, Neostigmine, Pyridostigmine, Edrophonium, Ambenonium, Demecarium
   - Irreversible: Echothiophate, Soman, Malathion, Parathion

Clinical uses of Parasympathomimetic drugs

1. Glaucoma (Carbachol, pilocarpine, echothiophate, physostigmine, demecarium)
2. Myasthenia gravis (Neostigmine, pyridostigmine, ambenonium, demecarium, edrophonium)
3. Alzheimer's disease – Tacrine, rivastigmine, galantamine, donepezil
4. Post operative Paralyticus ilues- Bethanichol, neostigmine
5. Post operative, post partum urinary retention, inadequate emptying of bladder in hypotonic, neurogenic and myogenic bladder conditions – Bethanechol, neostigmine
6. Atropine poisoning – Physostigmine

Ans: **(b) Receptor antagonism:** In this case the effects of an agonist are antagonized by the presence of an antagonist competing for the same receptor site, while the agonist shows both affinity and efficacy, the antagonist exhibits only affinity but no afficacy. The actions of antagonist can be overcome by increasing the concentration of the agonist and the feature is known as competitive antagonism.

Examples of receptor antagonism include

H1 receptor	-	Pheniramine
Opioids (μ) receptor		Naltrexone,
Neostigmine (nAch) receptor	-	Atracurium
Physostigmine (mAch) receptor	-	Atropine

c) Irreversible antagonism/ non-competetive antagonism

Here the agonist is unable to regain its full effect despite an increase in its concentration and not fully able to minimise the effects of the antagonist. In this case the antagonist binds irreversibly to the same site as the agonist and reduces the binding of the agonist

Example**:** Antagonism between adrenaline and phenoxybenzamine (for the α-receptor sites)

Physiological antagonism (Acting through different mechanisms)	–	Nitrates	–	Adrenaline

Ans: **(c) Limitations of opioids as analgesics**

Opioids are potent analgesics but there are certain limitations for their use. Respiratory depression is a dose related adverse effect of opioids. They also cause light-headedness, dizziness, sedation, nausea, vomiting and sweating. Opioids also cause euphoria, tolerance, drug abuse, physical and psychic dependence and addiction. Opioids can cause constipation and miosis. They are contraindicated in elderly and pediatric patients and use in head injury cases. They are not effective in nociceptive pain.

Ans: **(d) Microsomal enzyme inducers with examples**

Microsomal enzyme system may be induced by a variety of drugs, substances present in the environment, insecticides and hydrocarbon pollutants. Inducing agents are lipid soluble substances and have long half-lives. A majority of drug metabolising enzymes are located in the lipophilic membranes of the endoplasmic reticulum of the liver. There are two main microsomal systems in the body, namely NADPH CPY_{450} Oxidase and NADPH CPY_{450} reductase. Microsomal drug oxidation requires P_{450} oxidase, P_{450} reductase, NADPH and molecular oxygen. $CYP3A_4$ is said to be the most prominent CYP isoform involved in drug metabolism both in terms of quantity present in the liver as well as the variety of drugs that are metabolized by it. Few examples of enzyme inducing drugs and the drugs affected and whose pharmacological actions are_decreased are shown below

1. Barbiturates Coumarin anticoagulants

2. Rifampicin — Phenytoin, oral contraceptives
3. Carbamazepine — Testosterone, oral contraceptives, doxorubicin

(Few examples of inhibiting agents and the affected agents with enhanced pharmacological action)

1. Allopurinol — Azathioprine, Mercaptopurine
2. Dicoumarol — Phenytoin
3. Phenylbutazone — Tolbutamide, Phenytoin

3. Answer the following questions:

a) Why long acting β-agonists should not be used alone in bronchial asthma

Ans: $\beta_2$agonists are the frontline drugs for acute treatment and prevention of bronchial asthma and COPD. According to their duration of action they are classified as short acting $\beta_2$agonists (salbutamol, terbutaline, pirbuterol) and long acting $\beta_2$agonists (salmeterol, and formoterol) and ultra long acting $\beta_2$agonists (Indacarterol, vilanterol). Long acting $\beta_2$agonists are likely to produce tolerance due to continued beta-receptor stimulation. A moderate or severe persistent asthma requires the use of corticosteroids followed by long acting $\beta_2$agonists. Usually, the single use of $\beta_2$agonists may not be effective to control the symptoms. They are combined with inhaled corticosteroids and anticholinergic drugs for the better control of the symptoms. But chronic use of long acting β_2 agonists alone in monotherapy can lead to continuous stimulation of β2 receptors that leads to tolerance for therapeutic effects with an overall increase in severe asthma incidence upto hospitalization, intubation or even mortality. But in combination therapy such incidences are far low.

b) Name the nasal decongestants. Give a note on their adverse effects

Ans: Xylometazoline, Oxymetazoline, Naphazoline and Tetrahydrozoline are the commonly used nasal decongestants. Burning, stinging, sneezing, dryness, local irritation and rebound congestion can occur with their use. In addition, Oxymetazoline can cause hypotension because of its $\alpha_2$agonist action (clonidine like action) preventing the release of NAD.

c) Give a note on $\beta_3$agonists

Ans: β_3 agonists are the drugs used to treat overactive bladder which act by relaxing detrusor muscle of the urinary bladder thereby decreasing the urinary urgency and incontinence. Vibegron and mirabegron are the β_3 agonists available for the treatment of overactive bladder. They are better alternatives to anticholinergics like oxybutynin, trospium as they do not produce anticholinergic related adverse effects, more so the cognitive decline. They also do not produce dementia unlike anticholinergics.

d) Explain why phenoxybenzamine is preferred to prazosin in pheochromocytoma

Ans: Pheochromocytoma is an adrenal medullary tumor that causes an increase of catecholamine release with the consequent pharmacological effects such as persistent elevated hypertension, tachycardia, sweating and other features of catecholamine excess. Surgical removal is the only option for the treatment. However, preoperative reduction of elevated blood pleasure and tachycardia are essential to reduce perioperative complication of a possible rise of blood pleasure for which α-blockers followed by beta blockers should be advocated. Phenoxybenzamine is a non selective α-blocker (α_1 and α_2) and prazosin is a selective α_1 blocker. The β- blockers that can be used include propranolol, carvedilol, and labetalol. During the perioperative period there is a possibility of rise of blood pressure in spite of preoperative treatment with α and β blockers. It can be controlled by phenoxybenzamine more effectively than with prazosin.

e) Enumerate the clinical uses of β blockers

Ans: β-blockers can be used in a variety of clinical conditions such as hypertension, cardiac arrhythmias, prophylaxis of angina, prophylaxis of migraine, anxiety disorders, pheochromocytoma, thyrotoxicosis, congestive heart failure, portal hypertension, glaucoma, alcohol withdrawal, dissecting aneurysm of aorta.

4. Fill in the blanks

a) The prostaglandin analog that is used in erectile dysfunction is ________________ (sildenafil)

b) Niacin flush can be prevented by __________________ (aspirin)

c) Hydroxychloroquine is preferred to chloroquine in rheumatoid arthritis because _______________ (toxicity is less common with the former)

d) --------------------(Indomethacin) is the most commonly used NSAID in gout

Answers to the Questions given by National Board of Examinations

Note: The questions given here might be for a higher level of examination. Since they are relevant to the subject at all levels and since most of them cover the clinical conditions, they are taken up in a broader perspective to upscale the knowledge of the students at graduate level also

1. Discuss the therapeutic status and role of beta-blockers in the treatment of heart failure.

Ans: Congestive heart failure (CHF) is a modified state of myocardial function in which the heart is not capable of delivering adequate blood into the body systems to meet the metabolic and functional requirements of the organs. Various conditions such as pressure (elevated blood pressure) and volume overload, loss of muscle mass, primarily muscle diseases (idiopathic cardiomyopathies), altered cardiac rhythm (cardiac arrhythmias), excessive peripheral demands such as present in anemias and nutritional deficiencies, ischemic heart disease, thyrotoxicosis, contribute to the reduced cardiac contractile function leading to cardiac failure.

However, several compensatory mechanisms come into play to cope up with the extra cardiac workload and to maintain the normal contractile function and that include primarily an enhanced sympathetic activity, activation of renin-angiotensin- aldosterone mechanism, which will result in increased preload, which in turn leads to myocardial hypertrophy. These compensatory mechanisms also lead to an increase in heart rate and cardiac contractility, expansion of extra cellular fluid volume with retention of salts and water. These compensatory mechanisms are continued for a limited period only before the heart is no longer able to maintain the status. This ultimately leads to decompensated heart failure which requires medical attention to reduce the morbidity, mortality and frequent hospitalizations.

There are many drug groups that could be used to partially or totally restore the cardiac function within the reasonable limits. The drug groups that can be effective to treat heart failure include 1)angiotensin converting enzyme inhibitors (ACE – inhibitors like lisinopril and others) 2)angiotensin receptor blockers (losartan, valsartan and others), 3)β- receptor blockers (carvedilol, metoprolol, and bisoprolol), 4)diuretics (loop diuretics), 5)cardiac glycosides (digoxin), 6)phosphodiesterase inhibitors (amrinone, milrinone, vesnarinone, enoximone), 7)vasodilators (sodium nitroprusside, glyceryl trinitrate), 8)aldosterone antagonists (eplerenone, fenerenone) and 9) sacubitril / valsartan combination and 10) SGLT-2 inhibitors(Empagliflozin, canagliflozin)

Therapeutic status and role of β-blockers in heart failure

β – blockers can be considered as second line drugs as far as their effectiveness is concerned in the treatment of heart failure. They are of much use in chronic congestive heart failure as combination drugs with more effective drugs like ACE-inhibitors and other groups of drugs.

The mechanism of action of β-blockers in congestive heart failure:

1. They attenuate the increased sympathetic activity leading to a decrease of heart rate, myocardial oxygen demand and improved exercise tolerance. Though the systolic function decreases initially, it improves over a time. There is an improved left ventricular ejection factor **(EF)** and left ventricular function.
2. They improve left ventricular structure and function with decrease in chamber size (**ventricular remodelling)** and an increase EF. This is because they decrease the chronic sympathetic activity

with a gradual reduction of cardiac β_1 receptor desensitization, cellular and molecular events, all of which are associated with cardiac remodelling.

3. They resensitize the cardiac β_1 receptor activity (decrease of down regulation of β_1 cell function as seen in CHF) thus improving myocardial contractility
4. The beneficiary effects of β-blockers are also due to their antiarrhythmic activity.
5. Carvedilol is of much use in this class as it blocks both α and β receptors and causes vasodilator effects and decrease in the afterload. In addition, it has antioxidant effect reducing the oxidative stress on the heart. The other β-blockers that are found effective intreating congestive heart failure include metoprolol, bisoprolol, and nebiolol.

2. How do you classify the insulin preparations according to their duration of action? Discuss the advantages of newer non-insulin antidiabetic drugs.

Ans: Insulin preparations can be classified as follows:

1. **Rapid acting insulins** – Lispro, aspart, glulisine

   When given subcutaneously these insulin preparations get converted to monomers, the active forms, getting converted from hexamers are absorbed very rapidly, reaching peak serum levels in less than 1hr in contrast to regular human insulin whose hexamers require more time to dissociate and become absorbed. These insulin preparations do not cause post pandreal hypoglycemia unlike regular insulin which requires longer time to reach peak levels and sustained action even after meals thus causing postpandreal hypoglycemia. Hence regular insulin is taken half an hour before meals.

2. **Short acting insulins** – Regular human insulin (crystalline insulin) is short acting insulin usually taken 30 minutes before meals, peak levels reaching at 2.5 – 5 hrs and the effects lasting more than 4 – 8 hours. The hexameric nature of regular insulin causes delayed onset of action when compared to rapid-acting insulins. This insulin is particularly useful to treat diabetic ketoacidosis.

3. **Intermediate acting insulins** – Lente insulin, NPH (Neutral Protamin Hegedorn) insulin.

   Lente insulin is a mixture of 30% of Semilente an amorphous precipitate of insulin with zinc ion to reduce solubility and pH adjusted to 7.4 and 70% Ultralente an insoluble crystal of zinc and insulin, PH adjusted to 5.5. Its onset of action is 1-2 hours and reaches peak levels 4-12 hrs later and has a longer duration of action of 18-24 hours.

   NPH is also known as isophane insulin and its onset of action is delayed by combining two parts of soluble crystalline insulin with one part of protamine zinc insulin. Conjugation of insulin molecule with either zinc or protamine or both will convert the normally rapidly absorbed parenterally administered insulin to a preparation with a longer duration of action. The onset of action, peak levels and duration of action are comparable to lente insulin. It is usually mixed with regular insulin and given at least twice daily for insulin replacement in type I diabetes.

4. **Long-acting insulins** – Humulin Ultralente, protamine zinc insulin (PZI), glargine, detemir, degludec

   Human ultra-Lente is crystalline insulin. It has an onset of action of 4-6 hrs, peak action of 16-18 hours and duration of action of more than 24 hours. Insulin glargine when injected in the neutral pH environment of subcutaneous tissue, forms micro precipitates that slowly release the insulin into circulation over a period of 24 hours, hence given once daily. It controls nocturnal (fasting) blood glucose levels better than NPH insulin.

   Insulin detemir is also a long-acting insulin preparation and because of modification of amino acid sequence of the basal insulin, it facilitates longer blood sugar control by an increase of self-aggregation in the subcutaneous tissue and reversible binding to albumin molecules. Unlike NPH and glargine, detemir insulin remains as a liquid depot after subcutaneous injection, providing a longer surface area of absorption. It has an onset of action of 1-2hr, peak action of 6-7hrs and duration of action of 20hrs. It is administered twice daily. Insulin degludec is ultra long acting insulin analog and self associates into multiple hexamers after subcutaneous injection and forms a depot from which it dissociates into monomers gradually and gets absorbed continuously into the circulation. It has a half life of nearly 42hrs. Insulin icodec a once-weekly based insulin has a long half-life of week and has a pharmacokinetic and pharmacodynamic profile suitable for once weekly injection. It is given subcutaneously is a weekly dose of 70 U and titrated or weekly basis depending upon the glycemic control.

Newer generation of Non-insulin antidiabetic drugs

In the recent past, quite a good number of newer generation of antidiabetic drugs have come in handy to treat diabetes more effectively and more safely with wider clinical applications other than treating diabetes. These groups of drugs have become favourable to treat diabetic patients with associated comorbidities like atherosclerotic vascular disease, congestive heart failure, chronic kidney disease and obesity (for weight reduction). They include the following classes of drugs:

1. GLP-I analogs like exenatide (ER, SR), dulaglutide, liraglutide, albiglutide, lixisenaside, semaglutide.
2. Dipeptidyl peptidase – 4 inhibitors (DPP-4 inhibitors) like sitagliptin, saxagliptin, linagliptin, alogliptin.
3. Sodium glucose co-transporter-2 (SGLT-2) inhibitors like dapagliflozin, canagliflozin, remogliflozin, empagliflozin.

1) GLP-I analogs/agonists(Glucagon-like peptide 1 analouges)

GLP-I agonists have anti-diabetic action by an increase of or augmentation of glucose dependant insulin secretion, increase of β-cell function, β-cell mass, reduced β-cell apoptosis, decrease of glucagon secretion, decreased glucose production in the liver by reducing hepatic gluconeogenesis and increased uptake of glucose by skeletal muscle and adipose tissue. GLP-I agonists are considered as incretins which are released in the small intestine and carried to the pancreatic β-cells the stimulation of which causes the release of insulin.

2) Dipeptidyl peptidase-4 inhibitors (DPP-4 inhibitors)

Dipeptidyl peptidase-4 enzyme is responsible for degradation of various biologically active peptides including endogenous GLP-I and GIP. By binding DPP-4, these drugs increase the levels of endogenous GLP-I and they in turn cause increased insulin secretion by an action on the pancreatic β-cells.

3) SGLT-2 inhibitors – (sodium-glucose co-transporter 2 inhibitors)

They act by inhibiting a carrier protein, sodium-glucose co-transporter 2 (SGLT-2) responsible for glucose reuptake in the proximal renal tubule thus facilitating its elimination in the urine which is followed by a decrease of blood glucose levels. They have an additional action of increased insulin sensitivity, uptake of glucose in muscle cells, decreased gluconeogenesis and improved first-phase insulin release from β-cells.

3. Outline the importance of therapeutic drug monitoring (TDM). Explain target level strategy in drug monitoring. Give examples of clinical conditions and drugs requiring monitoring.

Ans: When a drug is being administered for a clinical condition there would be not only the desired pharmacological and clinical effects but also some undesirable adverse effects which are dependent on plasma levels of the drug. Monitoring of plasma levels is not necessary with the drugs with a high therapeutic index. But in the case of drugs with narrow margin of safety and narrow therapeutic index, drug monitoring (monitoring of drug plasma levels) is essential. This is in order to know whether the desired optimal therapeutic range has been reached and maintained over the treatment period and also for individualizing the dose and thus adjust the dose to avoid any adverse effects that the drug may produce. TDM is particularly indicated when the dosage regimens of the drug are continued over extended periods and which require lifelong use. TDM is also indicated when there is a possibility of fluctuations in the blood concentrations due to drug-drug interactions when multiple drugs are given simultaneously. TDM is necessary to correlate the dose given and the desired response it produces, and to adjust the dose in the presence of any organ insufficiency or disease and in conditions like renal failure, hepatic failure and cardiac insufficiency and further to avoid drug use that is likely to cause direct organ toxicity. TDM also helps to know about patient compliance with the dosage regimen and whether the therapeutic response is adequate or the dosage adjustments needed to avoid undesirable adverse effects.

Examples of clinical conditions and drugs requiring monitoring

1) Psychotic disorders – Desipramine, imipramine, amitriptyline, nortriptyline, lithium
2) Cardiac disorders – Digoxin, disopyramide, quinidine, flecainide, amiodarone
3) Microbial disorders – Gentamicin, tobramycin, kanamycin, vancomycin
4) Convulsive disorders – Phenytoin, carbamazepine, ethosuximide, sodium valproate
5) Graft rejections – Immunosuppressants – cyclosporine, sirolimus, tacrolimus
6) Malignancies – Methotrexate, bleomycin, 5-FU
7) Asthma, COPD – Bronchodilators – Theophylline
8) Pain management – Salicylates
   And inflammatory conditions

4. Discuss the pharmacological approaches for treatment of tobacco dependence and withdrawal

Ans: Nicotine addiction is the second leading cause of death worldwide and also the preventable cause of death. Nicotine addiction (of any tobacco products) can cause accelerated heart rate, increased blood pressure, and weight loss. In addition to its physical effects, nicotine exerts a strong behavioural influence. It may increase alertness and also can stimulate a frantic, almost manic picture. Speech may also be accelerated in line with the behaviour. Cessation on continued use can contribute to irritability, which is smoothened by a fresh dose of nicotine use.

Nicotine addiction can best be explained by any two of the features like longer periods of tobacco consumption, persistent desire or unsuccessful efforts to cut down the use of tobacco, a craving or strong desire or urge to use tobacco, continued tobacco use despite having persistent or recurrent social or interpersonal problems (arguments with others about tobacco use), giving up of important social, occupational, or recreational activities, continued use of tobacco (cigarette smoking) despite knowing that it can cause several morbid and fatal clinical conditions like bronchitis, persistent cough, bronchial asthma, COPD, lung cancer, peripheral artery disease, cardiovascular diseases and several mental and psychological disorders. Cigarette smoking during pregnancy can lead to miscarriage, still birth, preterm labor, fetal growth retardation, and congenital anomalies. Nicotine is not carsinogenic by itself but in concert with other ingredients present in the tobacco which number about 5000 carsinogenic compounds out of which 73 potential carsinogenic(genotoxic) have been identified to have carcionogenic effect. Tobacco smoke containing these chemicals which include heavy metals like nickel, tin, and lead cause oxidative stress on the repitory pathways and damage the lungs and other respiratory components.

Nicotine withdrawal and the treatment choices

Nicotine is the ingredient primarily responsible for tobacco addiction. Nicotine acts on reward pathway and causes both physical and psychological dependence. Withdrawal from nicotine may cause unpleasant adverse effects, including anxiety, irritability, difficulty concentrating, anger, fatigue, drowsiness, depression and sleep disruption. The aim of treating nicotine dependence is to reduce cravings and reduce withdrawal symptoms.

Nicotine replacement therapies after smoking cessation reduce withdrawal symptoms. Several nicotine replacement therapies are available.

1. **Nicotine polacrilex** is a chewing gum which is available in 2mg and 4mg proportions. Usually, 2mg pieces are to be used by individuals who smoke less than a pack per day and 4mg pieces are to be used for individuals who smoke one pack or more per day. These chewing gums are to be used at 1 hourly interval for 2 weeks and later can be reduced gradually over the next 3 months.
2. **Transdermal nicotine patches** are available for replacement therapy which is well tolerated.
3. **Nicotine nasal spray** and inhaler preparations are also available.
4. **Buproprion an antidepressant drug** is also effective for smoking cessation and is used in persons who have not responded adequately to nicotine gums and nicotine patches. The oral dose of bupropion is 150mg once a day for 3 days increased to twice a day, followed by 150mg once a day.
5. The other drug used in smoking cessation is **varenicline** which is a partial agonist selective for α-4, β-2 nicotinic Ach receptors. Its action is thought to result from activity at nicotine receptor subtype, where its binding produces agonist activity while simultaneously preventing nicotine binding (dose dependent agonist and antagonist action on nicotine receptor types)
6. E-cigarettes (Vapes) are the electronic nicotine delivery systems containing nicotine which are battery operated devices. They heat a liquid to create aerosols that are inhaled by the users. They also contain additives, flavours, and chemicals which are harmful to health. Nicotine content varies from zero to vey high levels. They are meant to wean away from smoking cigarettes that containe nicotine which is highly addictive.

5. Discuss clinically applicable classification of glucocorticoids with appropriate examples. Enumerate the side effects and drug interactions of chronic use of glucocorticoids.

Ans: The classification of corticosteroids based on clinical applications is not practical in view of their uses in different conditions which are all based on their antiinflammatory actions. However, the following classification may be adopted to meet the criteria.

1	Rheumatic fever, rheumatic arthritis, rheumatoid arthritis, osteoarthritis, Polymyalgia rheumatica including local intra-articular and intralesional therapy	Prednisolone, triamcinolone, methyl prednisolone, dexamethasone, betamethasone, hydrocortisone
2	Bronchial asthma (Oral, inhalational, IV preparations)	Budesonide, beclomethasone, hydrocortisone, prednisolone, fluticasone, flucinolide, triamcinolone, mometasone
3	Dermatological conditions (Topical application)	Alcometasone, Betamethasone, Dexamethasone, fluticasone, clobetasol, halcinolide, fludrocortisone
4	Malignancies (Acute lymphatic leukemia in children, Hodgkin's disease)	Prednisolone, Dexamethasone
5	Inflammatory bowel disease (ulcerative colitis, crohn's disease – particularly in acute exacerbations	Hydrocortisone (rectal anemata), prednisolone

Table *Contd...*

6	Connective tissue disease (Lupus erythematosus, vasculitis, polymyositis)	Prednisolone, betamethasone, Triamcinolone, Dexamethasone
7	Nephrotic syndrome	Prednisolone
8	Immunosuppression (for organ transplantation)	Prednisone and methylprednisolone
9	Allergic disorders including anaphylactic shock, angioneurotic edema, hay fever, serum sickness, urticaria, contact dermatitis and other types of acute and chronic allergic disorders	Methyl prednisolone, dexamethasone, betamethasone, triamcinolone, Fluoromethalone, difluprednate
10	Occular diseases (uveitis, allergic conjunctivitis, keratoconjunctivitis)	Dexamethasone, fluocinolone – Topical drops, ointments
11	Acute adrenal insufficiency	Hydrocortisone
12	Cerebral edema	Dexamethasone

Adverse effects of corticosteroids – Hyperglycemia and insulin resistance, myopathy and muscle wasting, development of diabetes on chronic therapy, immune suppression and eventual bacterial and viral infections, GI system adverse effects like nausea, vomiting, gastric irritation, and peptic ulcer, ocular complications like subcapsular cataracts, osteoporosis and spontaneous fractures; water, electrolyte retention, and metabolic effects that can cause edema, hypokalemia; growth retardation in children, neuropsychiatric disorders, and inhibition of gonadotropin synthesis.

Drug interactions of glucocorticoids: The blood levels of several drugs are decreased with the simultaneous use of glucocorticoids and effected drugs include aspirin, coumarin anticoagulants, insulin, INH, oral hypoglycemic agents, and lithium. The blood levels are increased with the drugs like cyclophosphamide, and cyclosporine when used with corticosteroids.

6. Discuss the pharmacology of reverse transcriptive inhibitors

Ans: HIV reverse transcriptase inhibitors are a class of drugs that block replication of viral genome by competitively inhibiting incorporation of native nucleotides (thymidine triphosphate, guanine triphosphate and adenine triphosphate) into DNA by inhibiting reverse transcriptase thereby preventing the conversion of viral RNA to DNA. These drugs block replication of new entrants and also have effect on the already infected cells. These group of drugs not only inhibit viral cellular and mitochondrial DNA polymerases and cellular kinases but also that of host cell (CD_4 cell) resulting in toxicity. There are three types of reverse transcriptors

1) Nucleoside reverse transcriptase inhibitors (NRTIs) – Zidovudine, stavudine, lamivudine, emtricitabine, zalcitabine, didanosine, abacavir
2) Nucleotide reverse transcriptase inhibitors – Tenofovir
3) Non – nucleoside reverse transcriptase inhibitors (NNRTIs) – Nevirapine, efavirenz, rilpivirine, delavirdine, etravirine
4) Protease inhibitors- Amprenavir, indinavir, lopinavir, ritonavir, saquinavir

Treatment guidelines to HIV infection

1) To effectively supress the virus, that is to reduce the viral load as quickly and as substantially as possible to undetectable levels and to keep it there as long as possible.
2) Restoration of CD_4 counts.
3) To improve patient survival rates
4) Drugs should be easy for administration and to follow the schedule, and have minimal adverse effects

5) Combination therapy – A single drug is not effective in supressing HIV on its own. It has to be taken in combination with other retroviral drugs to combat the disease. This is done usually by a combination of three drugs belonging to three different classes of different mechanisms of action. This combination prevents drug resistance, duration treatment and also the possible adverse effects apart from the synergistic effect.

The combination usually consists of two NRTIS (Abacavir, lamivudine, zidovudine, delavirdine, etravirine, nevirapine) and protease inhibitors (indinavir, saquinavir, amprenavir).

7. What ae the selective COX – 2 inhibitors? Discuss briefly their advantages over non – selective COX inhibitors. What are the evidences for the cardiovascular risk of selective COX – 2 inhibitors? What was the basis of banning COX – 2 inhibitors

Ans: Selective COX – 2 inhibitors (celecoxib, rofecoxib, etoricoxib, valdecoxib) selectively inhibit COX – 2 which is predominantly inducible immediately after injury, and upregulated by a variety of inflammatory stimuli – cytokines like interleukins – 1, 2, TNFα, bacterial lipopolysaccharides, mitogens and reactive O_2 intermediates. COX – 2 is predominantly present in macrophages, monocytes, fibroblasts, chondrocytes, all of which are involved in inflammatory reactions. It is absent in platelets, stomach, kidney and endothelium. Non – selective and relatively COX – 1 selective cyclooxygenase inhibitors (Salicylates, ibuprofen, ketorolac, piroxicam, diclofenac, aceclofenax, naproxen, indomethacin inhibits both COX – 1 and COX – 2 and they produce adverse gastrointestinal adverse effects like nausea, gastric irritation, heart burn, gastritis, gastric ulcer and renal disorders which limits their use for inflammatory conditions. However, drugs like aspirin have antiplatelet action which in lacking with selective COX – 2 inhibitors. The GI adverse effects of non – selective COX (COX-1 and COX-2) inhibitors are due to the inhibition of cytoprotective PGs (PGI_2, PGE1 and PGE_2) which protect GI mucosa against erosion and the development of GI symptoms. However, selective COX-2 inhibitors do not affect the synthesis of cytoprotective prostaglandins and hence do not produce GI adverse effects in contrast to non-selective COX inhibitors.

However, selective COX – 2 inhibitors are likely to cause adverse cardiovascular evens like hypertension, arrhythmias, peripheral edema, MI, stroke and death. The CV risk is more in patients of MI, CHF and renal disease. They are definitely contraindicated in patients with high CV risk. Rofecoxib is a banned drug. At present valdecoxib, etoricoxib, parecoxib are the only COX – 2 inhibitors in clinical use.

8. Mention antiemetic drugs acting on vomiting center and chemoreceptor trigger zone Enumerate drugs used for chemotherapy induced vomiting, motion sickness, and hyperemesis gravidarum

Ans: Antiemetic drugs acting on CTZ and vomiting center include the following

1) Dopamine receptor antagonists – Prochlorperazine, chlorpromazine, droperidol, metoclopramide, domperidone.
2) H_2 receptor antagonists – Dimenhydrinate, cyclizine, meclizine, diphenhydramine
3) 5 – HT_2 receptor antagonists – Ondansetron, granisetron, tropisetron, dolasetron.
4) Anticholinergic agents – Hyoscine (Scopolamine)
5) NK1 receptor antagonists – Apripilant, Fosaprepilant
6) Miscellaneous agents acting by different mechanisms – Cannabinoids (Nabilone), dexamethasone, dronabinol.

Chemotherapy induced vomiting can be managed with 5 – HT_3 receptor antagonists like ondansetron, granisetron, palonosetron, dolasetron, tropisetron and Ramosetron. 5 – HT_3 receptor are distributed centrally in the area prostrema, nucleus tractus solitarius, cerebral cortex and hippocampus, and peripherally in the gut mucosa, vagal nerve endings, and spinal afferent nerve endings. Antagonism of 5 – HT_3 receptor can prevent the emesis that follows the increased 5 – HT_3 concentration which usually occurs after chemotherapy or radiation therapy.

The other drugs that could be given for the condition include cannabinoids like Dronabinol, Nabilone and neurokinin (NK_1) receptor antagonist like Apripitant, Fosapripitant used either alone or in combination with corticosteroids like dexamethasone

Drugs used for travel or motion sickness include scopolamine which can be given orally or as trandermal patch (0.25-0.5 mg); and dimenhydrate(50mg), hydroxyzine(25mg), meclizine(25mg), and promethazine (12.5-25 mg) which are H1 antagonists given orally useful to treat travel sicknes.

Drugs used to treat hyperemesis gravidarum include pyridoxine (10mg) given in combination with doxylamine (10 mg) three times a day. The other drugs used in the condition include diphenhydramine (25-50 mg given three times a day)), prochlorperazine (25 mg given twice daily), promethazine (12.5-25 mg given 3 times a day), and metoclopramide (10 mg given three times aday).

9. Enumerate clinically used haemopoietic growth factors. Discuss their pharmacology and adverse effects?

Ans: Erythropoietin, darbepoietin, methoxy polyethyleneglycol epoetin beta are the growth factors that stimulate erythroid proliferation and differentiation by interacting with specific erythropoietin receptors on red cell progenetors and cause an increase of RBC. They are used in the treatment of anemia associated with chronic renal failure, cancer related anemia, anemia in AIDS patients, preoperative anemia to reduce the requirement of blood transfusion, anemia of prematurity, HIV infection, primary bone marrow disorders, myelodysplasia and secondary anemias like aplastic anemia and anemia of multiple myeloma.

Discussion of the role of erythropoietin in anemia associated with chronic renal failure

Erythropoietin produced in the kidneys stimulates erythroid proliferation in the bone marrow and increases the levels of RBC in the circulation. In chronic renal disease the production and activation of erythropoietin is decreased causing anemia. Endogenous erythropoietin production is controlled by a sensor mechanism present at the molecular level. Hypoxia – inducible factor (inducible factor liberated in response to hypoxia **-HIF - 1α**) causes activation of erythropoietin expression and increased erythropoiesis. The state of hypoxia is vital for the activation of erythropoiesis through erythropoietin. HIF propyl hydroxylase is an enzyme that is responsible for the breakdown of HIF - 1α. **Vadadustat** is an oral HIF propyl hydroxylase inhibitor that inhibits the breakdown of HVFIα and thereby causing an increase of erythropoietin and is used in anemia associated with CKD.

The other hemopoietic growth factors include myeloid growth factors (rHuG – CSF **filgrastim, pegylated filgrastim**) – granulocyte macrophase colony stimulating factor (rHuGM – CSF **sargramostim**). These colony stimulating factor are used in cancer chemotherapy – induced neutropenia, acute myeloid leukemia, congenital, cyclic or idiopathic neutropenia, and myelodysplasia. These colony stimulating factors are also used for patients undergoing high – dose chemotherapy and requiring autologous stem cell transplantation in tumor treatment.

Thrombopoietin administration leads to an increase of platelets and used clinically wherever an increase of platelets is required. **Interleukin – II (oprelvekin)** is indicated for the prevention of severe thrombocytopenia and for a reduction of the need for platelet transfusions following myelosuppressive chemotherapy in patients with nonmyeloid malignancies.

All the hemopoietic growth factors are potentially toxic, for example with erythropoietin use there would be rapid increase of hematocrit and hemoglobin levels, hypertension and thromboembolic complications, a functional or absolute iron deficiency and allergic, hypersensitivity reactions. IL – II can causes CVS effects such as tachycardia, palpitation, vasodilation and syncope.

10. Discuss briefly the basic etiopathologies of Alzheimer's disease (AD), what is the role of oxidative stress? Mention the current approach for management of Alzheimer's disease.

Ans: Alzheimer's is a neurodegenerative disease of the CNS which is presented by a decline of behavioural and cognitive abilities enough to interfere with activities of daily living and also the most common type of dementia. It is a disease of aging and the other risk factors or predisposing factors of Alzheimer's disease include traumatic head injury, depression, cardiovascular and cerebrovascular disease, family history of dementia, smoking and increased homocysteine levels,

Pathophysiology: Alzheimer's disease is characterised by an accumulation of extracerebellar amyloid plaques and intracellular neurofibrillatory tangles which are associated with neuronal destruction particularly in cholinergic neurons. **Plaques** develop in the hippocampus, the area that helps in memory function and in other areas of cerebral cortex that are involved in thinking and making decisions. Amyloid deposition occurs around meningeal and cerebral vessels and grey matter. Gray matter deposits are multifocal and coalesce to form miliary structures called plaques. **Neurofibillatory tangles** are fibrillatory intracytoplasmic structures in neurons formed by a protein called **tau.** The primary function of tau protein is to stabilize axonal microtubules. Microtubules run along neuronal axons and are essential for intracellular transport. Microtubule assembly is held together by tau protein. In Alzheimer's disease due to **aggregation of β – amyloid**, there is hyperphosphorylation of tau which then causes the formation of aggregates. Tau aggregates form twisted paired helical filaments known as neurofibrillary tangles which occur in the hippocampus and then in the cortex.

There are mainly two types of AD - familial and sporadic forms. The familial form is the result of mutations of one of the genes (amyloid precursor protein, presenilin 1 or presenilin 2). The sporadic form which is more common occurs usually after 65 years of age. The development of β – amyloid plaques and neurofibrillary tangles are thought to be intricately related to the cause and development of the disease. Synaptic degeneration, hippocampal neuronal loss, and aneuploidy (Presence of abnormal number of chromosomes in the neuronal cells) are the predominant pathological changes causing AD. It is possible that inflammation around plaques destroys neighbouring neurons.

Management of Alzheimer's disease: There is no cure for Alzheimer's disease. Only symptomatic treatment is available.

1) Cholinesterase inhibitors (Donepezil, Rivastigmine, galantamine act by increasing the level of Acetylcholine which plays an important role in memory, learning, and cognitive functions. Donepezil and galantamine are rapid, reversible inhibitors of acetylcholinesterase. Rivastigmine is a slow, reversible inhibitor of both acetylcholinesterase and butyrylcholinesterase. Donepezil is usually preferred of all because of once daily – dosing (5mg – 10mg). Galantamine is available as twice daily (4mg x 2, increased up to 12 mg twice a day) tablets. It cannot be used in end – stage renal disease or severe hepatic dysfunction. Rivastigmine is available as oral and transdermal patch forms and given in daily dose of 4.6mg Side effects of cholinesterase inhibitors include bradycardia, cardiac conduction defects and syncope all due to increased vagal activity.
2) Partial (N – methyl D – aspartate (NMDA) antagonist (Memantine): Memantine blocks NMDA receptors and slows intracellular calcium accumulation and given in daily doses of 5mg increased to 10mg/day.
3) Melatonin – Current studies suggest that melatonin is a prospective drug for the prevention and cure of AD. It is a tryptophan derivative synthesized mainly by the pineal gland. In patients with AD, decreased melatonin levels in serum and CSF and loss of diurnal rhythms are observed. Melatonin has been shown effective in preventing damage caused by exposure to amyloid beta protein
4) Selegiline is a MAO_B inhibitor and has shown improvements in cognition, behaviour, and mood and is a second line drug to treat AD because of drug interactions with sedatives, antipsychotics and antidepressants.

Answers to the Questions given by Rajiv Gandhi University of Health Sciences 2020 (February)

1. Classify anti – hypertensive drugs. Discuss in detail about the management of hypertensive emergency and urgency. Which anti – hypertensives are to be avoided in pregnancy and why?

Ans: Antihypertensive drugs may be classified according to their sites of action and the following categories are included

1. Centrally acting – clonidine, moxanidine, α – methyldopa, guanabenz, guanfacine, imidazole receptor agonists (rilmenidine, moxanidine).
2. Adrenergic neuron blockers – Guanethidine, guanadrel, bretylium, reserpine
3. Ganglion blockers – Trimetaphan, mecamylamine, pempidine
4. Adrenergic receptor blockers – α – blockers – prazocin and its derivatives
   B – blockers such as propranolol, metoprolol, and others
5. Calcium channel blockers – Nifedipine, verapamil, amlodipine, diltiazem
6. ACE inhibitors – Enalapril, lisinopril, Ramipril
7. Angiotensin receptor blockers – Losartan, Valsartan, Telmisartan.
8. Vasodilators –Arteriodilators – hydralazine, minoxidil, dizoxide, fenoldopam
9. Arteriovenodilators- Nitrates, Sodium nitroprusside
10. Diuretics – Frusemide, hydrochlorthiazide, aldosterone antagonists – Eplerenone, finerenone, spironolactone, amiloride.
11. Renin antagonists – Aliskiren

Hypertensive emergency and urgency

Hypertensive emergency is a condition of acute and sudden elevation of blood pressure which is the result of sudden and rapid withdrawal of antiadrenergic drugs like clonidine or β – adrenergic blockers. The condition may also arise due to an imbalance in the functioning of autonomic nervous system, sudden states of rage, anxiety, grief, and similar conditions of unexpected emotional states.

Hypertensive urgency is one type of hypertensive emergency in which blood pressure increases gradually and hypertension – mediated organ damage is present or evident in organs such as heart, kidney, brain, vascular system, and lungs. This needs immediate attention for rapid control of blood pressure. Hypertensive emergencies include hypertension associated with vascular damage termed as chronic hypertension, and hypertension associated with altered hemodynamic states such as heart failure, stroke, or dissecting aneurysm. Pheochromocytoma induced hypertensive crisis also forms part of hypertensive emergency. In hypertensive crisis/emergency nausea, vomiting, headache, chest pain, abnormal cardiac rhythms, nosebleeds, dyspnea, fainting can occur. The most common presentations of hypertensive emergencies are central ischemia, pulmonary edema, hypertensive encephalopathy and heart failure.

Management of hypertensive emergencies: Blood pressure should be lowered slowly over a period of minutes to hours with an antihypertensive agent. Hypertensive emergencies differ from hypertensive urgency in that they are treated parenterally, while in urgency it is recommended to use oral antihypertensives to reduce the risk of ischemia. Labetalol, esmolol, calcium channel blockers like nicardipine, clevidipine; vadodilators like nitropruside, nitroglycerine, hydralazine, dizoxide, fenoldopam and α_2 agonists like clonidine are the preferred drugs to treat hypertensive emergencies on controlled administration of the drugs concerned with monitoring of blood pressure periodically and adjusting the dose as per requirements.

ACE inhibitors and AT**1** receptor blockers are to be avoided in all trimesters of pregnancy, as they are likely to cause fetopathy, neonatal renal failure, and fetal death: β–blockers are also avoided as they cross placental barrier and are associated with several adverse effects, such as delayed intrauterine growth, respiratory depression, neonatal bradycardia, and hypoglycemia, particularly when the treatment is started early on in the pregnancy (12 – 24 weeks). The other drugs to be avoided during pregnancy include diuretics alone except in combination with other safe drugs as they are likely to cause fetal electrolyte disturbances and a reduction in maternal blood volume. Similarly, calcium channel blockers (Amlodipine) are also avoided as their use is likely to cause maternal hypotension and fetal hypoxia. Methydopa is the most preferred drug for treating gestational and chronic hypertension in combination with diuretics. Labetalol is the other alternative. Intervention is usually needed when diastolic blood pressure is around 100 mmHg and the drugs are given in lower doses particularly in patients with associated diabetes, renal disease or target organ damage. It is to be noted that no antihypertensive drug is safe during 1st trimester of pregnancy (the period of fetal organogenesis).

2. Write short notes on

1) Discuss in detail about Phase II biotransformation reactions with suitable examples

Phase II biotransformation reactions also know as **conjugation reactions** that involve endogenous substrate such as glucuronic acid, sulfuric acid, acetic acid or amino acid that combines with the newly incorporated functional group of phase I reaction and the resultant product becomes highly ionized and rapidly eliminated

Important Phase II reactions include

Glucuronide – morphine, acetaminophen, diazepam

Acetylation – Sulfonamides, INH, clonazepam, dapsone

Glutathione – Ethacrinic acid

Glycine – Acetyl salicylic acid, benzoic acid, nicotinic acid

Sulfate – Estrone, acetaminophen, methyldopa

Methylation – Dopamine, adrenaline, pyridine, thiouracil

2) Enumerate 2nd generation H_1 antagonists and their uses. Discuss the differences between 1st and 2nd generation antihistamines.

Ans: The second generation H_1 antagonists include fexofenadine, loratadine, desloratadine, levocarbastine, rupatadine, azelastine, cetirizine, levocetirizine.

Uses of second generation H_1 antagonists are the same as those used for by the 1st generation H1 antagonists. They are quite useful is managing seasonal rhinitis, conjunctivitis, and common cold to relieve sneezing, rhinorrhea, and itching of the eyes, nose and throat. They are also used for utricaria, contact dermatitis, napkin rash, atopic dermatitis, eczema, drug – induced skin rashes, and allergic cough. However, either 1st generation or 2nd generation H1 antagonists are not effective to counter the effects of anaphylactic reaction for which glucocorticoids are the preferred drugs

The difference of 1st and 2nd generation H_1 antagonists

	1st generation		2nd generation
1.	They are lipophilic compounds, easily cross the blood: brain barrier, enter CNS and cause sedation	1.	They are hydrophilic polar compounds, do not cross blood: brain barrier and do not cause sedation or drowsiness
2.	They block both central and peripheral H_1receptors	2.	They selectively block the peripheral H_1receptors
3.	They have short – half liver and need to be given 3 times /day	3.	They have long half- life and need to be given once daily
4.	They produce anticholinergic effects such as dryness of mouth, tachycardia	4	They do not cause adverse anticholinergic effects

3) Discuss the mechanism of action, uses and techniques of local anesthetics

Ans: Local anesthetics are a class of drugs which reversibly block impulse conduction along the axons and other excitable membrane areas that facilitate Na^+conduction for the propagation of action potential. They block the voltage – gated Na^+ channel which contains the receptor site for the agents, thought to be located at its cytoplasmic (inner portion) thereby preventing the permeability or flux of Na^+ into the excitable membrane.

1. **Surface anesthesia**: Local anesthetics are used to anaesthetize local areas for the relief of pain caused by minor burns; pruritis due to dermatoses or hemorrhoids. **Pramaxine/pramocaine** is used to facilitate sigmoidoscopic examinations. Local anesthetics can be applied to the skin, ear, eye, nose, mouth as well as other mucous membranes to anesthetize local areas for different clinical purposes.
2. **Local infiltration**: This involves extravascular placement of local anesthetics in the area to be anesthetized. Minor surgical produces can be undertaken by this technique. Lidocaine, prilocaine and mepivacaine are mainly used for this purpose.
3. **Nerve block anesthesia (Conduction anesthesia**)– Local anesthetics like lignocaine can be injected into tissues surrounding individual peripheral nerves (ulnar, radial or intercostal nerves) to block nerve conduction and to facilitate surgical procedures pertaining to those areas.
4. **Epidural or Extradural anesthesia**: Here the local anesthetics are placed in the epidural place between the dura matter and the periosteum lining the vertebral column. This is used in obstetric practice for undertaking caesarian section or control of labor pains.
5. **Spinal anesthesia**: Here the local anesthetics are injected into lumbar subarachnoid space and this is useful to undertake surgical procedures below the lumbar spine such as involving lower abdomen, pelvic region, and lower limbs.
6. **Intravenous anesthesia:** This is useful in providing analgesia for minor surgical procedures. It is also known as IV regional anesthesia or **Bier's block**. It is an anesthetic technique on the body extremities where a local anesthetic is injected IV (as closely as possible to the area of surgical procedure) and the area isolated from circulation to provide a bloodless field by applying a proximal double-cuffed pneumatic tourniquet. It is safe and does not require the use of any general anesthetic

4) Compare and contrast conventional and atypical antipsychotic drug

Ans: Conventional antipsychotics (antidepressants) have different mechanisms of action acting primarily on 5 – HT receptor subtypes. The examples include

1) **Tricyclic compounds**
   a. Tertiary amines – Amitryptiline, Imipramine, doxepin, clomipramine
   b. Secondary amines – Amoxapine, desipramine, maprolitine, nortryptiline, protryptiline
2) **Selective 5 – HT uptake inhibitors** – Citalopram, fluoxetine, fluvoxamine, paroxamine, Sertaline, paraoxetine
3) **MAO inhibitors** – Selegiline, rasagiline

Atypical antidepressants – Clozapine, loxapine, olanzapine, quetiapine, molindone, risperidone, ziprasidone, aripiprazole

Miscellaneous atypical antipsychotics: Bupropion, duloxetin, mirtazapine, trazadone, nefazodone, velnafaxine

Conventional antidepressants produce sedation, antimuscarinic action, and 5 – HT receptor blockade as well NAD blockade.

Atypical antipsychotics have affinity for both D_2 and 5-HT_{2A} receptors and block them and alleviate both positive and negative symptoms of schizophrenia while typical antipsychotic drugs block only D_2 receptors. They do not have antimuscarinic action, and produce minimal or moderate 5-HT and NAD blockade.

5) **Discuss the role of vasodilators in acute heart failure**

Ans: Vasodilators like sodium nitroprusside, nitroglycerine reduce both preload and afterload thereby reduce the cardiac workload and oxygen consumption and thus increasing the cardiac output. Sodium nitroprusside is given IV as infusion and has an onset of action of 30 seconds and the dose given is usually 0.25 – 1.5 mcg/kg/min.

Nitroglycerine (glyceryl trinitrate) is the most preferred vasodilator drug for treating acute congestive heart failure because it has anti – ischemic effect and less likely to produce coronary steal than nitroprusside. It is given in doses of 10 – 20 mcg/min and increased by 10mcg/min every 2 -3 min as per the progress in relief of symptoms of congestive heart failure.

6) **Discuss the mechanism of action, uses and adverse effects of spironolactone.**

Ans: Spironolactone is an aldosterone antagonist and acts by binding to the mineralocorticoid receptors in the renal tubules (distal collecting tubules) and acts as competitive inhibitor of aldosterone. It decreases Na^+ reabsorption and decreases K^+elimination, both the actions leading to natriuresis and K^+retention. It has very limited diuretic action when used alone because the distal Na^+/K^+exchange, the site where it acts accounts for reabsorption of only 2% of filtered Na^+.

It is used in hypertension, Congestive heart failure in combination with diuretics.

The adverse effects produced by spironolactone include hyperkalemia, progestational and antiandrogenic effects like gynecomastia.

III. Write short notes on

1. **Define bioavailability, why is it less when the drug is given orally?**

Ans: Bioavailability of a drug is defined as its net fraction or amount that reaches the circulation in an unchanged form given by any route. It can also be defined as the extent to which and the rate at which the active moiety of a drug enters the systemic circulation thereby gaining access to the site of action and resulting in the desired pharmacological response. Whereas the bioavailability is 100% when the drug is given intravenously, and it varies considerably when given orally or by any other routes as it requires the drug to be first absorbed into the system to varying extents which may reduce bioavailability.

Bioavailability also depends upon the rate of absorption and first – pass metabolism when given orally. It is also likely to get reduced by local conditions (acidic pH, alkalinity, gastric mucosal patency)

2. Why is pralidoxime not used as antidote for carbamate anticholinesterases poisoning?

Ans: Oximes such as pralidoxime and diacetyl monoxime containing oxime group(=NoH)have high affinity for the phosphorous atom and these drugs are able to hydrolyze the phosphorylated enzyme complex when it is not aged. Organophosphorus compounds are irreversible cholinesterase inhibitors, bind to the active site of the enzyme (cholinesterase) and prevent the accessibility of Ach to AchE. The covalent phosphorous enzyme bond is extremely stable and hydrolyzes in water at a very slow rate of hundreds of hours, thereby increasing the accessibility of Ach in higher levels to the tissues causing muscular paralysis. While oximes act on the phosphorylated enzyme complex, they do not have action on carbamolated enzyme complex formed by the action of carbamates such as physostigmine and neostigmine.

3. Mention the adverse effects of theophylline

Ans: The common adverse effects of theophylline include heartburn, abdominal pain, nausea and vomiting due to gastric irritation consequent to and increase in gastric acidity. The CNS manifestations include headache, anxiety, tremor, and insomnia. If higher levels of theophylline are reached in the blood, seizures and cardiac arrhythmias can result.

4. List four differences between buspirone and benzodiazepines

Ans:

Benzodiazepines	Buspirone
Benzodiazepines have GABA-ergic/GABA mimitic activity and facilitate opening of cl^- channel indirectly. Benzodiazepines have hypnotic, sedative, antianxiety, muscle relaxant, anticonvulsant properties. They are likely to impair motor or driving skills and potentiate the actions of CNS depressants like alcohol, sedative hypnotic drugs, and likely to ptoduce tolerance and dependence.	It acts through central 5-HT, A and D_2 receptors as agonist and has no abuse liability, unlike diazepam and other benzodiazepines. It does not impair motor or driving skills and does not potentiate the depressant actions of alcohol, sedative hypnotic drugs. It is a non – benzodiazepine anxiolytic drug and has no hypnotic or euphoritic effects. It also does not have anticonvulsant or muscle relaxant effects.

5. Mention four common drug interactions in an alcohol individual

Ans:

1) CNS depressants such as opioids, hypnotics, tranquilizers can potentiate the CNS depressant effects
2) Antihistamines, reserpine, methyldopa, and clonidine can cause severe depression in the presence of alcohol.
3) Vasodilators (hydralazine and nitroglycerine) can cause additive orthostatic hypotension.
4) Alcohol potentiates the adverse effects of aspirin (GI bleeding) sulfonylureas (hypoglycemia) and oral anticoagulants (bleeding).
5) INH and acetaminophen can cause hepatic toxicity in chronic alcoholics because of their increased conversion to toxic metabolites.
6) Ketoconazole, chlorpropamide, metronidazole, tolbutamide can cause a disulfiram like effect in chronic alcoholics.

6. Adenosine

Ans: It is given IV as bolus to terminate reentrant supraventricular arrhythmias and their conversion to sinus rhythm. It has very short half – life (10 seconds) and hence given as bolus. It's mechanism of action involves activation of inward rectifier K^+ current and inhibition of calcium current. This results in hyperpolarization and suppression of Ca^+ dependent action potentials. It causes shortening of AP duration.

When given IV, it inhibits SA nodal conduction and increases AV nodal refractory period due to blockade of Ca^+current. Intracellular cyclic AMP accumulation is decreased with reduced sym- pathetic activity.

Section 1 - MCQs and Quizzes

The MCQs and Quizzes are selected mainly to make the student to quickly recollect the topic taught earlier and the knowledge gained by other methods and to try to make a good selection of the given choices made out of their reasonable comprehension and judgement. They are not intended to go deep into the details. However the core subject is covered to the extent possible

1. Which of the following is the most accurate statement?
   - (a) α-adrenoceptor sympathomimetic agonists are used to reduce mucous membrane congestion
   - (b) α-adrenergic agonists are used to treat bronchial asthma
   - (c) β-adrenergic agonists are used to reduce surgical bleeding
   - (d) β-adrenergic agonists are used to prolong local anaesthesia
2. A 25-year-old man is noted to be in septic shock. A low-dose dopamine is administered and that results in which one of the following?
   - (a) Decrease of cardiac output
   - (b) Decrease in systolic blood pressure
   - (c) Increase in renal blood flow
   - (d) Produces significant peripheral vasoconstriction
3. A 35-year old man is prescribed labetalol for hypertension. Its' effect on the cardiovascular system is the result of its action as an antagonist at which one of the following
   - (a) α-adrenoceptors
   - (b) β-adrenoceptors
   - (c) Both α-and β-adrenoceptors
   - (d) Cardiac D_1 receptors
4. The inclusion of a spiranolactone with a thiazide diuretic in a regimen to treat hypertension is done to achieve which one of the following?
   - (a) Reduce hyperuricemia
   - (b) Reduce Mg^+ less
   - (c) Decrease the loss of Na^+
   - (d) Reduce K^+ loss
5. Carbidopa reduces which one of the following?
   - (a) The activity of dopa-decarboxylase activity is the CNS
   - (b) The L-dopa dose necessary to achieve a therapeutic effect
   - (c) The severity of L-dopa associated dyskinasias
   - (d) The time to onset of L-dopa's therapeutic effect
6. Which one of the following drugs used to manage seizures that requires a significant dose adjustment with continuous administration over a period?
   - (a) Carbamazepine
   - (b) Diazepam
   - (c) Ethosuximide
   - (d) Phenytoin
7. Choose the antibiotic used for cancer chemotherapy
   - (a) Cytarabine
   - (b) Doxorubicin
   - (c) Gentamicin
   - (d) Etoposide
8. Which one of the following anti enzymes in a beta lactamase inhibitor?
   - (a) Clavulanic acid
   - (b) Sulbactam
   - (c) Tazobactam
   - (d) All of the above

9. Immunosuppressive effect of glucocorticoids is caused by
   (a) Reducing the concentration of lymphocytes (T and B cells) and inhibiting function of tissue macrophages and other antigen-presenting cells
   (b) Decreasing the production of prostaglandins
   (c) Decreased fibroblast function
   (d) Decreased release of lipolytic and proteolytic enzymes
10. Which one of the following H_1 antagonists does not cause sedative effect
   (a) Dimenhydrinate
   (b) Cyclizine
   (c) Loratadine
   (d) Cyproheptadine
11. Which one of the following statements about estrogens is true
   (a) Estrogens are required for normal sexual maturation and growth of the female
   (b) Estrogens decrease the rate of resorption of bone
   (c) Estrogens increase the coagulability of blood.
   (d) All of the above
12. Which one of the following GLP-1 receptor agonist given orally in once daily and weekly doses to treat diabetes and obesity
   (a) Exenatide
   (b) Liraglutide
   (c) Lixisenatide
   (d) Semaglutide
13. Triptans act through which one of the following mechanisms to treat migraine
   (a) Activation of 5-HT_{1B} and 5-HT_D receptors on presynaptic trigeminal nerve endings to inhibit the release of vasodilating peptides CGRP and substance P
   (b) Inhibition of Synthesis of leukotrienes
   (c) Inhibition of synthesis of histamine
   (d) Inhibition of nociceptive responses in the afferent pathways in CNS.
14. Which one of the following is used in thrombosis related to heparan – induced thrombocytopenia?
   (a) Direct thrombin inhibitor like lepirudin/argatroban
   (b) Warfarin
   (c) Rivaroxaban
   (d) Streptokinase
15. Which one of the following nitrates and nitrite drugs is used for prevention of anginal attack?
   (a) Nitro-glycerine 2% transdermal patch
   (b) Nitro-glycerine oral sustained – release preparation
   (c) Isosorbide mononitrate
   (d) All the above
16. Which one of the following drug groups useful in angina that increases myocardial oxygen delivery, decrease oxygen demand or requirements and decrease cardiac work load?
   (a) Β-adrenergic blockers
   (b) Calcium channel blockers
   (c) Potassium channel openers
   (d) Fatty acid oxidation inhibitor (Ranolazine)
17. Which one of the following statements is true of β-adrenergic blockers in cardiovascular conditions?
   (a) Beneficial effects of these agents are related primarily to their hemodynamic effects – decrease of heart rate, blood pressure, and contractility
   (b) They increase the permeability of K^+ channels (ATP – dependent) that results in stabilizing the membrane potential of excitable cells.
   (c) They act on central sympathetic activity in the brain stem
   (d) They decrease the transmembrane Ca^+ currents resulting in vascular relaxation and reduce cardiac contractility
18. Dopamine receptor agonist activity can be explained by all of the following mechanisms except
   (a) D_1 receptor activation in renal, mesenteric and coronary vascular bed causing

vasodilation, increase in GFR, renal blood flow and Na^+ elimination

(b) In higher dose, it has predominant action on cardiac β_1 receptors releasing NAD from cardiac nerve cells, which contributes to positive inotropic action

(c) In still higher doses, it causes α_1-receptor activation that causes peripheral vasoconstriction and a rise of blood pressure

(d) All the above

19. Non contraceptive clinical uses of progestins include all of the following except
    (a) Habitual or recurrent abortions/ miscarriages
    (b) Abnormal uterine bleeding
    (c) As Ovulation inducing agents
    (d) Menopausal syndrome

20. Which one of the following drugs is a LTD_4 (leukotriene D_4) receptor) blocker?
    (a) Ibuprofen
    (b) Zafirlukast
    (c) Zileuton
    (d) diclofenac

21. Which one of the following antibiotic combination is the choice to treat septic shock?
    (a) Vancomycin + piperacillin + Tazobactam
    (b) Dicloxacillin or cephalexin or clinda-mycin
    (c) Ampicillin + Sulbactam
    (d) Cotrimoxazole

22. The most common adverse effect of ethambutol is
    (a) Optic neuritis (retrobulbar neuritis)
    (b) Hepatitis
    (c) Peripheral neuritis
    (d) Renal damage

23. Tacrolimus and Sirolimus are
    (a) Immunomodulators/immune boosters
    (b) Immunosuppressants
    (c) Antiinflammatory drugs
    (d) Drugs used for psoriasis

24. The action of parathyroid hormone is
    (a) It increases absorption of calcium through intestines
    (b) Mobilizes calcium from bone in higher doses (osteoclastic action) and increases bone formation (osteoblastic action) in low doses
    (c) Increases reabsorption of Ca+ from the kidney
    (d) All the above

25. The drug of choice in an cute attack of bronchial asthma for a quicker drug response is
    (a) Levalbuterol or Levosolbutamol nebulization
    (b) Ipratropium
    (c) Theophylline or aminohylline
    (d) corticosteroids

26. Norplant (levonorgestrel/implant) is used for
    (a) Osteoporosis
    (b) Hormone replacement therapy
    (c) Long acting contraceptive
    (d) Disfunctional uterine bleeding

27. Say 'Yes' or 'No' to the following statements
    (a) Niacin causes an appreciable increase in HDL – C levels [ ]
    (b) N – acetylcysteine, bromhexine are antitussive agents [ ]
    (c) Warfarin is extensively bound to plasma albumin and has small volume of distribution[ ]

28. Fill in the blanks
    (a) Budersonide is used by_______route in bronchial asthma
    (b) Amphotericin B is used by_______route to treat fungal infections
    (c) Emetine given subcutaneously is used to treat___________.

29. Cross match the following

1) Zidovudine	a) Parkinsonism
2) Naltrexone	b) HIV infection
3) Pergolide	c) Alcohol addiction
4) Colchicine	d) Acute attack of gout

30. Cross match the following

1) Benzodiazepine	a) Acute congestive heart failure
2) Sodium nitroprusside	b) glaucoma
3) Methazolamide	c) Anxiety states
4) vigabatrine	d) partial seizures

Answers to MCQs

1) a	2) c	3) c	4) d	5) b
6) a	7) b	8) d	9) a	10) c
11) d	12) d	13) a	14) a	15) d
16) a	17) a	18) d	19) c	20) b
21) a	22) b	23) b	24) d	25) a

26) c

27) (a. Yes) (b. No) (c. Yes)

28) (a. Inhalation) (b. IV) (c. hepatic amoebiasis)

29) (1. b) (2. c) (3. a) (4. d)

30) (1. c) (2. a) (3. b) (4. d)

Section 2 - MCQs and Quizzes

1. Receptor mediated endocytosis is facilitated by which one in one of the following drugs
   (a) Carvedilol
   (b) Glibenclamide
   (c) Iron
   (d) Amlodipine
2. The dose adjustments of which one of the following is determined by creatinine clearance
   (a) Gentamicin
   (b) Gabapentine
   (c) Miconazole
   (d) Cytarabine
3. One of the following has potential and clinically significant drug interactions
   (a) Rivaraxaban
   (b) Danaparoid
   (c) Warfarin
   (d) Dalteparin
4. Allopurinol can influence the metabolism of which one of the following and increase its toxicity
   (a) Mercaptopurine
   (b) Phenobarbital
   (c) Rifampicin
   (d) Clonazepam
5. One of the following transdermal patch is useful to relieve postoperative pain
   (a) Ketoprofen
   (b) Meloxicam
   (c) Fentanil/ buprenorphine
   (d) methylprednisolone
6. All of the following undergo entero-hepatic clearance except
   (a) Vecuroneum
   (b) Cephaperazone
   (c) Morphine
   (d) Ethinylestradiol
7. Elimination of excess dose of acetylsalicylic acid can be facilitated by
   (a) changing the pH of the urine
   (b) Hemodialysis
   (c) IV normal saline
   (d) oral consumption of water
8. Succinylcholine can cause all the actions except
   (a) Depolarizing neuromuscular block
   (b) Reparatory paralysis during anesthesia
   (c) Increase intraocular pressure
   (d) Sustained muscle relaxation for longer periods
9. Probenecid has one of the following additional actions apart from being a uricosuric drug
   (a) potent anti-inflammatory action
   (b) competitive inhibitor of renal tubular secretion of penicillin
   (c) colchicine like effect
   (d) xanthine oxidase inhibition
10. All of the following have potent renal toxicity except
    (a) Vancomycin
    (b) Streptomycin
    (c) Gold salts
    (d) Ampicillin
11. All of the following have potent teratogenic effect except
    (a) Isotretinoin
    (b) Cytotoxic drugs
    (c) Thalidomide
    (d) Chloramphenicol

12. All of the following drugs produce parkinsonism or extrapyramidal effects except
    (a) Butyrophenones
    (b) Phenothiazines
    (c) Venlafaxine
    (d) Domperidone
13. One of the following shows lupus syndrome or lupus like drug effects
    (a) Hydralazine
    (b) Statins
    (c) Steroids
    (d) INH
14. CYP3A4 isoenzyme present in grapefruit juice can increase the pharmacological actions all of the following drugs except
    (a) Protease inhibitors
    (b) HMG-CoA inhibitors
    (c) Calcium channel blockers
    (d) warfarin
15. Which One of the following acts by inhibiting cholesterol absorption by enterocytes of the small intestine
    (a) Ezetimibe
    (b) Rosuvastatin
    (c) colestepol
    (d) Gemfibrozil
16. One of the following is an irrational combination for clinical use
    (a) Sulfonamides + penicillin
    (b) Lidocaine + epinephrine
    (c) Lopinavir + Ritonavir
    (d) Sulfadiazine + Pyrimethamine
17. Selegiline is a
    (a) Mao_A inhibitor
    (b) Mao_B inhibitor
    (c) HMGcoA inhibitor
    (d) ACE inhibitor
18. The transport of Choline from plasma into neurons in the synthesis of acetylcholine is facilitated by
    (a) Na^+ dependent carrier system
    (b) Ca^+ dependent carrier system
    (c) increased cell membrane permeability
    (d) Affinity for intracellular Acetyl CoA
19. Which one of the following statements is not correct
    (a) Nadolol has the highest half-life among Beta blockers
    (b) Propranolol undergoes first pass metabolism
    (c) E_{max} signifies the efficacy of a drug
    (d) A sublingual drug is poorly absorbed into systemic circulation
20. Which one of the following does not act through a specific receptor
    (a) Dizoxide
    (b) Carvedilol
    (c) Insulin
    (d) Vasopressin
21. All the following drugs require therapeutic drug monitoring except
    (a) Lithium
    (b) Digoxin
    (c) Theophylline
    (d) Frusemide
22. Hemolytic anemia due to glucose 6-phosphate dehydrogenase deficiency can be caused by which one of the following
    (a) Primaquine
    (b) Penicillin-G
    (c) Chloramphenicol
    (d) INH
23. The target site of action for steroids is
    (a) G-protein coupled receptors
    (b) Ligand-gated ion channels
    (c) Nuclear receptors
    (d) Kinase linked receptors
24. Tachyphylaxis can be produced by all of the following drugs except
    (a) Amphetamine
    (b) Adrenaline
    (c) Tyramine
    (d) Ephedrine
25. Anaphylactic Shock is
    (a) Type-2 reaction

(b) Type – 3 reaction
(c) Type -1 reaction
(d) Type-4 reaction

26. Fill up the blanks
   (a) __________is the antagonist for warfarin
   (b) Dopamine is given exclusively by ___ route
   (c) Mannitol is a ____________diuretic
   (d) cumulative graph of the frequency distribution curve is known as _____________
   (e) LD50/ED50 is expressed as __________________
   (f) The levels of blood concentration at various intervals is represented as _____________
   (g) mAch, α2, and Opioids act through ___________ type receptors
   (h) Better entry of penicillin into CNS can be seen is ___________

27. Cross match the following

1) Digoxin	a) HMG-CoA
2) Protamine	b) Thiazide diuretic
3) Bumetanide	c) Cumulative drug
4) Atorvastatin	d) Heparin

28. Cross match the following

1) Nitroglycerine	a) Aldosterone antagonist
2) Eplerenone	b) H_1 blocker
3) Rizatryptan	c) Unstable angina
4) Desloratadine	d) Migraine

29. Fill up the blanks
   (a) Dyskinasea as a side effect is produced by ___________
   (b) Cyclosporine A is mainly used for ____________
   (c) Methotrexate is a _____________ antagonist
   (d) Ondansetron is an _____________ drug

30. Fill up the blanks
   (a) Ceftriaxone is mainly indicated for ____________
   (b) The drug of choice for methicillin resistant penicillin allergic staphylococcus aureus infections is ____________________

Answers to MCQs

1) c	2) a	3) c	4) a	5) c
6) a	7) a	8) d	9) b	10) d
11) d	12) c	13) a	14) c	15) a
16) a	17) b	18) a	19) d	20) a
21) d	22) a	23) c	24) b	25) c

26) (a. Vitamin K) (b. IV) (c. Osmotic) (d. Bell shaped curve) (e. Therapeutic Index) (f. Dose response curve) (g. G_i) (h. meningitis)

27) (1. c) (2. d) (3. b) (4. a)

28) (1. c) (2. a) (3. d) (4. b)

29) (a.Levodopa) (b. Immunosupression) (c. Folate) (d. Antiemetic)

30) (a. Gonococcal urethritis or typhoid fever) (b. Vancomycin)

Section 3 - MCQs and Quizzes

1. Which one of the following is used commonly for the prevention of nausea and vomiting associated with malignancy or radiation therapy?
   (a) Ondansetron
   (b) Metoclopramide
   (c) Promethazine
   (d) Cyproheptadine
2. All of the following are the common adverse effects of oral contraceptives on long term use except
   (a) Nausea, vomiting, anorexia and increase episodes of migraine
   (b) Stroke/ venous thromboembolism
   (c) Breakthrough bleeding
   (d) Unfourable bone mineral density
3. All the following are non-psychiatric indications of antipsychotics except
   (a) Preoperative medication
   (b) Nausea and vomiting
   (c) Neurolept anesthesia
   (d) Degenerative disorders
4. Which one of the following is the non-conventional drug used to treat Alzheimer's disease
   (a) Rivastigmine
   (b) Galantamine
   (c) Melatonin
   (d) Memantine
5. Which one of the following is used most commonly and also the first line drug for absence seizures
   (a) Ethosuximide
   (b) Diazepam
   (c) Zonisamide
   (d) Felbamate
6. Which one of the following is not a disease – modifying antirheumatic drug (DMARDs)?
   (a) Methotrexate
   (b) Methylprednisolone
   (c) D – Penicillamine
   (d) Hydroxychloroquine
7. Which one of the following is used to treat an acute attack of gout?
   (a) Sulfinpyrazone
   (b) Probenecid
   (c) Colchicine
   (d) Allopurinol
8. Which one of the following ergot alkaloids has affinity for dopamine receptors?
   (a) Dihydroergotamine
   (b) Ergonovine
   (c) Bromocriptine
   (d) Lysergic acid diethylamide
9. All the antipsychotic drugs owe their action due to
   (a) 5 – HT_2A receptor blockade
   (b) Predominant D_2 receptor blockade
   (c) Activation of GABA receptor
   (d) α_1 – receptor blockade
10. Phenytoin is used in all the following clinical conditions except
    (a) Grand mal epilepsy
    (b) Absence seizures
    (c) Digitalis induced cardiac arrhythmias
    (d) Partial seizures / focal seizures
11. Which one of the following is used as adjutant to L-dopa-carbidopa combination to control end-of-dose akinesia?
    (a) Apomorphine

(b) α – methyldopa
(c) Cabergoline
(d) Cholinergic antagonists

12. All the statements of succinylcholine are true except
(a) It causes apnea
(b) Its actions are antagonized by butyrylcholinesterase
(c) It is a short acting skeletal muscle relaxant
(d) Its actions can be antagonized by neostigmine

13. All are true of Ramelteon(Melatonin agonist), a new generation sedative hypnotic except
(a) Lack of abusive liability
(b) Lack of rebound insomnia on discontinuation
(c) It does not impair psychomotor or cognitive function
(d) Tolerance develops sooner

14. Oxytocin acts primarily by which one of the following mechanisms
(a) Through autonomic innervation of the uterus
(b) By a direct action on the smooth muscle of the uterus
(c) Exclusively acting by the release of PGE_2 and $PGE_{2\alpha}$
(d) By enhancing the estrogen effect

15. A 38-year old woman is given ibuprofen for her compliant of dysmenorrhea, but she complains of gastritis. She was given a medication to arrest her gastric problem. Which one of the following would suitably work for her gastric problem
(a) PGE_1 analog
(b) PGE_1 antagonist
(c) PGE_2 analog
(d) PGI antagonist

16. Which one of the following salicylates is used to treat inflammatory bowel diseases, ulcerative colitis and Crohn's disease?
(a) Diflunisol
(b) Acetyl salicylic acid
(c) Sodium salicylate
(d) Olsalazine

17. Which one of the following is a potential adverse effect of aceclofenac other than GI effects?
(a) Uterine contractions and induction of abortion
(b) Acute and chronic kidney injury
(c) Acute CVS dysfunction
(d) Excerebration of existing bronchial asthma

18. Which one of the following is not a contraindication of morphine?
(a) Hypoxia and reduced respiratory reserve
(b) Head injury
(c) Perioperative analgesia
(d) Supraventricular tachycardia and atrial fibrillation

19. Adalimumab and infliximab used in rheumatoid arthritis act by which one of the following mechanisms?
(a) $TNF\alpha_1$ and $TNF\alpha_2$ receptors blockade
(b) Leukotriene synthesis inhibition
(c) Suppression of 'T' lymphocyte function
(d) Inhibition of migration and phagocytic activity of macrophages

20. Combination of aldosterone antagonists and ACE inhibitors is likely to cause
(a) Hypokalemia
(b) Hyperkalemia
(c) Hyponatremia
(d) Decrease of glomerular filtration rate (GFR)

21. All are true of preoperative preparation of a patient of pheochromocytoma except
(a) Phenoxybenzamine (10mg orally twice daily for 7 to 10 days)
(b) Propranolol (20 mg twice daily) at least 3 days after initiation of phenoxybenzamine

(c) A high sodium diet a few days after the initiation of phenoxybenzamine to manage volume contraction which is more likely to occur

(d) Ketamine 15 mg IV before surgery

22. Chloroquine, Quinine, Mefloquine act by which one of the following mechanisms for antimalarial effect
   (a) By binding to toxic heme and preventing its conversion to nontoxic hemozoin in the food vacuoles of the parasite
   (b) Inhibiting folate synthesis in the parasite
   (c) By binding to 30S ribosomal subunits inhibiting protein synthesis
   (d) Formation of cytotoxic complexes in the parasite leading to damage to membrane damage

23. Which of the following adrenergic drug used to treat glaucoma
   (a) Apraclonidine
   (b) Phenylephrine
   (c) Methoxamine
   (d) Midodrine

24. A 55-year old woman is being treated for rheumatoid arthritis. As her condition is becoming worse, a new drug is added. After 6 months, she notes night sweats, weight loss, chronic cough and chest radiograph shows cavity lesion (probably due to tuberculosis as an opportunist infection). Which drug of the following might have been prescribed to her for RA?
   (a) Gold salts
   (b) D – Penicillamine
   (c) Adalimumab
   (d) Hydroxychloroquine

25. AT1 receptor antagonists have all the following advantages over ACE inhibitors except
   (a) They are equally potent antihypertensives
   (b) They do not have any effect on bradykinin metabolism and hence do not produce dry cough and angioedema
   (c) No special contraindication in elderly or in patients with renal impairment
   (d) They are as effective as ACE inhibitors in congestive heart failure and also to provide renal protection

26. Clinical uses of ergot alkaloid include all the following except
   (a) Postpartum hemorrhage
   (b) Migraine
   (c) Coronary artery disease
   (d) Hyperprolactinemia

27. Cross match the following

i) Valsartan	a) Bronchial asthma
ii) Verapamil	b) Hypertension
iii) Tiotropium	c) Supraventricular tachycardia
iv) Dobutamine	d) Acute congestive heart failure

28. Cross match the following

i) Prazosin	a) α_1 selective blocker
ii) Muscarinic M_2 receptors	b) Skeletal muscle
iii) Nicotine Ach receptor	c) Myocardium
iv) Isosorbide	d) Angina pectoris

29. Say **'True'** or **'False'** of the following statements
   (a) Lithium can cause renal tubular impairment and produce diabetes insipidus [ ]
   (b) Fenoldopam causes fall of blood pressure and used in hypertensive emergency because it acts through α – receptor blockade [ ]

30. Fill up the blanks
   (a) Indapamide is a________________ diuretic
   (b) Lidocaine is used to treat--------------- apart from being a local anesthetic

Answers to MCQs

1) a	2) d	3) d	4) c	5) a
6) b	7) c	8) c	9) b	10) b
11) a	12) d	13) d	14) b	15) a
16) d	17) b	18) c	19) a	20) b
21) d	22) a	23) a	24) c	25) d

26) c

27) i→b; ii→c; iii→a; iv→d

28) **i →a; ii→c; iii→b; iv→d**

29) a→True b→ False

30) a→ Loop b→ Ventricular arrhythmias

MCQs given in the Dr. MGR Medical University 2022 (Twenty in Number)

1. The insulin preparation of choice in diabetic ketoacidosis is
   (a) Lente insulin
   (b) A 30:70 mixture of plain and isophane insulin.
   (c) Isophane insulin.
   (d) Regular insulin.
2. Red man syndrome (flushing) is caused by
   (a) Vancomycin
   (b) Teicoplanin
   (c) Polymyxin
   (d) Clindamycin
3. Danazol produces all the following side effects in premenopausal women except
   (a) Hot flushes
   (b) Weight gain
   (c) Acne
   (d) Irregular menstrual periods
4. Pirenzepine is used for
   (a) Glaucoma
   (b) b. Asthma
   (c) c. Peptic ulcer
   (d) d. Motion sickness
5. Pulmonary Fibrosis is seen with
   (a) Bleomycin
   (b) Cisplatin
   (c) Methotrexate
   (d) Actinomycin D
6. Oxytocin antagonist among the following
   (a) Ritodrine
   (b) Methergine
   (c) Atosiban
   (d) Isoxsuprine
7. Which of the following is a 5 α reductase inhibitor useful in benign prostate hypertrophy and male pattern baldness
   (a) Flutamide
   (b) Prazosin
   (c) Minoxidil
   (d) Finasteride
8. The following drug is used for Hyperprolactinemia
   (a) Clonidine
   (b) Yohimbine
   (c) Bromocriptine
   (d) Haloperidol
9. Metronidazole is used for all except
   (a) Amoebiasis
   (b) Giardiasis
   (c) Trichomonas vaginalis
   (d) Malaria
10. Agent which is used in NSAID induced gastric ulcer
    (a) PGE 1 agonist
    (b) PGE 2 agonist
    (c) PGD2 Agonist
    (d) PGF2 alpha agonist
11. Most epileptogenic Carbapenem
    (a) Doripenem
    (b) Imipenem
    (c) Meropenem
    (d) Ertapenem
12. Select the drug that is active against both HIV and Hepatitis B virus
    (a) Indinavir
    (b) Efavirenz

(c) Didanosine
(d) Lamivudine

13. Thyroid storm management includes all except
(a) Propylthiouracil
(b) Surgery
(c) Steroids
(d) Lugol's iodine

14. Antipseudomonal penicillin
(a) Methicillin
(b) Ampicillin
(c) Piperacillin
(d) Penicillin G

15. Bisphosphonates are beneficial in the following condition except
(a) Paget's disease
(b) Rickets
(c) Senile osteoporosis
(d) Osteolytic bony metastasis.

16. The most frequent side effect of oral Ampicillin is
(a) Diarrhoea
(b) Nausea and vomiting
(c) Constipation
(d) Sedation

17. The following drug is a radical curative in vivax malaria
(a) Chloroquine
(b) Primaquine
(c) Quinine
(d) Mefloquine

18. Drug which prolongs QT interval is
(a) Domperidone
(b) Metoclopramide
(c) Cisapride
(d) Omeprazole

19. Lumefantrine is an
(a) Antimalarial
(b) Antifungal
(c) Antimycobacterial
(d) Antiamebic

20. Antiulcer drug which acts by inhibiting gastric acid secretion
(a) Lactulose
(b) Aluminium hydroxide
(c) Sucralfate
(d) Ranitidine

Answers to MCQs given in the Dr. MGR Medical University 2022

1) d	2) a	3) c	4) c	5) a
6) c	7) d	8) c	9) d	10) a
11) b	12) d	13) b	14) c	15) b
16) a	17) b	18) c	19) a	20) d

Section 4 - MCQs and Quizzes

1. The bioavailability of an oral preparation of a new drug is assessed in crossover study with the following observations. What would be the bioavailability of the new drug being assessed?

Route	IV	Oral
Dose	20mg	50mg
C_{max}	2mg/L	0.5ml/L
AUC	60mgh/L	30mgh/L

   (a) 80%
   (b) 60%
   (c) 20%
   (d) 10%

2. What would be the half-life of a drug when its volume of distribution is 100L, clearance 2ml/min?
   a) 31.5 hrs
   b) 60.2 hrs
   c) 56.2 hrs
   d) 27.2 hrs

3. All the following can cause potential nephrotoxicity except
   (a) Cisplatin
   (b) Gentamicin
   (c) Cyclosporine
   (d) Carbapenems

4. Apart from supportive treatment, which one of the following is more effective and appropriate to treat methanol poisoning?
   (a) IV administration of bicarbonate
   (b) IV administration of mannitol
   (c) IV administration of ethanol
   (d) Hemo dialysis

5. All the following are used as preanesthetic agents except
   (a) Skeletal muscle relaxants
   (b) Analgesics
   (c) Sedatives and antianxiety drugs
   (d) Anticholinergic drugs

6. Which one of the following fluoroquinolones is effective against methicillin- resistant, methicilin susceptible staphylococcus aureus, pseudomonas aeruginosa, anaerobic and other Gram negative infections and inhibits both topoisomerase IV and DNA hyrase
   (a) Ciprofloxacillin
   (b) Gatifloxacin
   (c) Delafloxacin
   (d) Lomefloxacillin

7. Bacterial resistance to β-lactam antibiotics can be due to all of the following except
   (a) Neutralization by the surface specific antibodies
   (b) Efflux of the antimicrobial agent
   (c) Inactivation of the antibiotic by β-lactamases
   (d) Structural modification of the penicillin binding proteins

8. Which of the following is the most effective tetracycline to treat community acquired pneumonia
   (a) Minocycline
   (b) Doxycycline
   (c) Demethylchlortetracycline
   (d) Tigecycline

9. Acyclovir or ganciclovir act by which one of the following mechanisms
   (a) Inhibition of viral DNA polymerase
   (b) Inhibition of viral reverse transcriptase
   (c) Inhibition of viral protease
   (d) Inhibition of viral DNA gyrase
10. Tetracyclines are useful in all the following clinical conditions except
   (a) Plague
   (b) Sexually transmitted diseases
   (c) UTI caused by pseudomonas
   (d) Chlamydial infections
11. Which one of the following is the prime indication of rifabutin
   (a) Prophylaxis of TB used alone or in combination with pyrazinamide
   (b) Disseminated Mycobacterium avium complex (MAC)
   (c) As a substitute to rifampin in the treatment of TB associated with HIV infection
   (d) As anti leprosy drug
12. Which one of the following is not a blood schizonticide of malarial parasite
   (a) Mefloquine
   (b) Primaquine
   (c) Halofantrine
   (d) Proguanil
13. The use of Ivermectin includes all the following except
   (a) Onchocersiasis
   (b) Lymphatic filariasis
   (c) Primary or secondary prophylaxis for treating Pneumocystis jiroveci in AIDS patients
   (d) Scabies
14. Acyclovir is not indicated in any of the following conditions except
   (a) Acute hepatitis C
   (b) Chronic hepatitis C
   (c) AIDS related Kaposi Sarcoma
   (d) Herpes simplex and varicella zoster infections, genital herpes, orolabial herpes, mucocutaneous herpes
15. Which one of the following is highly beneficial to treat cryptococcal and coccidioidal meningitis because of its high penetration into CNS
   (a) Voriconazole
   (b) Fluconazole
   (c) Itraconazole
   (d) Ketoconazole
16. Which one of the following is highly effective to treat chorioepithelioma, hydatiform mole
   (a) 5 – Fluorouracil
   (b) Azathioprine
   (c) Methotrexate
   (d) 6 – Mercaptopurine
17. Which one of the following anti malignancy drugs causes cardiotoxicity
   (a) Mitomycin C
   (b) L – Asparaginase
   (c) Procarbazine
   (d) Daunorubicin (Adriamycin)
18. Which one of the following mechanisms is responsible for the pharmacological action of taxanes (Paclitaxel, docetaxel)
   (a) Promote microtubule polymerization, inhibit depolymerization and stabilization of microtubules
   (b) Inhibition of enzyme dihydrofolate reductase
   (c) Inhibition of purine synthesis
   (d) Inhibition of topoisomerase – 1 (TOP 1)
19. Which one of the following is an important indication for the combination of a penicillin and an aminoglycoside
   (a) Urinary tract infections
   (b) Typhoid fever
   (c) Meningococcal meningitis
   (d) Enterococcal endocarditic

20. As a patient being treated for gouty arthritis, which one of the following is more likely to cause hyperurecemia and limiting the use of anti gout drugs?
    (a) Pyrazinamide
    (b) INH
    (c) Ethambutol
    (d) Rifampicin
21. Meningococcal carrier state is eradicated by which one of the following
    (a) Azithromycin
    (b) Sparfloxacin
    (c) Minocycline
    (d) d)Amoxicillin
22. Which one of the following statement is not correct?
    (a) IV infusion of regular insulin is useful in the treatment of diabetic ketoacidosis
    (b) Lente insulin is a mixture of insulin, zinc and protamine
    (c) Insulin lispro and aspart are rapid-acting insulins
    (d) Glargine insulin is the longest acting insulin and give once daily
23. Danazol is indicated for which one of the following clinical conditions?
    (a) Contraception
    (b) Endometriosis and menorrhagia
    (c) Dysfunctional uterine bleeding
    (d) Prostatitic malignancy
24. Which one of the following antiplatelet drugs acts on platelet P_2 Y_{12} receptor and used in delayed PCI procedure after MI?
    (a) Prasugrel
    (b) Abciximab
    (c) Aspirin
    (d) Eptifibatide
25. N – acetylcysteine is indicated in all the following conditions except
    (a) Paracetamol toxicity
    (b) Contrast agent- associated nephrotoxicity
    (c) As a mucolytic agent
    (d) As antitussive drug
26. Interferon α-2b indications include all the following except
    (a) Chronic hepatitis B
    (b) Hairy cell leukemia
    (c) Prostatic malignancy
    (d) AIDS related Kaposi Sarcoma
27. Cross match the following

1) Heparin	a) Iron toxicity
2) Vitamin K	b) Diabetes mellitus
3) Desferrioxamine	c) Binding to antithrombin
4) Rosiglitazone	d) Antidote to oral anticoagulants

28. Cross match the following

1) Erythropoietin	a) A selective estrogen receptor modulator
2) Raloxifene	b) Chronic renal failure
3) Ipratropium	c) Gastric acid secretion
4) Misoprostol	d) Chronic bronchial asthma

29. Fill up the blanks
    (a) Esomeprazole decrease gastric acid secretion by ______________________
    (b) Exenatide acts as ______________ to increase insulin secretion.
30. Mention the following statements as 'True' or 'False'
    (a) In pregnancy – associated hypothyroidism, serum thyroxine binding globulin levels are increased resulting in a decrease of serum FT3 and FT4 levels decreased.(   )
    (b) Glucocorticoids cause hypoglycemia and increase insulin sensitivity. (   )

Answers to MCQs

1) Reasoning: Oral bioavailability (absolute bioavailability) of a drug is expressed by the formula)

$$100\times\left(\frac{\text{AUC P}_o}{\text{AUC IV}}\right)\times\left(\frac{\text{Dose IV}}{\text{Dose P}_o}\right)$$

AUC: Area Under The Concentration-Time Curve in the question all the readings are given and applying the formula, we get

Ans) $100\times\left(\frac{30}{60}\right)\times\left(\frac{20}{50}\right)=20\%$

Hence the oral bioavailability of a drug is only 20% in comparison to its IV bioavailability of 100%

2) Reasoning: The half-life ($t_{1/2}$) of a drug can be calculated as follows

$$t_{1/2}=0.693\times\frac{vd}{CL}$$

Here Vd = 100L; clearance (total clearance) is 2 ml/min,

Ans) $t_{1/2}=0.693\times\frac{100}{2}=31.50$ hours

3) d	4) c	5) a	6) c	7) a
8) d	9) a	10) c	11) b	12) b
13) c	14) d	15) b	16) c	17) d
18) a	19) d	20) a	21) c	22) b)
23) b	24) a	25) d	26) c	

27) i-→c; ii→d; iii→a; iv→b

28) i→b;ii→a; iii→d; iv→c

29) 1. Inhibiting proton pump (H^+/K^+/ATPase) 2. GLP-I agonist

30) 1→ True 2→False

Section 5 - MCQs and Quizzes

1. The primary mechanism of action of heparin as anticoagulant is
   (a) Inhibition of factor Xa
   (b) Activation Of antithrombin III
   (c) Inactivation of factor VII, X, II
   (d) Direct inhibition of thrombin
2. The ultra duration of action of thiopental is due to
   (a) Rapid redistribution
   (b) Rapid metabolism in the liver
   (c) Extensive protein binding with little bioavailability
   (d) Rapid renal elimination
3. Desmopressin is indicated in all the following conditions except
   (a) Central diabetes insipidus
   (b) Nephrogenic diabetes insipidus
   (c) Esophageal varices
   (d) Nocturnal enuresis
4. The initial excitatory responses of ethyl alcohol are due to
   (a) Decrease of function of inhibitory centres in the brain (inhibition of inhibitory functions)
   (b) Activation of excitatory glutamate receptors (NMDA receptors)
   (c) Inhibition of GABA receptor mediated action
   (d) Conversion to an excitatory metabolite
5. Allopurinol is effective in gouty arthritis because of
   (a) Inhibition of renal tubular reabsorption of uric acid
   (b) Enhancement of renal uric acid elimination
   (c) Inhibition of biosynthesis of uric acid
   (d) Inhibition of Phagocytosis and inflammatory mediators
6. The predominant anti- inflammatory and immunosuppressant effects of glucocorticoids include all except
   (a) Inhibition of chemo active substances like bradykinin
   (b) Inhibition of synthesis of cytokines and Pro-inflammatory cellular actions
   (c) Inhibition of synthesis of arachidonic acid derivatives
   (d) Inhibition of synthesis of TNFα
7. Which one of the following describes the first- pass effect (metabolism at a specific site before the drug reaches the target site)?
   (a) Drug inactivation leading to poor oral bioavailability
   (b) b)Slow Absorption of the drug through the duodenum
   (c) Drug given orally is metabolised by the liver and at other sites before entering the circulation
   (d) Rapid transit of the drug from the intestines before it is adequately absorbed
8. When a drug is injected IV and found to be highly bound to plasma proteins, which one of the following is more likely to be increased as a result of
   (a) Distribution of the drug to tissue sites
   (b) Drug interaction
   (c) Renal elimination
   (d) Hepatic metabolism
9. Lidocaine is the most effective agent in which one of the following conditions
   (a) Atrial fibrillation
   (b) Supra ventricular tachycardia

(c) Rapid control of ventricular arrhythmias due to MI
(d) Tachyarrhythmias due to anxiety

10. Carbonic Anhydrase inhibitors are indicated in all of the following clinical conditions except
    (a) Glaucoma
    (b) Urinary alkalinization
    (c) Epilepsy
    (d) Pulmonary edema

11. Midazolam is indicated in all the following conditions except
    (a) Preoperative medication
    (b) Induction of anesthesia
    (c) Maintenance of anesthesia as a supplement to opioids or inhaled general anesthetics
    (d) To facilitate postoperative analgesic effect

12. Pramoxine, a surface local anesthetic is used in which one of the following conditions
    (a) To relieve pain due to burns or pruritus due to dermatosis when applied to the skin
    (b) To facilitate sigmoidoscopy examination
    (c) To anesthetise the upper airway before direct laryngoscopy
    d) To anesthetise nasal and tracheal mucosa

13. The most effective drugs to treat positive symptoms of schizophrenia are
    (a) Atypical or 2nd generation antipsychotic drugs
    (b) Selective 5-HT uptake inhibitors
    (c) Tricyclic antidepressants
    (d) MAO inhibitors

14. A 34-year old man is prescribed Bisoprolol for hypertension. The effect on the cardiovascular system is a result of its action as an antagonist at which one of the following sites
    (a) α-Adrenoceptor
    (b) β_1- Adrenoceptor
    (c) D_1 receptors
    (d) Both α and β - Adrenoceptor

15. Which one of the following is the least likely clinical use of β- Adrenoceptor blockers?
    (a) Peripheral artery disease
    (b) Hypertension
    (c) Cardiac arrhythmias
    (d) Ischemic heart disease

16. A 55-year old man with congestive heart failure is noted to be taking furosemide each day. Which one of the following is most likely to be found in the serum?
    (a) Decreased potassium levels
    (b) Decreased uric acid levels
    (c) Elevated magnesium levels
    (d) Low bicarbonate level

17. Which one of the following is the most effective agent for converting paroxysmal atrial tachycardia to normal sinus rhythm?
    (a) Adenosine
    (b) Digoxin
    (c) Lidocaine
    (d) Phenytoin

18. Sacubitril/Valsartan is the drug of choice in which of the following clinical condition
    (a) Congestive heart failure
    (b) Cardiac arrhythmias
    (c) Ischemic heart disease
    (d) Pulmonary edema

19. Melatonin and the Ramelteon are the drugs used for
    (a) Sleep disorders/ Insomnia
    (b) Gonadotropin dysfunction
    (c) Preanesthetic medication
    (d) Menopausal syndrome

20. Which one of the following general anesthetics is contraindicated in patients with seizure disorders as evidenced by occurrence of jerks during the period of anesthesia ?
    (a) Enflurane
    (b) Desflurane
    (c) Isoflurane
    (d) Sevoflurane

21. What is Tizanidine?
    (a) An α_2 agonist used as centrally acting skeletal muscle relaxant
    (b) A local anesthetic
    (c) A halogenated general anesthetic
    (d) A curare derivative
22. Apomorphine is mainly used for
    (a) Regular treatment drug for parkinsonism
    (b) For temporary relief of 'off symptoms of akinesia in patients on dopaminergic therapy
    (c) Prolactin-dependant menstrual cycle disorders
    (d) Initial therapy for mild form of parkinsonism
23. Which one of the following is used to distinguish cholinergic and myasthenic crisis?
    (a) Azathioprine
    (b) Physostigmine
    (c) Edrophonium
    (d) Prednisolone
24. PCSK9(proprotein convertase subtilisin/ kexin type9) inhibitor Evalocumab a cholesterol lowering agent, acts by which one of the following mechanisms?
    (a) Inhibition of absorption of cholesterol in the small intestine
    (b) Inhibition of synthesis of cholesterol
    (c) By bile acid sequestering
    (d) Facilitating recycling of LDL-receptor in the hepatocytes allowing rapid removal of cholesterol from circulation
25. Phenytoin and local anesthetics have which one of the following common property
    (a) Blockade of K^+ channels
    (b) Blockade of Na^+ channels
    (c) Blockade of 'T' type of Ca^+ channels
    (d) Blockade of Cl^2 channels
26. Albendazole and Mebendazole are used in all the following conditions except
    (a) Ascariasis, hook worm, Enterobious infections
    (b) Hydatid cyst
    (c) Visceral larva migrance
    (d) Amoebiasis
27. Match the following

i. Anticholinergic drugs	a) Dopaminergic neurons
ii. Perioperative analgesia	b) Preanesthetic medication
iii.Methotrexate	c) Rheumatoid arthritis
iv.Substantia nigra	d) Fentanyl

28. Match the following

i. Voriconazole	a) IV general anesthetic
ii Propofol	b) Aspergills infections
iii. dopamine	c) Congestive heart failure
iv. Benzhexitol	d) Drug induced parkinsonism

29. Fill up the blanks
    (a) The major adverse effect of antipsychotic drug is ____________
    (b) Nalbufine is the antagonist of ____________
30. Say True or False
    (a) Allopurinol is a uricosuric drug( )
    (b) Suvorexan is an orexin receptor antagonist used in insomnia( )

Answer to MCQs

1) b	2) a	3) b	4) a	5) c
6) a	7) c	8) b	9) c	10) d
11) d	12) a	13) a	14) b	15) a
16) a	17) a	18) a	19) a	20) a
21) a	22) b	23) c	24) d	25) b

26) d

27) i→b; ii→d; iii→c; iv→a

28) i→b; ii→a; iii→c; iv→d

29) a→ Parkinsonism/Extrapyramidal effects b→ morphine

30) a-False, b-True

MCQs of the Tamilnadu Dr. MGR University March 2022 (New MCI guidelines)

1. Essential drugs are
   (a) Life saving drugs
   (b) Drugs that meet the priority health care needs of the population
   (c) Drugs that are used in medical emergencies
   (d) Drugs that are listed in the pharmacopoeia of a country
2. The loading dose of the drug is governed by its
   (a) Renal clearance
   (b) Plasma half-life
   (c) Volume of distribution
   (d) Elimination rate constant
3. Pseudocholinesterase differs from true cholinesterase in that
   (a) It hydrolyses acetylcholine at slower rate
   (b) It is more susceptible to inhibition by physostigmine
   (c) It doesn't hydrolyse acetylcholine
   (d) It is the only form of circulating cholinesterase
4. Bromhexine acts by
   (a) Inhibiting cough centre
   (b) Depolymerizing mucopolysaccharides present in sputum
   (c) Irritating gastric mucosa and reflexly increasing bronchial secretion
   (d) Desensitizing stretch receptors in lung
5. The following general anesthetic has poor muscle relaxation
   (a) Ether
   (b) Halothane
   (c) Nitrous oxide
   (d) Sevoflurane
6. The antiepileptic drug that is effective in manic depressive illness also is
   (a) Phenobarbitone
   (b) Ethosuximide
   (c) Phenytoin
   (d) Carbamazepine
7. The major limitation to the use of clozapine for treatment of schizophrenia is
   (a) Its inability to benefit negative symptoms of schizophrenia
   (b) Its potential to cause agranulocytosis
   (c) It produces hyperprolactinemia
   (d) High incidence of extra pyramidal symptoms
8. Select the most suitable antiarrhythmic drug for ventricular arrhythmia due to digoxin toxicity
   (a) Lidocaine
   (b) Propranolol
   (c) Verapamil
   (d) Quinidine
9. Glyceryl trinitrate is administered by following routes except
   (a) Intravenous
   (b) Intramuscular
   (c) Oral
   (d) Sublingual

10. Reversible loss of taste sensation can be a side effect of the following anti-hypertensive drug
    (a) Prazosin
    (b) Verapamil
    (c) Propranolol
    (d) Captopril
11. The following drug is a poor inhibitor of prostaglandin synthesis in peripheral tissues but more active in brain
    (a) Mefenamic acid
    (b) Ketorolac
    (c) Paracetamol
    (d) Nimesulide
12. Prolonged lithium therapy can cause
    (a) Parkinsonism
    (b) Goiter
    (c) Diabetes mellitus
    (d) Gout
13. Which of the following drug is a potassium channel opener?
    (a) Nicorandil
    (b) Hydralazine
    (c) Amiloride
    (d) Glibenclamide
14. Indication of desmopressin include the following except
    (a) Nephrogenic diabetes insipidus
    (b) Neurogenic diabetes insipidus
    (c) Bleeding due to hemophilia
    (d) Bedwetting in children
15. The following is not a valid indication for parenteral iron therapy
    (a) Inadequate response to oral iron due to patient non compliance
    (b) Anemia during pregnancy
    (c) Anemia in a patient with active rheumatoid arthritis
    (d) Severe anemia associated with chronic bleeding
16. The primary mechanism by which heparin inhibits coagulation of blood is
    (a) Inhibition of factor XII a and XIII a
    (b) Activation of antithrombin III with inhibition of factors IX and XI
    (c) Inhibition of factor Xa and thrombin mediated conversion of fibrinogen to fibrin
    (d) Direct inhibition of prothrombin to thrombin conversion
17. Select the fibrinolytic drug that is antigenic
    (a) Streptokinase
    (b) Urokinase
    (c) Alteplase
    (d) All
18. Which of the following hypolipidemic drug is most effective in increasing HDL cholesterol level and lowering serum triglyceride?
    (a) Cholestyramine
    (b) Fenofibrate
    (c) Pravastatin
    (d) Nicotinic acid
19. Tranexamic acid is used in following condition
    (a) Organophosphorus compound poisoning
    (b) Barbiturate poisoning
    (c) Excessive bleeding due to fibrinolytic drugs
    (d) Bleeding due to heparin overdose
20. The following drug is neither analgesic nor anti-inflammatory and do not have uricosuric effect, but highly efficacious in acute gout
    (a) Naproxen
    (b) Colchicine
    (c) Prednisolone
    (d) Sulfinpyrazone

Answers to MCQs given by Dr. MGR Medical University

1) c	2) c	3) a	4) b	5) c
6) d	7) b	8) a	9) b	10) d
11) c	12) b	13) a	14) a	15) b
16) b	17) d	18) d	19) c	20) b

Section 6 - MCQs and Quizzes

1. Genetic differences in enzyme activity can modify the responses of all the following drugs except
   (a) INH
   (b) Procainamide
   (c) Hydralazine
   (d) Penicillin
2. The actions of which one of the following drugs is not affected in the presence of preexisting liver disease
   (a) Acetaminophen
   (b) Warfarin
   (c) Pyrazinamide
   (d) Betalactam antibiotics
3. All the following drugs produce peripheral neuritis except
   (a) INH
   (b) Disulfiram
   (c) Alcohol
   (d) Cisplatin
4. Dimercaprol is effective in all the following poisoning cases except
   (a) Lead
   (b) Arsenic
   (c) Mercury
   (d) Iron
5. Except one, all the following are true that drug disposition varies greatly in pregnancy due to
   (a) Reduced gastrointestinal mobility leading to delayed absorption
   (b) An increase in extracellular fluid volume with an increase of volume of distribution
   (c) Fall in plasma albumin levels and an increase of the acid glycoprotein with lesser protein binding.
   (d) Microsomal enzyme system is inactivated with resultant slow metabolism
6. The sympathomimetic actions of cocaine and tricycle antidepressants are due
   (a) Post ganglionic sympathetic nerve stimulation
   (b) Inhibition of metabolism of adrenaline and nor-adrenaline
   (c) Blockade of reuptake of nor-adrenaline form nerve endings
   (d) displacement of nor-adrenaline from storage sites
7. Allopurinol acts by inhibiting
   (a) HMG – CoA reductase
   (b) MAO-B
   (c) Xanthine oxidase
   (d) Carbonic anhydrase
8. Which one of the following cholinergic drugs can resist the action of cholinesterase enzyme?
   (a) Carbachol
   (b) Acetylcholine
   (c) Methacholine
   (d) Muscarine
9. Aqueous passive diffusion of drugs requires all the following parameters except
   (a) Requires energy
   (b) Requires the presence of concentration gradient
   (c) High Lipid to aqueous partition coefficient
   (d) Drug molecules less than 150-200MW
10. One of the following is used for arresting the preterm labor/premature labor
   (a) Clonidine
   (b) Ritodrine

(c) Pindolol
(d) Dobutamine

11. All the effects of α_2 receptor agonist activity are true except
(a) Inhibition of norepinephrine release
(b) Decrease of aqueous humor synthesis
(c) Increase of myocardial contractility
(d) Mediation of platelet aggregation

12. Which one of the following effects is not caused by sympathomimetic drugs?
(a) Oxytocic effect
(b) Positive chronotropic effect
(c) Positive inotropic effect
(d) Positive dromotropic effect

13. All the following drugs can be used in hypertensive emergency except
(a) Clevidipine
(b) Labetolol
(c) Hydralazine
(d) Valsartan

14. Which one of the following is not a cardioselective Beta blocker?
(a) Carvedilol
(b) Bisoprolol
(c) Esmolol
(d) Metoprolol

15. Prazocin, terazocin, doxazocin belong to a class of
(a) β– receptor agonists
(b) Selective α_1 – receptor blockers
(c) Non – selective α_1 – receptor blockers
(d) Ganglion blockers

16. All of the following are used for overactive bladder except
(a) Oxybutynin
(b) Tropsium
(c) Tolterodine
(d) Clidinium

17. All the following drugs are used to treat travel sickness except
(a) Scopolamine
(b) Dimenhydrinate
(c) Doxepin
(d) Diphenhydramine

18. Which one of the following anticholinergic drug is used in acute MI associated with vagal discharge and decreased SA or AV nodal conduction?
(a) Cyclopentolate
(b) Homatropine
(c) Atropine
(d) Ipratrropium

19. All are true of M_2 receptor activation on CVS except
(a) Bradycardia
(b) Decreased AV nodal conduction
(c) Decreased force of contraction
(d) Tachycardia

20. Apraclonidine is a drug used to treat
(a) Glaucoma
(b) .Hypertension
(c) Congestive heart failure
(d) Ischemic heart disease

21. Methadone is the drug of choice for
(a) Morphine abstinence syndrome
(b) Alcohol withdrawal syndrome
(c) LSD withdrawal syndrome
(d) Barbiturate habituation

Fill up the Blanks

22. Non-depolarizing muscle relaxants block receptors-------at the neuromuscular junction.
23. Neostigmine, Pyridostigmine and Revastigmine are mainly used in _________.
24. _________________is the action of muscarinic drugs on bronchial tree.
25. Monoamine oxidase and catechol – o – methyltransferase are the enzymes responsible for _______________.
26. Diltazem and verapamil are the drugs mainly used for ________________________.
27. Dissociative anesthesia characterized by catatonia, amnesia and analgesia is produced by____________________.

28. Doxazocin, Alfuzocine, Tomsulosin are the drugs used for ___________________.

29. Cross match the following

a)Yohimbine	1. Antispasmodic action
b)Timolol	2. α_2 antagonist
c)Ipratropium	3. Glaucoma
d clidinium	4. Bronchial asthma

30. Cross match the following

(a) Ramipril + thiazide	1. Slow inactivation and more prolonged muscle relaxation
(b) Body surface area in m^2 / 1.7 × adult dose	2. Hypertension
(c) Atypical pseudocholi-nesterase	3. Dose calculation in children
(d) Phosphodiesterase	4. Cyclic AMP

31. Cross match the following

(a) Eplerenone	1. Bronchial asthma
(b) Flurazepam	2. Aldosterone antagonist
(c) Tiotropium	3. Travel sickness
(d) Diphenhydramine	4. Sedation

Answers to MCQs

1) d	2) d	3) b	4) d	5) d
6) c	7) c	8) a	9) a	10) b
11) c	12) a	13) d	14) a	15) b
16) d	17) c	18) c	19) d	20) a

21) a 22) Nicotinic acetylcholine

23) Myasthenia gravis

24) Bronchoconstriction

25) Metabolic degradation of catecholamines

26) Atrial fibrillation to reduce the ventricular rate

27) Ketamine

28) Benign prostatic hyperplasia

29) (a-2) (b-3) (c-4) (d-1)

30) (a-2) (b-3) (c-1) (d-4)

31) (a-2) (b-4) (c-1) (d-3)

Section 7 - MCQs and Quizzes

1. The feature of zero – order kinetics is
    (a) The rate of elimination is directly proportional to the drug concentration
    (b) The drug undergoes initial metabolism in the intestines and liver
    (c) A constant amount of drug is eliminated in unit time
    (d) The drug undergoes extensive metabolism with small fraction of bioavailability.
2. Efficacy of a drug means
    (a) The intrinsic activity of a drug that can produce maximal response
    (b) The activity or response a drug produces per unit weight
    (c) Ability to counter the effects of an antagonist at the same receptor site
    (d) Can produce the responses in spite of extensive metabolism
3. Termination of action of adrenergic drugs is mediated by all the following mechanisms except
    (a) Reuptake by active transport (uptake 1) from the synaptic cleft
    (b) Metabolism by monoamine oxidase (MAO) located in mitochondria
    (c) Metabolism by catechol – o – methyl transferase (COMT)
    (d) Prevention of release from the adrenergic nerve endings
4. Reserpine acts by which one of the following mechanisms
    (a) preventing the uptake and storage of catecholamines in the granules
    (b) Blocking metabolic degradation
    (c) Blocking adrenergic neuronal transmission and preventing release of noradrenaline
    (d) Blocking the ganglionic transmission
5. The main action of adrenergic β_1 receptor is
    (a) Contraction of the smooth muscle
    (b) Lipolysis
    (c) Increase in heart rate, contractility, and conduction
    (d) Relaxation of the smooth muscles.
6. The relaxation of bronchial smooth muscle is mediated by
    (a) β-2 receptors
    (b) $H_{.1}$ receptors
    (c) β -1 receptors
    (d) α_{-2} receptors
7. All of the following are true of side effects of non-selective β-blockers except
    (a) CNS stimulation
    (b) Increased airway resistance
    (c) possibility of hypoglycemia when used with antidiabetic drugs
    (d) Bradycardia and cardiac depression
8. One of the following is used in bipolar affective disorder that also can cause renal tubular impairment that leads to diabetes insipidus
    (a) Clozapine
    (b) Risperidone
    (c) Lithium
    (d) Escitalopram
9. Bethanechol is used in all the following conditions except
    (a) Glaucoma
    (b) Urinary retention in the absence of obstruction

(c) Postoperative ileus
(d) Gastric atony and retention after vagotomy

10. Which one of the cholinesterase inhibitors crosses the blood brain barrier and used in atropine poisoning?
(a) Neostigmine
(b) Pyridostigmine
(c) Physostigmine
(d) Edrophonium

11. Which one of the following can be reactivated by oximes?
(a) Rivastigmine
(b) Ecothiophate
(c) Donepezil
(d) Neostigmine

12. Which one of the following is used to diagnose a case of myasthenia gravis?
(a) Pyridostigmine
(b) Neostigmine
(c) Edrophonium
(d) Donepezil

13. Timolol, Betaxolol, Levobunalol, Metipranolol all have one common use
(a) Cardiac arrythmias
(b) Hypertension
(c) Sinus tachycardia
(d) glaucoma

14. Which one of the following β – blockers is used to treat supraventricular arrhythmias when given IV
(a) Nebiolol
(b) Carvedilol
(c) Esmolol
(d) Labetalol

15. Which one of the following is a selective α1 blocker used in the treatment of benign prostatic hyperplasia and hypertension?
(a) Phentolamine
(b) Bunazocin
(c) Tolazolin
(d) Phenoxybenzamine

16. All the following can be used for attention deficit hyperactivity disorder except
(a) Methamphetamine
(b) Automoxetin
(c) Ephedrine
(d) Methylphenidate

17. Which one of the following α_2- receptor agonist can be used in ICUs to provide prolonged sedation, procedural sedation, and general anesthesia during diagnostic investigations?
(a) Dexmeditomidine
(b) Clonidine
(c) Guanfascine
(d) Guanabenz

18. The synergistic action of levodopa and carbidopa is by virtue of
(a) Inhibition of peripheral decarboxylase metabolism of levodopa
(b) Facilitating the central metabolism of levodopa to dopamine
(c) Lesser plasma binding and easy entry to dopaminergic areas
(d) Preventing further conversion of dopamine to nor-adrenaline

19. Which one of the following route of administration is used for diagnostic contrast media for angiography, myelography, CT scan?
(a) Intravenous route
(b) Intraarterial route
(c) Subcutaneous route
(d) Intrathecal route

20. Which one of the following statements is not correct?
(a) A sublingual drug undergoes extensive first pass metabolism
(b) Propranolol undergoes first – pass metabolism
(c) E_{max} signifies the efficacy of the drug
(d) Nadolol has the highest half – life among β – blockers

21. All the following are potential cardiotoxic drugs except
    (a) Emetine
    (b) Methotrexate
    (c) Doxorubicin
    (d) Astemazole

22. Cross match the following

1) Esterification of drugs	a) Ethinyl estradiol
2) Poor absorption of fat – soluble vitamins	b) Pre-systemic drug metabolizing enzyme
3) Cytochrome P450 3A, 3A4	c) Medroxy-progesterone
4) Enterohepatic Circulation	d) Liquid Paraffin

23. Cross match the following

1) Pilocarpine	a) Bronchial asthma
2) Glycopyrrolate	b) Nasal decongestant
3) Xylometazoline	c) Reduction of gastric secretions and prevent regurgetation
4) Ipratropium	d) Glaucoma

24. Cross match the following

1) Ritodrine	a) Congestive heart failure
2) Prazocin	b) Uterine relaxant
3) Dihydro-ergotamine	c) Acute attack of migraine
4) Dobutamine	d) Hypertension

25. Cross match the following

1) Fenoldopam	a) Testosterone
2) Botulinum Toxin	b) Blepharospasm
3) Muscarinic M2 receptor	c) Myocardium
4) Transdermal Patch	d) Hypertensive emergency

26. Cross match the following

1) Benztropine	a) vasopressor and rise of BP
2) Atenolol	b) Drug induced parkinsonism
3) Isoprenaline	c) Stokes – Adams syndrome
4) Mephen-teramine	d) Hypertension

27. Fill up the blanks
    (a) The neurotransmitter released in substantia nigra, globus pallidus, putamen and caudate nucleuses__________________.
    (b) Myopathy is an important adverse effect of__________________.

28. Fill up the blanks
    (a) The process of transport or passage of a drug through the cell membrane against a concentration gradient and is energy dependent is known as____________.
    (b) Anticholinesterases cause miosis due to ________________.

29. Fill up the blanks
    (a) The antipsychotic drug (bipolar depression) that requires regular therapeutic monitoring is ________________.
    (b) The principal parasympathetic nerve supply to the heart is mediated through________________.

30. Say **<u>Yes</u>** or **<u>No</u>** to the following statements
    (a) Apraclonidine is the drug used to treat hypertension [ ]
    (b) Retinoic acid, Vitamin D and steroids act through nuclear receptors [ ]

31. Say **<u>Yes</u>** or **<u>No</u>** to the following statements
    (a) The dose of a drug in dose – response curve is represented on abscissa (x-axis) [ ]
    (b) Noradrenaline convention to adrenaline is mediated by dopamine – β – hydroxy lase [ ]

Answers to MCQs

1) c	2) a	3) d	4) a	5) c
6) a	7) a	8) c	9) a	10) b
11) b	12) c	13) d	14) c	15) b
16) c	17) a	18) a	19) b	20) a 21) b

22) 1→ c; 2→d; 3→b;4→a

23) 1→ d; 2→c; 3→b;4→a

24) 1→ b; 2→d; 3→c;4→a

25) 1→ d; 2→b; 3→c;4→a

26) 1-b; 2d: 3c; 4a

27) a) Dopamine b) Statins/Steroids

28) a) Active transport b) Contraction of Constrictor pupillae

29) a) Lithium b) Vagus nerve

30) a) No b) Yes

31) a) Yes b) No

Section 8 - MCQs and Quizzes

1. Probenecid is effective in treating gout because it decreases which one of the following?
   (a) Inflammation in affected joints
   (b) Production of uric acid
   (c) Reabsorption of uric acid
   (d) Secretion of uric acid
2. Which of the following describes the action of allopurinol
   (a) Inhibits metabolism of purines to uric acid and lower uric acid levels
   (b) Inhibits prostaglandin synthesis
   (c) Inhibits uric acid reabsorption
   (d) Interferes with cytokine production
3. Telmisartan acts to decrease which one of the following
   (a) AT-1 receptor activity
   (b) Bradykinin production
   (c) Production of angiotensin II
   (d) Renin production
4. Which one of the following is a limiting adverse effect of ACE Inhibitors?
   (a) Acidosis
   (b) Hyperkalemia
   (c) Hypernatremia
   (d) Hypokalemia
5. Digoxin increases cardiac contractility by directly engaging with which one of the following?
   (a) Increasing membrane stabilization
   (b) Activating L-Type Ca^{+}channels
   (c) Inhibiting myocardial Na^{+}/Ca^{+} – ATP ase (sodium pump) and preventing Ca^{2+}efflux
   (d) Inhibiting cardiac Phosphodiesterase
6. Which one of the following drugs may be used to increase cardiac output in a patient with pulmonary edema on a short term basis secondary to MI
   (a) Metoprolol
   (b) Verapamil
   (c) Dobutamine
   (d) Captopril
7. Which one of the following is the most accurate statement regarding digoxin?
   (a) Decreased mortality in patients with congestive heart failure with normal sinus rhythm
   (b) Increase vagal tone and decreases AV nodal conduction
   (c) Lengthens the action potentials and increase the refractoriness of the heart
   (d) Useful in the treatment of Wolff-Parkinson-white syndrome
8. Which one of the following drug is used most commonly to treat ventricular tachycardia after MI
   (a) Sotalol
   (b) Metoprolol
   (c) Lidocaine
   (d) Digoxin
9. Which one of the following anti arrhythmic drug has long half-life and has cumulative effects in the lung, cornea and skin and responsible for its adverse effects
   (a) Procainamide
   (b) Sotalol
   (c) Amiodarone
   (d) Lidocaine

10. Which one of the following causes orthostatic hypotension in the initiation of therapy and later diminishes
    (a) Prazosin
    (b) Atenolol
    (c) Captopril
    (d) Telmisartan
11. The inclusion of spiranolactone with a thiazide in a regimen to treat hypertension is done to achieve which one of the following?
    (a) Reduce hyperuricemia
    (b) Reduce Mg^+ loss
    (c) Decrease the loss of Na^+
    (d) Reduce K^+ loss
12. Which one of the following drugs would be the best to treat moderate hypertension in a diabetic patient with mild proteinuria?
    (a) Ramipril
    (b) Propranolol
    (c) Hydrochlorothiazide
    (d) Nifedipine
13. A 35-year-old man is diagnosed with essential hypertension. He is started on a blood pressure control medication and after 4 weeks of treatment he reports with dry unproductive cough, angioedema and hyperkalemia. Which one of the following is the most likely agent used
    (a) Captopril
    (b) Nebivolol
    (c) Amlodipine
    (d) Atenolol
14. Lovastatin reduces the plasma cholesterol by which one of the following processes
    (a) HMG-COA reduction and inhibition of cholesterol biosynthesis
    (b) Inhibition of $APOB_{100}$ biosynthesis
    (c) Interfering with bile acid reabsorption
    (d) Inhibiting cholesterol absorption
15. Which one of the following is the usual and predominant effect of niacin?
    (a) Decrease of LDL
    (b) Increase of HDL
    (c) Decrease of triglycerides
    (d) Decrease of total cholesterol
16. Myalgia, rhabdomyolysis, mild altered liver function tests are seen with which one of the following drugs used to treat hyperlipidemia over a period and in higher doses
    (a) Fenofibrate
    (b) Simvastatin
    (c) Ezetimibe
    (d) Evalocumab
17. The therapeutic effect of haloperidol, at least in part, is by its blockade of which one of the following receptors
    (a) α-adrenoceptors
    (b) Dopamine D_2 receptors
    (c) 5-HT_2 recepttors
    (d) Control muscarinic receptors
18. Mechanism of action of fluoxetine is by virtue of
    (a) Preventing reuptake of 5-HT by the post junctional nerve terminal by inhibiting serotonin transporter
    (b) Inhibition of MAO_B
    (c) Activation of noradrenaline reuptake
    (d) Facilitation of NMDA receptor
19. The antidepressant effect and use in nicotine dependence is brought about by which one of the following antidepressants
    (a) Desipramine
    (b) Trazadone
    (c) Buproprion
    (d) Amitryptiline
20. Carbidopa reduces which one of the following
    (a) The activity of dopa-decarboxylase in CNS
    (b) The L-dopa dose necessary to achieve the therapeutic effect
    (c) The severity associated with dyskinesia
    (d) The time to onset a L-dopa's therapeutic effect
21. Which one of the following is the most common limiting adverse effect of L-dopa
    (a) Depression
    (b) Dyskinesia
    (c) Sedation
    (d) Orthostatic hypotension

22. Blockade of T-type calcium channels is the major mechanism of action for which one of the following drugs used to manage seizures
    (a) Ethosuximide
    (b) Phenytoin
    (c) Carbamazepine
    (d) Diazepam

23. Nystagmus, ataxia, confusion, hirsutism and gingival hyperplasia are usually seen with which one of the following antiseizure drugs?
    (a) Carbamazepine
    (b) Ethosuximide
    (c) Phenytoin
    (d) Valproic acid

24. The relief of pain by morphine is brought about by all the mechanisms except
    (a) Inhibition of excitatory transmitters acting on receptors on the terminals of primary afferent sensory neurons in the spinal cord
    (b) Inhibition of pain transmission in the ascending path ways from the spinal cord to higher centres in the CNS
    (c) Activation of descending inhibitory neurons to the spinal cord
    (d) Inhibition of release of inflammatory mediators in the CNS

25. Minimal development of tolerance to the continued use of morphine occurs with which one of the following effects
    (a) Miosis and constipation
    (b) Euphoria
    (c) Nausea and vomiting
    (d) Sedation

26. By which one of the following receptors benzodiazepines bind to produce the pharmacological effects
    (a) 5-HT_1 receptors
    (b) $GABA_A$ receptors
    (c) D2 receptors antagonizing their effects
    (d) α-adrenoceptors antagonizing their effects

27. Cross match the following

1) Clonazepam	a) Edema associated with congestive heart failure
2) Indapamide	b) Inflantite spasms
3) cotrimoxazole	c) Infection by pneumocystis joroveci
4) Valsartan	d) Hypertension

28. Cross match the following

1) Olanzapine	a) Prolactin-dependant menstrual cycle disorders like amenorrhea, oligomenorrhea
2) Escitalopram	b) Antidepressant
3) Entacapone	c) COMT inhibitor
4) Bromocriptine	d) Schizophrenia

29. Say '**Yes**' or '**No**' to the following statements
    (a) Buspirone is a selective anxiolytic drug without sedative and euphoritic effects-------
    (b) Loop diuretics act at proximal convoluted tubule ---------

30. Say '**Yes**' or '**No**' to the following statements
    (a) Quinidine acts as antiarrhythmic drug by blocking K^+ channels in the heart --------
    (b) Botulinum toxin is used to treat blepharospasm and strabismus-------

Answers to MCQs

1) c	2) a	3) a	4) b	5) c
6) c	7) b	8) c	9) c	10) a
11) d	12) c	13) a	14) a	15) b

16) b	17) b	18) a	19) c	20) b
21) b	22) a	23) c	24) d	25) a

26) b

27) i-b, ii-a, iii-c, iv-d

28) i-d, ii-b, iii-c, iv-a

29) i- Yes, ii-No

30) i- No, ii-Yes

Section 9 - MCQs and Quizzes

1. All the following are metabolized by N – acetylation (by conjugation) except
   (a) sulphonamides'
   (b) INH
   (c) Dapsone
   (d) Salicylic acid
2. Which one of the following acts as a **selective** **β_3** agonist for overactive bladder
   (a) Mirabegron
   (b) Oxybutynin
   (c) Trospium chloride
   (d) Tolterodine
3. Which of the following $\alpha 2$ – agonist is used in the treatment of attention – deficit hyperactivity disorder (ADHD)
   (a) Dexmedetomidine
   (b) Clonidine
   (c) Apraclonidine
   (d) α - methydopa
4. Gonodotropin releasing harmones (GNRH) Leuprolide, Nafarelin (for LH suppression) are used in all the following conditions except
   (a) Assisted reproductive techniques (IVF)
   (b) Endometriosis
   (c) Prostatic cancer
   (d) Contraception
5. Which one of the following drugs not useful in the treatment of intermittent (peripheral) claudication and Raynaud's phenomena?
   (a) Phentoxyphylline
   (b) Asprin /Clopidogrel
   (c) Cilostazol (Phospho – diesterase inhibitor)
   (d) Felodipine
6. All the following mechanisms of adrenergic drugs play a role in the treatment of glaucoma except
   (a) Decrease in aqueous synthesis
   (b) Enhancement of uveoscleral outflow
   (c) Inhibition of synthesis of carbonic anhydrase
   (d) Increase of trabecular meshwork outflow reducing episcleral venous pressure
7. All the following drugs exhibit antiarrhythmic action by prolongation of action potential duration and repolarization except
   (a) Amiodarone
   (b) Sotolal
   (c) Dronedarone
   (d) phenytoin
8. All the following are GP IIb/IIIa (Glycoprotein GP IIb/IIIa) inhibitors used as antiplatelet drugs except
   (a) Prasugrel
   (b) Abciximab
   (c) Eptifibatide
   (d) Tirofiban
9. All the following drugs are used in osteoporosis except
   (a) Bisphosphonates
   (b) Selective estrogen receptor modulators
   (c) Teriparatide (PTH fragment)
   (d) Glucocorticoids
10. Ornidazole is useful in all the following conditions except
    (a) Amoebiasis
    (b) Giardisis
    (c) Tichomoniasis
    (d) H. pylori infection

11. All the following are mechanisms of action of theophylline except
    (a) Activation of adenyl cyclase
    (b) Adenosine receptor antagonism
    (c) Inhibition of phosphodiesterases
    (d) Inhibition of leukotriene pathway
12. Which of the following statement is correct?
    (a) Antihistamine agents are used for allergic rhinitis and have antagonism for both H_1 and H_2 receptors.
    (b) Antihistamines are generally used to treat bronchial asthma
    (c) Antihistamines are the preferred agents in the treatment of acute anaphylactic shock
    (d) Second generation antihistamines have less sedating and anticholinergic side effects compared to first generation agents
13. Which one of the following is not the clinical use of ondansetron?
    (a) Pregnancy associated Nausea and vomiting
    (b) Nausea and vomiting associated with surgery(Post-operative)
    (c) Nausea and vomiting associated with radiation and chemotherapy (Nausea and vomiting due to Cancer).
    (d) Migraine headache
14. Which one of the following would be the best drug to reduce prolactin levels in patient with pituitary tumor?
    (a) Bromocryptine
    (b) Ergonovine
    (c) Methysergide
    (d) Ergotamine
15. Which one of the following is the advantage of specific COX_2 inhibitors?
    (a) Decreased GI adverse effects
    (b) Decreased vasoconstrictor activity
    (c) Increased anti – inflammatory effects
    (d) More tolerability in patients of bronchial asthma
16. All the following drugs produce teratogenic effects except
    (a) Cephalosporins
    (b) Isotretinoin
    (c) Methotrexate
    (d) Tetracyclines
17. Which one of the following statement is not correct with regard to addition of epinephrine to a local anesthetic?
    (a) Localization of the anaesthetic effect due to vasoconstrictor action
    (b) Prolongation of the anaesthetic effect
    (c) Delayed onset of action.
    (d) Slow absorption and minimize systemic toxic effects
18. All are true of the effects of Phenytoin and phosphenytoin except
    (a) They are used in absence seizures
    (b) Show initial first order kinetics followed by zero order kinetics
    (c) Used to treat status epilepticus
    (d) The predominant antiepileptic action is due to blockade of Na+ channels reducing repetitive neuronal firing
19. All the effects of gabapentin and pregabalin are true except
    (a) They are useful in tonic and clonic seizures.
    (b) They are used in neuropathic pain and post herpetic neuralgia
    (c) They reduce the brain glutamate levels which is responsible for the antiepileptic action
    (d) Bind with α - 2δ(delta) submit of $Ca^{2}+$ channels in the brain areas
20. The atypical antipsychotics differ from typical antipsychotics in that
    (a) They block both **D_2** and **5-HT2A** receptors and alleviate both positive and negative symptoms of psychosis.
    (b) They block only **D_2** receptors and alleviate only positive symptoms

(c) They do not cause extrapyramidal symptoms

(d) They do not cause sedation and hypotensive effects

21. Sacubitril (neprilysin inhibitor) and valsartan (**AT_1** receptor blocker) combination is useful in acute cases of congestive heart failure because

(a) There is an increase of ANP, BNP, CNP and an increase of diuresis, natriuresis and vasodilatation.

(b) There is a decreased effect of aldosterone

(c) It inhibits the release of NE from the adrenergic nerve endings

(d) It has agonist action on central α2 receptors

22. The mechanism of action of baclofen is

(a) GABA agonist action

(b) Depolarization of the motor end plate

(c) Competitive antagonism of ach at the motor end plate

(d) Antagonism of glutamate

23. Which of the following prostaglandins oppose the actions of TXA2 on the platelets

(a) PGI_2 and PGD_2

(b) $PGF_{2\alpha}$

(c) PGE_2

(d) PGD_2

24. Which one of the following is not an immunomodulator drug that stimulates immunity?

(a) Levamisole

(b) Thalidomide

(c) Cyclosporin

(d) Lenalidomide

25. Aprepitant and fosaprepitant (**Neurokinin-1**antagonists) are the drugs used for

(a) Delayed nausea and vomiting caused due to radiation and cancer chemotherapy

(b) Nausea and vomiting due to motion/travel sickness

(c) Nausea and vomiting due to migraine

(d) Nausea and vomiting associated with vertigo

26. The uses of bisphosphonates include all the following except

(a) Treatment of osteoporosis in postmenopausal women

(b) Hypercalcemia of malignancy

(c) Paget's disease

(d) osteomalacia

27. Cross match the following

1) Androgens	a) Prostatic cancer
2) Danazol	b) Benign prostatic hyperplacia
3) Doxazocin	c) Endometriosis and menorrhagia
4) Flutamide	d) Positive nitrogen balance and muscle development

28. Cross match the following

1) Budesonide	a) Female infertility
2) Gonadorelin	b) Bronchial asthma
3) Vinblastin	c) Breast cancer
4)Diethylcarbamazine	d) Filariasis

29. Fill in the blanks

(a) Fluconazole is especially useful for cryptococcal and coccidioidal meningitis because ______________

(b) Zidovudine acts by-------------

30. Say '**Yes**' or '**No**' to the following statement

(a) Pretomanid in combination with bedaquilin and linezolid used for the treatment of a specific type of highly – multidrug resistant tuberculosis of lungs ----------

(b) Methenamine mandelate is quite effective for the treatment of an acute urinary tract infection '----'

(c) Dextropropoxyphene is a commonly used antitussive drug '----'

Answers to MCQs

1) d	2) a	3) b	4) d	5) d
6) c	7) d	8) a	9) d	10) d
11) d	12) d	13) d	14) a	15) a
16) a	17) c	18) a	19) a	20) a
21) a	22) a	23) a	24) c	25) a

26) d

27) 1-d→ ;2→c ;3→b; 4→a

28) 1→b; .2- a; 3→c ;4→d

29) a. high penetration into CSF; b. Inhibition of HIV reverse transcriptase

30) a.Yes; b.No; c.Yes

Section 10 - MCQs and Quizzes

1. Acetyl salicylate and phenobarbitone are better absorbed from stomach because they are
   (a) Weak acid and remain ionized in gastric PH.
   (b) Strong acids fully ionized in gastric PH
   (c) Weak acids remain non – ionized in gastric PH
   (d) Weak bases which are ionized at gastric PH
2. Which one of the following crosses the blood - brain barrier to be useful to treat the adverse effects of atropine poisoning
   (a) Physostigmine
   (b) Neostigmine
   (c) Ambenonium
   (d) Pyridostigmine
3. Which one of the following general anesthetic has blood-gas partition of 0.47 and MAC of 107, poor solubility and rapid onset of action
   (a) Nitrous oxide
   (b) Ether
   (c) Halothane
   (d) Enflurane
4. One of the important adverse effects of prazocin is
   (a) Increased urinary voidance
   (b) Reflex tachycardia
   (c) Hypertrichosis
   (d) Postural hypotension
5. Ethyl alcohol is given in methanol poisoning because
   (a) Ethanol diverts the metabolism of methanol and prevents formation of formic acid
   (b) It competitively inhibits the effects of methanol on CNS and
   (c) It facilitates rapid removal of methanol through urine, respiration and other routes
   (d) It protects the possible hepatotoxicity of methanol
6. All the following drugs are effective to control status epilepticus except
   (a) Phenytoin and phosphenytoin IV
   (b) Lorazepam IV
   (c) Midazolam as a buccal patch
   (d) Sodium valproate
7. Ethyl alcohol is likely to produce a disulfiram – like effect with which one of the following
   (a) Metronidazole
   (b) INH
   (c) Nitro-glycerine
   (d) Barbiturates
8. A beta – blocker and nifedipine can be used to treat hypertension because
   (a) Pedal edema of nifedipine can be prevented
   (b) Reflex sympathetic activity of nifedipine can be prevented and enhance the therapeutic effect
   (c) Facilitation of better pharmacokinetic properties
   (d) Better agnoistic action
9. Which one of the following statements is not correct?
   (a) Coumarin anticoagulants act by inhibiting factors 11_a, V11,1X, and X
   (b) Most drugs are absorbed in ionized from
   (c) Blood brain barrier is deficient in the chemoreceptor trigger zone
   (d) Ketamine is a NMDA antagonist

10. Most of the drugs cross biological barriers by
    (a) Active transport
    (b) Passive diffusion
    (c) Carrier mediated transport
    (d) Pinocytosis/ endocytosis
11. Which one of the following is not contraindicated during pregnancy?
    (a) Diethylstilbestrol
    (b) Retinoic acid
    (c) Warfarin
    (d) Macrolides
12. All are genetically explained and bear a pharmacogenetic basis for drug action except
    (a) G6PD deficiency
    (b) N – acetyl transferase
    (c) Butyrylcholinesterase
    (d) Aromatic hydroxylation
13. Which one of the following acts as a SGLT-2 receptor antagonist to treat diabetes mellitus?
    (a) Empagliflozin
    (b) Semaglutide
    (c) Linagliptine
    (d) Colesevelam
14. Which one of the following drug combinations is the choice to treat constipation in geriatric populations and those with diabetic gastroperesis?
    (a) Lactitol+ Ispaghula
    (b) Methycellulose+ Magnesium sulphate
    (c) Senna+ lactulose
    (d) Sodium picosulfate +liqid paraffin
15. Which one of the following COX2 inhibitors has a long half – life (22 hours) and given in once daily doses(60 mg)
    (a) Celecoxib
    (b) Rofecoxib
    (c) Etoricoxib
    (d) Valdecoxib
16. Which one of the following antituberculosis drugs can be used to treat for prophylaxis of meningococcal and H. influenza meningitis in the carrier state?
    (a) Ethambutol
    (b) Rifampicin
    (c) Ethionamide
    (d) INH
17. All are true of the therapeutic uses of heparin except
    (a) As a substitute to warfarin
    (b) Thromboembolic disorders such as DVT, PE, Postoperative DVT
    (c) Unstable angina or non – ST segment elevation or non - Qwave MI
    (d) Renal dialysis procedure
18. Which one of the following in useful for rapid control of Ventricular arrhythmias due to MI, or those that occur post cardioversion and due to inhalational general anaesthetics?
    (a) Esmolol
    (b) Lidocaine
    (c) Amiodarone
    (d) Metoprolol
19. Which one of the following is a pure antagonist of opioid receptors?
    (a) Butorphanol
    (b) Pentazocine
    (c) Naltrexone
    (d) Nalbuphine
20. Sulfonylureas release insulin at the cellular levels by
    (a) Promoting Na^+ influx
    (b) Blocking the glucagon receptor
    (c) Blockade of inward rectifier K^+ channel
    (d) Promoting Ca^{2+} efflux
21. Thyroid storm can be treated with all of the following except
    (a) Propranolol
    (b) Radiolabeled iodine
    (c) Hydrocortisone
    (d) Propylthiouracil
22. For synergistic effect of sulphamethoxazole with which one of the following drugs is added
    (a) Trimethoprim
    (b) Chlortetracycline
    (c) Erythromycin
    (d) Pyrimethamine

23. Leishmaniasis can be effectively treated with all of the following drugs except
   (a) Pentamidine
   (b) Sodium stiboglyconate
   (c) Meglumine
   (d) Ivermectin

24. Which one of the following is effective in the treatment and prophylaxis of Influenza A and B?
   (a) Oseltamivir
   (b) Efavirenz
   (c) Nevirapine
   (d) Lopinavir

25. Amikacin is found to be effective in all the following clinical conditions except
   (a) Septicemia and nosocomial infections
   (b) Complicated UTI
   (c) Skin and soft tissue infections
   (d) Viral meningitis

26. All the following are active against Pneumocystis jiroveci (Pneumocystosis) except
   (a) Atovaquone
   (b) Pentamidine
   (c) Co-trimoxazole
   (d) Paromomycin

27. Progestins can be used in all the following conditions except
   (a) Menopausal syndrome
   (b) Habitual/Threatened abortion
   (c) Abnormal uterine bleeding
   (d) Dysmenorrhea

28. Cross match the following

1) Hydroxy cobalamine	a) Steroids
2) Calcitriol	b) Vitamin D deficiency
3) Acarbose	c) Megaloblastic anemia
4) Immuno-suppression	d) Diabetic mellitus

29. Cross match the following

1) Tetracyclines	a) Herpes simplex
2) Lamivudine	b) Systemic fungal infections
3) Amphotericin – B	c) Hepatitis B infection
4) Acyclovir	d) cholera

30. Fill in the blanks
   (a) The site of action of antimalarial primaquine is ________________
   (b) The drug of choice in the life-threatening staphylococcal infections such as septicemia,, cellulitis, and endocarditis is________________.

31. Say 'Yes' or 'No' to the following statements
   (a) Clozapine is used in schizophrenia ( )
   (b) Maximal Na^+ conservation does take place at distal convoluted tubule ( )
   (c) Diltiazem and verapamil can be used in ventricular arrhythmia ( )

Answers to MCQs

1) c	2) a	3) a	4) d	5) a
6) d	7) a	8) b	9) b	10) b
11) d	12) d	13) a	14) a	15) c
16) b	17) a	18) b	19) c	20) c
21) b	22) a	23) d	24) a	25) d
26) d	27) d			

28) 1—c; 2—b; 3—d; 4—a

29) 1---d: 2—c; 3---b; 4---a

30) a)Hypnozoites (hepatic) forms of the parasite b) Clindamycin

31) a) Yes; b) No ; c) No

Section 11 - MCQs and Quizzes

1. Which of the following best describes the cellular action of adrenaline?
   (a) Activation of adenylyl cyclase
   (b) Decreased activity of cAMP – dependent protein kinase
   (c) Increased intracellular store of ca^{z+}
   (d) Inhibition of the activity of phospholipase
2. Adrenaline – mediated β_1 - adrenoceptor activation results in which one of the following?
   (a) Constriction of the bronchial smooth muscle
   (b) Gastrointestinal relaxation
   (c) Dilatation of the pupils
   (d) Increased heart rate
3. The clinical uses of morphine include all the following except
   (a) Pre-anesthetic medication
   (b) b. Adjuvant to general anesthesia
   (c) c. Epidural and intrathecal anesthesia
   (d) d. Somatic pain
4. A person going on a sea travel and given scopolamine for its prevention most likely to suffer from
   (a) Bradycardia
   (b) Drowsiness
   (c) Miosis
   (d) Urinary urgency
5. Cholinesterase inhibitors like neostigmine can antagonize and reverse the action of which one of the following
   (a) Cisatracurium
   (b) Succinylcholine
   (c) Both A & B
   (d) Neither A & B
6. A 35-year-old man undergoes surgery for a hernia repair. After the surgery he complains of muscle aches and an increase of body temperature which the anesthetist considers it to be due to the administration of the skeletal muscle relaxant. Which of the following is the most accurate statement?
   (a) The agent also causes hypokalemia
   (b) The agent acts as an antigen to induce the adverse effects
   (c) The patient likely had malignant hyperthermia
   (d) The agent might alter the central thermoregulatory mechanisms.
7. All the following are characteristic of aminoglycosides except
   (a) Demonstrate concentration-dependent killing of sensitive organisms
   (b) Have post-antibiotic effect and can be given in once daily doses
   (c) Their dose needs to be adjusted based on renal function
   (d) They are used as first line drugs in combination with other drugs to treat tuberculosis
8. Muscarinic 2 (**M_2**) receptors are predominantly seen in
   (a) CNS
   (b) Myocardium
   (c) Bronchi
   (d) Intestines
9. In the synthesis of catecholamines, aromatic – L – amino acid decarboxylase facilitates the conversion of
   (a) Tyrosine to DOPA
   (b) DOPA to Dopamine

(c) Dopamine to noradrenaline
(d) Noradrenaline to adrenaline

10. All of the following are effective against Salmonella typhi infection except
(a) Cefuroxime
(b) Amoxacillin
(c) Cotrimoxazole
(d) Quinolones

11. One of the following β – blockers has both α – and β – receptor blocking actions
(a) Carvedilol
(b) Celiprolol
(c) Betaxolol
(d) Pindolol

12. Which one of the following ergot preparations is commonly used to control postpartem hemorrhage?
(a) Dihydroergotamine
(b) Ergonovine
(c) Bromocriptine
(d) Cabergoline

13. Which one of the following prostaglandins is used to cause therapeutic/ medical termination of pregnancy?
(a) Carboprost tromethamine
(b) Brimatoprost
(c) Alprostadil
(d) Iloprost

14. Which one of the following opioids is used as adjuvant to general anesthesia?
(a) Alfentanil
(b) Tramadol
(c) Buprenorphine
(d) Oxycodone

15. Which one of the following IV general anesthetic used for induction of anesthesia in persons with raised intracranial pressure?
(a) Ketamine
(b) Propofol
(c) Etomidate
(d) Thiopental sodium

16. Which one of the following skeletal muscle relaxants is having ultra- short duration of action and used for investigative purposes usually
(a) Mivacurium
(b) Atracurium
(c) Succinylcholine
(d) Rapa curium

17. Which one of the following macrolides given in once daily doses of 500 mg
(a) Clarithromycin
(b) Azithromycin
(c) Roxithromycin
(d) Erythromycin

18. Benzodiazepines, barbiturates, Gabapentine have which one of the following mechanisms of action
(a) Binding to the GABA receptor and facilitate Cl^- conductance
(b) Inhibition of NMDA receptor subtype
(c) Blockade of K^+ channels
(d) Potentiate the action of inhibitory neurotransmission mediated by glycine

19. Which one of the following benzodiazepines is useful for induction and maintenance of anaesthesia?
(a) Lorazepam
(b) Diazepam
(c) Midazolam
(d) Estazolam

20. A patient with hypertension is being treated with an agent that has agonist action on central presynaptic α2 – receptors and the agent is
(a) Minoxidil
(b) Clonidine
(c) Prazocin
(d) Guanethidine

21. The plateau of the cardiac action potential in non-pacemaker cardiac cell is caused by
(a) A slow inward and outward flux of ca^2
(b) Rapid outflux of K^+

(c) Na^+ and Ca^{2+}channel inactivation
(d) Inactivation of K^+ rectifier currents

22. The action of digoxin on the heart includes all the following except
(a) An increased chronotropic effect in the failing heart
(b) An increased systolic force of contraction
(c) A prolongation of AV nodal conduction
(d) A reduction of end – diastolic filling pressure

23. Latanoprost is useful in the treatment of glaucoma as it causes
(a) An increase of uveoscleral outflow
(b) Decrease of aqueous humor synthesis
(c) Miosis due to contraction of constrictor pupillae muscle
(d) Inhibition of dilatorpupillae muscle

24. The predominant adverse effect of ganglion blockers is
(a) Orthostatic hypotension
(b) Bradycardia and decrease of cardiac output
(c) Dry mouth
(d) Urinary hesitancy

25. All the following are true of phenothiazines, butyrophenones and reserpine, except
(a) Deplete central dopamine levels
(b) Cause hypotension
(c) Cause sedation and catatonia
(d) Commonly used antiemetics

26. Cross match the following

1) Diazoxide	a) Nitrogen retention and increase of muscle mass
2) Insulin	b) Hypertensive emergency
3) Estradiol	c) Kinase – linked receptor
4) Testosteron	d) Hormone replacement therapy

27. Cross match the following

1) Norgesteral	a) Endometriosis
2) Tamoxifen	b) Contraception
3) Mifepstone	c) Therapeutic abortion
4) Danazol	d) Breast cancer

28. Cross match the following

1) Clonazepam	a) Kappa – receptor agonist, an analgesic
2) Oxcarbazepine	b) Myoclonic jerks
3) Nalmephene	c) Alcohol withdrawal
4) Pentazocine	d) Complex partial seizures

29. Say '**Yes**' or '**No**' to the following statement
(a) COX – 2 predominantly inducible and produced immediately after an inflammatory stimulus_________.
(b) Paracetamol has anti-inflammatory actions and hence used in osteoarthritis_________.

30. Say' **Yes'** or '**No**' to the following statement
(a) Acetylsalicylic acid in smaller doses inhibits platelet aggregation_________.
(b) Ethosuximide is the drug of choice to treat tonic – clonic seizures_________.

Answers to MCQs

1) a	2) d	3) d	4) b	5) a
6) c	7) d	8) b	9) b	10) b
11) a	12) b	13) a	14) a	15) d
16) c	17) b	18) a	19) c	20) b
21) a	22) a	23) a	24) a	25) d
25) d	26) 1-b; 2-c; 3-d; 4-a		27) 1-b; 2-d; 3-c; 4-a	
28) 1-d; 2-b; 3-c; 4-a		29) a- Yes; b)- No	30) a-Yes ; b-No	

Section 12 - MCQs and Quizzes

1. A 35 - year old woman is being treated with gentamicin for a urinary tract infection. The gentamicin plasma level is 4μg/ml shortly after initial IV administration of an 80mg dose of the drug. The distribution volume of gentamicin is
   (a) 5L
   (b) 8L
   (c) 10L
   (d) 20L
2. All the following statements are true of Dexmedetomidine except
   (a) α_2 receptor agonist
   (b) Used as sedative in intubated and mechanically ventilated patients in ICU wards
   (c) Perioperative analgesic
   (d) Used as skeletal muscle relaxant
3. All are true of succinylcholine adverse effect except
   (a) Hyperkalemia
   (b) Increased intraocular pressure
   (c) Paralysis of intercostal and diaphragmatic muscles
   (d) Delayed onset of action
4. Which of the following routes of drug administration produces the most rapid absorption
   (a) Inhalation
   (b) Intravenous
   (c) Oral
   (d) sublingual
5. Most drugs gain entry to cells by
   (a) Passive diffusion with zero – order kinetics
   (b) Passive diffusion with first – order kinetics
   (c) Active transport with zero – order kinetics
   (d) Passive diffusion through membrane pores
6. A boy aged 11 years is brought to emergency room who was reported to be 'crazy' after eating seeds from a plant unintentionally. He was incoherent with dry and hot skin, pupils dilated and unresponsive to light. His blood pressured recorded was 160/100 mmg Hg and pulse rate of 110/min. His body temperature was 100^0F. What would be the presumptive diagnosis based on the clinical findings? Poisoning due to
   (a) Datura stramonium
   (b) Strychnous lethalis
   (c) Aconitine
   (d) Cannabis
7. Tachyphylaxis of ephedrine or tyrosine is due to
   (a) Blockade of pre-junctional adrenoceptors
   (b) Inhibition of impulse conduction in sympathetic nerves
   (c) Reduced stores or depletion of available transmitter
   (d) Compensation of cholinergic responses
8. Cardiovascular effects of a new drug (X) that activates autonomic receptors are shown in the table below. The most probable receptor affinities of drug (X) are likely be due to which of the following.

Parameter	Control	Drug(X)
Systolic BP	120mm Hg	110 mm of Hg
Diastolic BP	85mm Hg	55mm of Hg
Heart rate	60/min	120/min

   (a) α_1 and α_2

(b) α_1, α_2, β_1
(c) β_1, β_2
(d) M_2

9. Digitals toxic manifestation include all the following except
(a) Hypokalemia
(b) Nausea and vomiting
(c) Extrasystoles and bigeminy
(d) Bradycardia and heart block

10. Which of the following neurons originate mainly in the substantia nigra and hypothalamus
(a) Dopaminergic
(b) Sertonergic
(c) GABAergic
(d) Noradrenergic

11. Which one of the following is not the characteristic of Phenytoin?
(a) First order kinetics
(b) Blockade of Use-dependent Na+ channels
(c) Gingival hyperplasia
(d) Has a half-life of 22 hours and reaches steady state concentration in 7-10 days

12. Which one of the following effect morphine and d – tubocurarine have in common?
(a) Increased bladder tone
(b) Histamine release
(c) Malignant hyperthermia
(d) ANS ganglion blockade

13. The effects of drug induced parkinsonism can be alleviated by which one of the following
(a) GABA agonists
(b) Anticholinergics
(c) Dopa agonists
(d) NMDA antagonists

14. Which one of the following is effective in the treatment of both major depressive disorder and obsessive compulsive disorder?
(a) Fluoxetine
(b) Trazodone
(c) Clonazepam
(d) Phenytoin

15. Two patients, one taking imipramine for anxiety disorder and the other chlorpromazine for psychotic disorder reported to a consulting physician for a common adverse effect. Which one of the following is most likely the adverse effect?
(a) Orthostatic hypotension
(b) Pupillary constriction
(c) Excessive salivation
(d) ↑ Seizure threshold

16. Labetalol a drug used in hypertension and hypertensive emergency differs from propranolol in that
(a) It is a selective cardiac β1 – receptor blocker
(b) Has both α and β receptor blocking action
(c) Has α1 – receptor blocking action
(d) Available only for IV use

17. Resistance of Mycobacterium tuberculosis to INH involves all the following mechanisms except
(a) Deletions or mutations of KatG gene for its conversion to active form by catalase –peroxidase enzyme
(b) Mutations in INHA, KasA, and ahp C, all involved in mycolic acid synthesis
(c) Reduced permeation into bacterial cell
(d) Mutations in the gene encoding for DNA – dependent RNA polymerase

18. A 7 – year old girl presents with pharyngitis and fever of 2 days duration and the microbiological findings reveal small, translucent beta – hemolytic colonies in the secretions collected locally. The girl was allergic to penicillin from the previous history of her treatment for otitis media. Which one would the most appropriate drug?
(a) Cefaclor
(b) Doxycycline
(c) Azithromycin
(d) Vancomycin

19. A person being treated for severe Gram – negative bacterial infection and has a creatinine clearance of 25mL/min. What should be the dose of Gentamicin
    (a) 3.5 mg/kg
    (b) 1.0 mg/kg
    (c) 4 mg/kg
    (d) 2.5 mg/kg

20. Several antibiotics are effective in single doses for the treatment of uncomplicated gonorrhea. Which one of the following drugs necessitates a 7 – 10 day course of treatment and to be highly effective?
    (a) Doxycycline+ceftrioxone
    (b) Ofloxacin
    (c) Azithromycin
    (d) Ceftriaxone alone

21. Despite its “age”, penicillin – G remains the drug of choice in the treatment of which one of the following infections caused by?
    (a) B.fragilis
    (b) T.pallidum
    (c) H.influenza
    (d) S.aureus

22. Highly active antiretroviral therapy(HAART) in HIV infection is associated with all of the following except
    (a) A decrease in viral mRNA copies/mL of blood
    (b) A possible increase in CD4 cell count
    (c) Re-emergence of infection
    (d) A reduced incidence of opportunistic infections.

23. Following an overdose of an over – the counter (OTC) drug, a young college student has marked GI distress and is lethargic and confused, with an elevated body temperature. Lab analysis of blood reveals ↑PCO3 - ↓HCO3 - ↓K+ and an anion gap acidosis. The most likely cause of these signs and symptoms is the toxic dose of
    (a) Acetaminophen
    (b) Acetylsalicylic acid
    (c) Naproxen
    (d) Indomethacin

24. A reasonable explanation for the therapeutic effect of ibuprofen and naproxen in primary dysmenorrhea is that these drugs cause
    (a) ↓PGE, $PGF_{2\alpha}$
    (b) ↓Leukotrein B
    (c) Inhibit phospholipase A2
    (d) Selective inhibition of COX_2

25. A chronic alcoholic develops hepatotoxicity with the use of acetaminophen, the reason for which is
    (a) Ethanol inhibits the metabolism of acetaminophen
    (b) Ethanol induces P450 that forms the toxic metabolite
    (c) Nutritional deficiency
    (d) The associated smoking in alcoholics sensitizes the liver due to nicotine present in the tobacco.

26. 6 – Merceptopurine (6 – MP), frequently used in malignancies, RA and other conditions is metabolized by xanthine oxidase. Major dose adjustments are needed in patients who are being treatment with
    (a) Acetylsalicylic acid
    (b) Allopurinol
    (c) Indomethacin
    (d) Sulfinpyrazone

27. Which one of the following antituberculosis drugs is having excellent sterilizing activity against semidormant bacteria (intracellular mycobacteria?
    (a) Pyrazinamide
    (b) Rifampicin
    (c) Ethambcitol
    (d) INH

28. Fill in the blanks
    (a) Methadone is the drug of choice for____________
    (b) Lithium is the drug choice for ________
    (c) Tolcapone and entacapone (COMT inhibitors) are used in the treatment of---------
    (d) Adalimumab, a TNF_α inhibitor is used in the treatment of______________

29. Cross match the following

a) Hydrocodone	1. Mineralocorticoid antagonist
b) Finerenone	2. Prolong repolarization in cardiac cells
c) Sotalol	3. Analgesic
d) venlafaxine	4. Atypical antidepressant

30. Say **'Yes'** or **'No'** to the following statement
    (a) Ethyl alcohol is used in methyl alcohol poisoning '--'
    (b) Triptans are contraindicated in patients with CV related diseases while treating migraine '--'
    (c) Sulfadoxine and pyrimethamine combination is used to treat an acute attack of falciparum malaria as alternative to Mefloquine '--'
    (d) The mechanism of action of Vinca alkaloids is by disruption of micro-tubules and inhibition of mitosis'--'

Answers to MCQs

1) d	2) d	3) d	4) a	5) b
6) a	7) c	8) c	9) a	10) a
11) a	12) b	13) b	14) a	15) a
16) b	17) d	18) c	19) b	20) a
21) b	22) c	23) b	24) a	25) b

26) b

27) a

28) a) Morphine withdrawal b) Manic depressive psychosis c) Parkinsonism d) Rheumatoid arthritis

29) a---3 ; b---1 ; c---2 ; d---4

30) a) Yes; b) Yes; c) No d) Yes

Clinical Case Study-1

A 32 year old man presents with palpitations and insomnia of recent origin. He reports being well until 7 months ago, when he started a new exercise regimen. Since then, he noticed intermittent palpitations described as fast, forceful, regular heart beats, both at rest and with exertion. He also noticed a poor sleep pattern. He lost 10 kg of body weight in the recent past and complains of weakness or fatigue. There is no apparent goiter and neither any ocular manifestations.

Physical examination shows apparent slight anxiety, but no clinical distress. His vital function are as follows - HR 122/min, BP of 142/61 Hg, and O_2 saturation of 98% and a BMI of 32.4. The palms of the patient are diaphoric and a slight tremor was seen. The clinical investigations showed an E.C.G with tachycardia but not irregular beats, TSH reading at 0.006 µg/ml, (reference range 0.5 - 4.7) FT level of 5.2 ng/dl (reference range (0.8 – 1.8). A low radioactive uptake(I^{131}), negative for antibody titers (thyroperoxidase or microsomal antigen, TSH receptor antibodies) and no or absent response to antithyroid drugs.

1. From the clinical picture and the presentation of laboratory findings what would be the most probable diagnosis of the patient?
2. How you justify the condition?
3. What would be the ideal treatment for the patient?
4. If it were to be Grave's disease, what would be treatment?

Ans:

1. From the clinical presentation and the signs and symptoms, a justifiable diagnosis of thyrotoxicosis can be made.
2. But as per the history of 7 months duration, and as per the laboratory findings (only traces of TSH, low or almost nil I^{131}uptake, nil presence of antibody titers) a condition of exogenous thyrotoxicosis/ Factitious thyrotoxicosis/ Subacute thyroiditis could be made out. This is substantiated by the absence of any goiter, short history. Absence of ophthalmic manifestations which are most affected or seen in Grave's disease.

   Grave's disease is an autoimmune disease and of long duration and develops over a period (insidious onset) unlike the present case of 7 months duration. In Grave's disease there would be enlargement of the thyroid gland which may be nodular also. Presence of antibodies is also suggestive of Grave's disease which can be substantiate by an increase of radioactive iodine uptake and an elevated FT4 or FTI, T_3 and FT_3 levels. Most importantly TSH levels in Graves disease would be 0 – 0.1 µU/ml.

   Exogenous thyrotoxicosis or factitious thyrotoxicosis/subacute thyroiditis is due to excessive use of thyroid preparations for an unclaimed or unsubstantiated use for weight loss, which may become a part of the other remedial measures used for the similar purpose. As mentioned before, the history of the case being short, and in the absence of any laboratory data the presentation is suggestive of Exogenous thyrotoxicosis
3. The treatment for this patient is withdrawal from use of thyroid preparations and also the use of β – blockers for a short term.
4. If the case were to be Grave's disease, anti-thyroid drugs like propylthiouracil, methimazole, carbemazole; radio labeled iodine (I^{131}) and surgical removal of the gland are the lines of treatment.

Clinical Case Study-2

A male patient aged 56 years with known hypertension, diabetes mellitus, and early renal dysfunction with a history of recurrent urinary tract infections not responding to cotrimoxazole and carboxy penicillins requires further change of a suitable antibiotic. He is on regular treatment for hypertension and diabetes. His blood pressure recorded was 160/90mmHg, serum creatinine levels are 2.6mg/100ml, GFR reading was 60ml/min. The urine culture showed the growth of P. aeruginosa sensitive to gentamicin.

1) How do you proceed to give the required dose of gentamicin and what is the basis for the same?
2) How do you adjust the dose?
3) Does the patient require a single dose or multiple doses?
4) What ae the possible adverse effects of gentamicin?
5) What is the normal duration of the treatment?

Ans:

1. Gentamicin is an aminoglycoside drug and has narrow margin of safety and therapeutic monitoring is required if the duration of treatment exceeds 7 days and if the patient shows associated renal dysfunction as in the present case.

   Renal function is usually assessed in terms of creatinine clearance/serum creatine levels and glomerular filtration rate (GFR expressed as ml/min/1.73m^2).

   The relationship of creatinine and GFR can be made out as follows

   (a) Creatinine 1 mg/100ml is the baseline with normal GFR
   (b) Creatinine 2 mg/100ml – GFR reduced by 50%
   (c) Creatinine 4 mg/100ml – GFR reduced by 70 – 80%
   (d) Creatinine 8mg/100ml – GFR reduced by 90 – 95%

   Chronic kidney disease (CKD) can be staged based on GFR as follows

   1) Stage 1– 120ml – 90ml – None
   2) Stage 2 – 89 – 60ml – mild
   3) Stage 3
      (a) – 59 – 45ml – Intermediate
      (b) – 44 – 30ml – Moderate
   4) Stage 4 -29 – 15ml– Severe
   5) Stage 5 – 14ml – Nil – Pre- terminal and dialysis required

      Based on the above observations and the clinical findings of the patient, gentamicin requirement would be 2.5- 3mg/kg/day given once daily, the usual requirement with normal range of creatinine and creatinine clearance(100mL/min) being 3-5 mg/kg/day.

1. Dose adjustments are required to avoid accumulation and toxicity of the drug in patients both with renal insufficiency and diabetes mellitus. The usual serum levels of gentamicin should be less than 1mcg/ml over a period of 18-24 hours following a dose of 5mg/kg of the drug is normal healthy people.
2. The patient requires a single daily dose as against twice daily doses given in normal healthy people.
3. The possible adverse effects of gentamicin include aggravation of the damage of the kidney function as in this patient. It can also cause cochlear damage causing hearing loss, muscle twitches.
4. The normal duration of treatment with gentamicin 5 to 7 days.

Clinical Case Study-3

A 35 year old businessman is brought to the department of psychiatry for his abnormal behaviour observed by his close relatives for the past 3 months. On enquiry it was found that he suffered heavy losses in business and that he felt he was cheated by his business partners. He is also under a state of abnormal, bizarre, disorganized and agitated behaviour when brought to the department. Occasionally he goes into a state of delusions, hallucinations, reality disorder and feelings of persecution. He was also observed earlier by his relatives to withdraw himself from social gatherings, and becoming emotionally upset.

His physical examination revealed no abnormality and from the symptoms presented a case of acute psychosis secondary to schizophrenia was made out by the psychiatrist and put on haloperidol on hospital admission.

1. What is the mechanism of action of haloperidol?
2. What mediates the extrapyramidal side effects of the antipsychotic drugs?
3. What are the other antipsychotic drugs that cause lesser extrapyramidal effects, less sedation and lesser hypotension compared to haloperidol?

Answers:

1. Haloperidol blocks D2 receptors in dopaminergic pathways of the brain and thereby limit the release of dopamine in the mesolimbic and mesocortical pathways that leads to the control of clinical features of schizophrenia.
2. Extrapyramidal effects or features like Parkinsonism are produced by haloperidol and other antipsychotic drugs, particularly with high potency drugs (maximum receptor blockade) like haloperidol, flufenazine and trifluoperazine.
3. The other antipsychotics that cause lesser extrapyramidal effects, less sedation and less hypotension include risperidone, quetiapine, ziprasidone, aripiprazole and lumateperone.

Clinical Correlation:

Schizophrenia is a chronic though disorder characterized by the presence of **positive symptoms** that include delusions, hallucinations (often in the form of voices) and reality disorders that include thought disorders (abnormal irrational thoughts, feelings of grandeur, persecution, feelings of being cheated upon, conspired against and jealously, abnormal, bizarre, disorganized and agitated behaviour. The **negative symptoms** include social withdrawal from persons and surroundings, emotional outbursts, and cognitive impairments.

The therapeutic benefits of antipsychotic drugs are by virtue of their blockade of D2 receptors in the dopaminergic pathways (mesolimbic and mesocortical areas of the brain). Excess release of dopamine in the dopaminergic areas has been linked to psychotic disorders, the blockade of which is responsible for the control of clinical features of schizophrenia. Atypical antipsychotic (clozapine, loxapine, olanzapine, quetiapine, risperidone, aripiprazole) have affinity for both D2 and 5-HT2A receptors, block them and alleviate both positive and negative symptoms of schizophrenia, while typical antipsychotics (Phenothiazines, Thioxanthenes and butyrophenones – haloperidol) block only D2 receptors at therapeutic doses and alleviate only positive symptoms. The dopamine receptor antagonist activity of antipsychotic drugs at multiple sites in CNS and throughout the body, contributes to the presence of numerous adverse effects. However, the availability of many atypical antipsychotics with more site specific activity resulted in lesser incidence of adverse effects. The adverse effects of antipsychotics in general include extrapyramidal effects, akathesia, acute dystonias, tardive dyskinasia, autonomic nervous system effects (both adrenergic and cholinergic blockade effects), metabolic and endocrine effects – weight gain, loss of libido, impotence and infertility, hyperprolactonemia)

Clinical Case Study-4

A 14 year male child is brought to the medical outpatient department with a complaint of feeling quite ill with headache, dizziness, nausea and a feeling of weakness. There is an increase of body temperature (104^0F) within next two days and also the development of rash on extremities and wrists. The other symptoms seen were stiffness of the neck, sensitivity to light, confusion and seizures. The attending physician ordered for complete blood picture, spinal fluid analysis which showed an increase in WBC count, the presence of Gram-negative diplococci in the spinal fluid with an elevated protein and decrease of glucose levels. An x- ray and CAT scan revealed pressure on the brain.

1. From the clinical presentation what could be the tentative diagnosis of the case?
2. What microorganisms could have caused the clinical symptoms?
3. What is the line of treatment of the case?
4. What are the preventive vaccines available for the condition?

Answers:

1. From the clinical presentation a case of meningitis can be made out. Meningitis is usually caused by a viral or bacterial infection. Differentiation between the two is important in order to know the line of treatment and also to estimate the possible severity and the damage it could cause if not attended to immediately.
2. Bacterial meningitis is caused by Neisseria meningitidis (meningococci), Streptococcus Pneumoneae (Pneumococcus), Haemophilus influenzae (Hi) and Streptococcus agalactiae (group B streptococcus GBS). Viral meningitis is caused by non-polio enteroviruses and the symptoms are similar to those seen in bacterial meningitis. Mild cases of viral meningitis resolve within 7-10 days. However bacterial meningitis is severe and can cause serious complications such as brain damage, hearing loss, or learning disabilities. Antibiotics would not be useful in viral meningitis and instead antiviral drugs along with conservative therapy may help in case of meningitis caused by viruses such as herpes virus and influenza virus.
3. The drugs that could be effective to treat an active case of bacterial meningitis include a 3rd or 4th generation Cephalosporin such as Ceftriaxone, Cefotaxime, Ceftizoxime, and Cefepime.

   The usual doses of the drugs used are

   (i) Ceftriaxone – 2gIV – 12th hourly for 7 – 10 days

   (ii) Cefotaxime – 1 to 2 g IV/IM – 8th hourly

   (iii) Ceftizoxime – 1 g IV – 8 – 12 hourly IV

   (iv) Vancomycin could be added with cephalosporins possibly to cover cephalosporin resistant *streptococcus pneumoniae*.

Causative organisms	Prophylactic vaccines for meningitis
1. Neisseria meningitis	Men-B Men ACWY
2. Haemophilus influenza	Hib
3. Streptococcus pneumoniae	PCVs (Polysacchride Vaccine) -PVC15 and PVC20 -Pneumococcal Poly saccharide Vaccine 23

Clinical Case Study-5

A 53 year old man reports in the emergency ward of severe substernal chestpain described as aching or feeling of pressure, dyspnea, restlessness, nausea and diaphoresis. The pain radiates to his left jaw, neck and left arm .. The patient has a history of hypertension, dyslipidemia, stage 3 chronic kidney disease, and an earlier episode of inferior myocardial infarction.. An exercise stress echocardiogram performed three months ago showed changes indicative of ischemia when the patient reached 96% of his predicted maximum heart rate. Clinical recordings showed blood pressure of 100mmHg/70mmHg, a heart rate at 56 beats/ min. ECG showed ST segment elevation most notable in V6, increased cardiac biomarkers like cardiac specific Troponin T (cTnl), and increased creatinine kinase isoenzyme levels, and cardiac wall motion abnormalities and reduced ejection fraction in echocardiogram.

The patient is currently taking aspirin 75 mg/day, lisinopril 40 mg/day, carvedilol 25mg twice per day, and atorvastatin 80 mg/day.

1) What would be the most probable diagnosis of the patient?
2) What lines of treatment should be followed for the condition?
3) Explain the mechanism of action of each drug used in the treatment

Ans:

1) From the clinical presentation of the case a firm establishment of acute myocardial infarction could be made out. The diagnosis is based on the laboratory findings and clinical investigations done.
2) The immediate treatment to the patient includes restoration of balance between oxygen supply and demand by providing continuous oxygen supply through nasal prongs or face mask. This is followed by IV administration of 2-4 mg of morphine or any other opioid analgesic to relieve the pain, buccal or sublingual aspirin or any chewable aspirin (160-325 mg), sublingual administration of 4 mg nitroglyserine at regular intervals given few times. The chances of recovery of the patent are very bright if the patient is brought to the hospital within 10-20 minutes after the complaint.

   This is followed by administration of unfractinated heparin (70-100 U/Kg) to those patients who are likely to undergo percutaneous coronary intervention (PCI- angiography and stent placement)) if facilities are available at the center. If PCI is to be done some time later, antiplatelet drugs like prasugrel, ticagrelar, elinogrel, abciximab, eptifibatide can be given a few days earlier to the procedure.

   If PCI is not contemplated, thrombolytic therapy should be given to facilitate revacularization/reperfusion of the occluded coronary artery branches. The drugs most commonly employed include alteplase(tPA), reteplase, tenecteplase, streptokinase and urokinase. Patients without ST segment elevation should not receive thrombolytic therapy.

   Once the patient is stabilized and normalized slowly confirmed by repeat of ECGs taken at regular intervals during the stay of the patient in the ICU, he can be shifted to the ward and follow up treatment started. This consists of IV nitoglycerine for 24-48 hours with simultaneous use of β-blockers like metoprolol or bisoprolol, antiplatelet drugs like aspirin and clopidogrel, ACE inhibitors like lisinopril or ramipril and statins like atorvastatin or rosuvastatin which are used very commonly as prophylactic drugs to prevent any possible episodes of the present type during post recovery period and later and continued on long term basis (almost as life-long drugs). Coronary artery bypass surgery (CABG) is considered if the episodes are continued in spite of the continued therapy and done after confirming by angiography

3) A) Buccal/sublingual or any chewable form of aspirin facilitates rapid inhibition of TXA2 preventing further platelet aggregation.

B) Sublingual nitroglycerine provides coronary vasodilatation, redistribution of coronary blood flow from non-ischemic areas to ischemic areas, reduces myocardial oxygen demand and also a decrease of preload and after load.

C) β-blockers decrease myocardial oxygen demand as they cause negative inotropic and chronotropic effects

D) Antithombotic drugs like heparin or antiplatelet drugs prevent the formation of new or evolving thrombus acting by different mechanisms

E) Thrombolytic drugs immediately lyse or dissolve thrombus and prevent recurrent thrombus and facilitate rapid restoration of patency of coronary blood vessels and hemodynamic function

F) ACE inhibitors like lisinopril, ramipril are useful in the early stages of recovery of MI to reduce the cardiac preload and after load and thereby reducing myocardial oxygen demand. They are also used as follow on therapy in post MI period as maintenance drugs

G) Statins like atorvastatin or rosuvastatin are given to decrease the lipid levels (LDL cholesterol, triglyserides) which are considered to facilitate atheromatous plaque in the coronary blood vessels and to facilitate thrombus formation with platelet aggregation.

Clinical Case Study-6

A 24 year old woman was admitted to hospital at 8.50 A.M for delayed maturity of pregnancy, her pregnancy gestation being 40 weeks and 1 day. The attending gynaecologist decided for the induction of labor for her because of post maturity and also in view of her pregnancy associated diabetes. Syntocinon/pitocin(Oxytocin) drip was started after the rupture of the membranes. The woman progressed well in labor and has a normal delivery of a female infant at 1:19 PM.

1) What are the requirements of syntocinon (oxytocin/Pitocin) for induction of labor and how do you prepare a solution that contains syntocinon and to start the IV drip?
2) What is the difference between induction of labor and augmentation of labor
3) What are the indications and contraindications for the induction of labor?
4) What complications would arise out of excess use of syntocinon dose?
5) What are the other pharmacological approaches available for induction of labor?

Ans:

1. A standard solution of oxytocin (syntocinon)s in prepared by adding 5IU (International units) to 500ml of normal saline. The preparation contains 10mu/ml. The initial dose is 1 to 2mU/min which is equal to 2 to 4 drops/minute. The dose can be gradually increased in increments of no more than 1 to 2 mu/ at 30 to 60 minute intervals until the labor is progressed to 5 – 10 Cm cervical dilation, and the contraction pattern has been established which is similar to normal labor. The dose can be reduced gradually by similar adjustments (as done for infusion at the beginning). If the uterine contractions are found to be too powerful the infusion can be stopped and soon there is a decrease of contractions. Infusion up to 6mu/min has been shown to produce oxytocin levels found in spontaneous labor at term.
2. Induction of labor is defined as the artificial process of initiating labor before spontaneous onset, using mechanical or pharmacological methods. Augmentation of labor, however, is the stimulation of uterine contractions once the women has spontaneously initiated labor, but the process is considered inadequate.
3. As a general rule, induction of labor is indicated when the benefits of delivery to the mother of the fetus outweigh the risks associated with induction of labor. That is to say that induction of labor is indicated when the continuation of pregnancy poses a risk to maternal and/or fetal health.
4. **The indications for induction of labor include**
   - Post – dated pregnancy
   - Pregnancy induced hypertension
   - Pre – eclampsia
   - Intrauterine growth retardation
   - Diabetes/gestational diabetes
   - Isoimmunization

- Maternal medical conditions (Cardiac, renal, lupus)
- Intrahepatic cholestasis of pregnancy
- Oligohydramnios
- Chorioamnionitis
- Premature rupture of membranes
- Fetal structural defects
- Intrauterine fetal death

Contraindications for Induction of Labor

- Placenta previa
- Transverse fetal lie (position)
- Umbilical cord prolapse
- Previous myomectomy and breaching cavity
- Active genetical infection
- Breach presentation
- Polyhydramnios

5. The most common complications with the use of oxytocin is hyperstimulation of the uterus which can cause fetal distress. Hence continuous fetal monitoring is required.
6. Dinoprostone (PGE2) is the prostaglandin most commonly used for cervical ripening. The PGE2 acts by three mechanisms – It alters the extracellular matrix of the cervix, increases the activity of smooth muscle of the uterus and finally it leads to gap junction formation necessary to coordinate the uterine contractions. Dinoprostone can be given as slow – release pessary containing 10mg, a vaginal tablet containing 3mg or gel containing 1 or 2 mg of dinoprostone. The standard guideline recommends the use of one cycle ofPGE2tablets or gel followed by a second dose if labor is not established or the use of slow-release pessary over 24 hours. The use of dinoprostone most likely results in vaginal delivery within 24 hours.

Clinical Case Study-7

A male patient aged 46 years is brought to the neurology department along with his friend when the former complained of a state of blankness, unaware of his surroundings and unresponsive to any communication. The patient also presented with automatisms which are purposeless and repetitive activities such as lip smacking, chewing, picking his shirt, hip thrusting, repeated recitations of a prayer and unwarranted laughing. The patient is not able to respond appropriately during seizure. He is unaware of dangers such as traffic, fire or slopes on the ground. The most notable point was amnesia and he has no memory of what had occurred during the seizure. The episodes of seizure varied from one to two in a day to once in 3 to 4 days. EEG shows unilateral or bilateral spikes or slow wave discharge over temporal lobe or frontotemporal regions both during seizures and in between.

1. What would be the probable diagnosis of the patient?
2. What are the possible drugs of choice to treat the condition?
3. What is the mechanism of action of carbmazepine and related drugs?

Ans: From the clinical presentation of the symptoms of the patient, he might be suffering from a focal type of epilepsy mostly a complex partial type as evidenced by brief loss of consciousness, presence of automatisms, a period of amnesia in the postictal period and the occurrence of periodic episodes ranging from one to two in a day to once in 3 to 4 days and the findings of EEG during and acute attack of seizure.

The drugs of choice for the treatment of this type of epilepsy (Temporal epilepsy) include carbamazepine with average daily dose of 800-1200mg, oxcarbazepine (600-2400mg/day), and eslicarbazepine (400-800mg/day)(the most preferred drugs as a first choice). The other drugs that also find favor for the treatment of complex partial seizures include lamotrigine, vigabatrine, topiramate, zonisamide, retigabine, gabapentine, and pregabalin.

3) Carbamazepine and related drugs facilitate anti-seizure activity by blocking Na+ channels and limiting repetitive neuronal firing of action potentials evoked by sustained depolarizations. They abolish maximum electroshock convulsions. In addition they increase potassium conductance and modulate the activity of high-voltage activated calcium channels.

Vigabatrin and felbamate are reserved for intractable epilepsy patients due to the potential of serious adverse events produced by any of the older antiepileptic drugs (carbamazepine and its derivatives)

Clinical Case Study-8

A 12-year girl presents to the emergency department with a sore throat and fever and was diagnosed with pharyngitis by group A β – hemolytic streptococcus. She was put on IM penicillin. Approximately 5 minutes later, she is found to be in respiratory distress and audibly wheezing. Her skin is mottled and cool. She is tachycardic and her blood pressure fallen to 70/30 mm Hg. She is diagnosed as having anaphylactic reaction to the penicillin and given adrenaline IM in a dose of 0.2 ml of 1:1000 solution.

1. What is the effect of adrenaline on the vascular system of the girl?
2. Which adrenoceptor primarily mediates the vascular response?
3. What effect will adrenaline have on her respiratory system?
4. Which adrenoceptor primarily mediates the respiratory system response?

Ans:

1. Effect of adrenaline on vascular system is vasoconstriction.
2. Adrenoceptor which primarily mediates the vascular response is α_1.
3. Effect of adrenaline on pulmonary system is bronchial relaxation.
4. Adrenoceptor which primarily mediates the pulmonary response is β_2.

Discussion:

Anaphylaxis is an acute, immune – mediated response (type 1 reaction) to an allergen (here penicillin) characterized by bronchospasm, urticaria, swelling of the soft tissues, vasodilation and hypotension and pallor of the skin. Adrenaline is the drug of choice used to treat this condition because it appears through the activation of $\alpha_1$and β_2 receptors increasing and restoring the blood pressure and causing bronchial relaxation, thus countering the pathophysiologic process underlying anaphylaxis. The other drugs which can cause this type of reaction (Type 1) include streptokinase, asparaginase, aspirin, dextrans, radio contrast media, vaccines, and local anesthetics. Adrenaline can be supplemented with dexamethasone or betamethasone given IV in doses of 2 – 4 mg. In addition, life support with maintenance of vital parameters also becomes necessary. Occasionally anaphylaxis can cause edema of the larynx and thus cause restricted airway patency for which emergency tracheostomy maybe needed. H_1 receptor antagonists have little effect in annulling the effects of type 1 reactions as many a types of allergic mediators are released apart from histamine for which H1 antagonists have no role to play.

Clinical Case Study-9

A 22 years old man is brought to the emergency department after being found on the side walk unresponsive. He is lethargic and does not answer questions. He has been given 1 ampoule of Dextrose IV without any result. On examination, his heart rate is 60 beats per minute, and respiratory rate is 8 perminute. His pupils are pinpoint and not reactive. There are many IV trace marks on his arms bilaterally. The emergency physician concludes that the patient has had a drug overdose.

a) What is the most likely diagnosis?
b) What is the most appropriate medication for this condition?
c) What other drugs may interact with the drug that the person supposed to have consumed
d) How do you explain the probable mechanism of action of the drug that the person might have consumed and the anti dote to be given?

Ans:

a) From the clinical presentation the most likely diagnosis is overdose of an opioid, like heroin
b) Most appropriate medication for this condition is naloxone
c) Opioids (morphine, heroin) are the most frequently abused drugs that cause tolerance and physical dependence followed by addiction. Certain individuals seek euphoria obtained from the IV injection of opioids such as heroin. There are others who use morphine, fentanyl and methadone for the relief of chronic pain and are more prone for overdose if treatment guidelines are not followed. There are three types of opioid receptors – mu (μ), kappa (κ) and delta (δ). This patient has the classic signs of opioid over dosage as manifested as somnolence, respiratory depression and miosis. Stimulation of (μ) receptors results in analgesia (supraspinal and spinal), respiratory depression, euphoria, tolerance and physical dependence. Psychological dependence is the compulsive desire of addicts to use morphine or heroine to experience euphoritic effects. Kappa receptors cause mostly spinal analgesia and sedation but not respiratory depression. Delta receptors bind endogenous opiates such as enkephilins, endorphins and dynorphins and modify pain sensation

   Naloxone is mainly used in the treatment of acute opioid overdosage and is given in an initial dose of 0.1 – 0.4 mg IV to effectively attenuate the effects of (μ) receptor agonism over a period of 1 – 3 minutes followed by a maintenance dose of 0.4 – 0.8 mg given IV. It is highly beneficial in patients with respiratory and CNS depression.
d) The other drugs which can enhance the actions of opioids include alcohol, benzodiazepines, barbiturates and phenothiazines.

Clinical Case Study-10

A male patient aged 36 years is brought to the emergency department with a complaint of restlessness, sleepiness, irritability, tremors, abdominal cramping, bone pains, diffuse muscle aching, nausea, rhinorrhea, diaphoresis, lacrimation, shivering, experiencing chills and cold flushes. He had a history of drug abuse for seeking pleasure euphoria and other feelings of personal satisfaction for many desires. As he could not get the drug as per his regular use, he had to cut short and abstain from the drug for the past few days. He had no other clinical history suggestive of panic attacks, use of benzodiazepines, and barbiturates.

1. From the presentation of the case what would be most possible diagnosis?
2. What are the opioids that can be misused?
3. If it were to be substance misuse of an opioid, what are the treatment guidelines?

Ans:

1. From the presentation of the case and the past history of the patient, a substance misuse of opioid usually in the form of heroin could be made out.
2. The opioids that could be misused include morphine, heroin, codeine, oxycodone, meperidine and fentanyl
3. Pharmacologic therapy for heroine addiction is focused on ameliorating withdrawal symptoms and reducing the cravings for the drug by replacing heroine with legally obtained opioid agonistslike methadone. Methadone is a long acting synthetic opioid agoinst that can be given once daily in doses of 10 – 20mg. It stabilizes the drug – abusing lifestyle, reduces criminal behaviors (if present and reported) and preventing the possible HIV transmission if the needles for use are exchanged between persons. Methadone is available at specialized methadone maintenance clinics which are legally approved for chronic misusers of heroine.

Buprenorphine is a μ - partial agonist that suppresses withdrawal symptoms and cravings similar to methadone. However, the property of partial agonism confers a "ceiling effect" at which higher doses of buprenorphine cause no additional benefits. This 'ceiling effect' affords a wider margin of safety than methadone, which can be lethal in overdose. Because of this safety profile, buprenorphine has a legal authorization for use for opioid withdrawal treatment.

Buprenorphine has been combined with naloxone in a 4:1 ratio to 6-7:1 ratio as sublingual or buccal film preparations in order to alleviate concerns that the injectable preparations might give rise to. Naloxone is an opioid antagonist.

Buprenorphine/Naloxone sublingual tablet formulation has higher bioavailability, a fast dissolve time, a small tablet size and a methanol flavor to encourage patient adherence with treatment. The drug combination is available as 2mg/0.5mg; 4mg/1mg; 8mg/2mg. The dosage is titrated according to a schedule starting with a dose of 4mg/1mg and gradually maintaining or increasing the dose in the next few days.

Clonidine and α^2 agonist that can effectively control the autonomic responses of opioid withdrawal such as nausea, vomiting, muscle cramps, sweating, tachycardia and hypertension.

Clinical Case Study-11

A 70 – year old man presents to the emergency department complaining of shortness of breath for the past 2 weeks. Earlier he used to walk everywhere, but now he becomes fatigued after a short stroll through a nearby shopping area. He also notes that he has felt his heart racing even when he is at rest. His past medical history is notable only for hypertension for which he takes amlodipine and frusemide. His blood pressure is 130/90 mm Hg, heart rate is 144 beats/minute, respiratory rate is 18/minute, oxygen saturation is 98% at room air and his body temperature is 37° C. His head and neck examination is unremarkable. His lungs are clear on auscultation. His heartbeat is irregular and rapid, without murmurs, rubs or gallops. He has no edema of the extremities or jugular venous distension but had a history of valvular heart disease which remained dormant for many years. Lab shows a normal CBC, normal electrolytes, BUN, creatinine, troponin and BNP. ECG showed an irregular tachycardia consistent with the diagnosis of atrial fibrillation (AF) with rapid ventricular response

1) What are the contributing factors or diseases associated with atrial fibrillation?
2) What are the treatment guidelines for acute and chronic management of atrial fibrillation?

Ans:

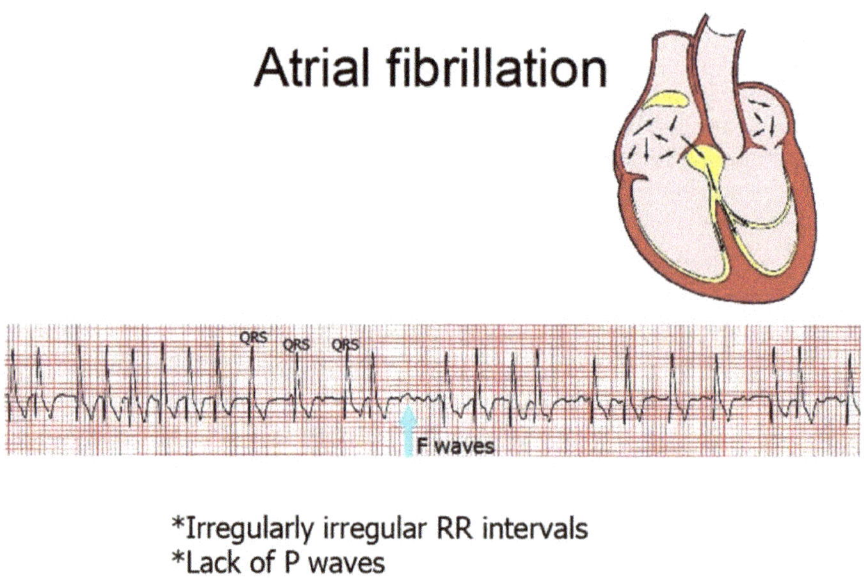

1) Contributing factors or diseases associated with AF include
   (a) CVS conditions like hypertension, coronary artery disease, cardiomyopathy, valvular heart disease, rheumatic heart disease, congenital heart disease, myocardial infarction, pericarditis;
   (b) Pulmonary conditions like pulmonary embolism, chronic obstructive pulmonary disease (COPD), obstructive sleep apnea
   (c) Systemic diseases like hyperthyroidism, metabolic syndrome
   (d) Postoperative conditions – cardiac surgery or any surgery.

2) The immediate task while treating this patient is to ensure cardiac rate control and or rhythm control, with or without anticoagulation. In the acute setting such as in the emergency department, ventricular rate control is the single most important goal of therapy. Slowing the ventricular response to AF has a number of positive hemodynamic effects including increasing diastolic filling time, improving stroke volume and cardiac output, and stabilizing blood pressure.

   In hemodynamically stable patients rate control can be achieved by

   1. Calcium channel blockers (verapamil, diltiazem). Diltiazem carries the lowest risk of hypotension because it has lesser vasodilatory effect compared to verapamil and also has least negative inotropic effect.
   2. β – blockers (metoprolol, atenolol) have more negative inotropic effect than diltiazem and carry a greater risk for hypotension, particularly in patients with borderline low blood pressure or poor LV function.
   3. Amiodarone is less effective than the effective rate control agents such as calcium channel blockers and β – blockers. Amiodarone is more effective in rhythm control.
   4. Digoxin has a role in rate control in sedentary patients or those with chronic CHF. It has no role for an acute rate control in emergency settings.

      Patients who are hemodynamically unstable should get immediate electrical cardioversion. Cardioversion can also be achieved through the use of antiarrhythmic drugs like amiodarone, dofetilide, and ibutilide, but the adverse effects like ventricular tachycardia, torsade de pointes, hypotension, bradycardia for most of the drugs and hepatotoxicity, hyper/hypothyroidism with amiodarone must be born in mind.

      Amiodarone, dronedarone, and propafenone and vernakalant are the commonly preferred drugs used for rhythm control of AF and with associated hypertension, and enlarged left atrium, heart failure or AF of more than 1 year duration.

3) Thromboembolic risk reduction: Patients with AF have a two to threefold risk of stroke than the general population. The risk is the same for patients with paroxysmal, persistent or chronic AF.

   Anticoagulant therapy which is to be instituted in such patients consists of warfarin with INR goals between 2 and 3. The usual dose of warfarin is between 2 to 4 mg/day depending upon INR ratio. Dabigatran, a directly acting thrombin inhibitor inhibiting the conversion of fibrinogen to fibrin is superior to warfarin. It reduces the rate of ischemic and hemorrhagic strokes, major bleeding, and overall mortality compared to warfarin. It is more effective and safer than warfarin and does not require regular monitoring of PT/INR and also less susceptible to diet and drug interactions and does not have narrow therapeutic swindow unlike warfarin. The dosage is 150mg twice a day. It has antidotes now available as activated prothrombin complex concentrate (25-50 units/kg/IV and indarucizumab (5g/IV). The other anticoagulant that can be used for preventing thromboembolic risk is apixaban that can be given in twice daily doses of 5 mg.

Clinical Case Study-12

A 77 year old man presents in the casualty department with complaints of frequent dizziness on standing from a seated position. He has Type-2 diabetes, stable coronary artery disease, and a benign prostatic hyperplasia. His current medications are finasteride 5mg, doxazosin 2mg, atenolol 50mg taken in two daily doses., simvastatin 40mg /day, metformin 1000mg/day, and aspirin 75mg/day.

His current blood pressure reading is 120/80 mm Hg, and heart rate 65 beats/minute. After standing for one to two minutes, his blood pressure recorded is 100/60 mm Hg and heart rate72 beats/minute. Examination of the heart and lungs is normal. An ECG showed no abnormality.

Which one of the following changes in this patient's treatment regimen would be most appropriate?

- Initiate fludrocortisone
- Discontinue finasteride
- Increase salt and water intake
- Discontinue doxazosin
- Discontinue atenolol

Answer: Discontinue doxazosin

Case study:

The medication change that should be made for an older man with coronary disease, benign prostatic hyperplasia, and type 2 diabetes who has postural dizziness, and who is taking finasteride, doxazosin and atenolol is to discontinue doxazosin.

Discussion:

Alpha – I adrenergic antagonists, which relax smooth muscle in the prostate and bladder neck are often prescribed for patients with benign prostatic hyperplasia. However, orthostatic hypotension is a relatively common side effect with two such agents – doxazosin and terazosin. Several other $\alpha 1$ – blockers (tamsulosin, alfuzosin and silodosin) are more selective for prostate tissue and are thought to cause less orthostatic hypotension.

Finasteride reduces prostrate size by inhibiting 5-α reductase and thereby preventing the conversion of testosterone to the active dihydrotestosterone (DHT) which blocks its action on the prostrate. This drug does not cause orthostatic hypotension.

Beta blockers like atenolol may contribute to hypotension through negative ionotropy in patients with decompensated heart failure or by causing excessive bradycardia in patients with conduction defects. However, they do not cause orthostatic hypotension. Because this patient has diabetes, he is at increased risk for orthostatic hypotension secondary to autonomic dysfunction. Increasing salt and water intake does not facilitate sustained blood pressure and initiating synthetic mineralocorticoid fludrocortisone would be appropriate treatment for selected patients only with autonomic orthostatic hypotension. However, these treatments should be considered for this patient only if his orthostatic hypotension does not resolve with the discontinuation of doxazosin.

Clinical Case Study-12A

A 70 year old man visited a cardiologist for consultation after he underwent an angioplasty preceded by an acute attack of MI and currently asymptomatic. Prior to MI he was not receiving any medications. He is not a smoker nor a diabetic. As a follow up therapy he was put on metoprolol 100mg/day along with aspirin 75mg + clopidogrel 75mg and atorvastatin 20mg/day.

1. To which classes of drugs they belong?
2. Explain the rationale of using each drug?

Ans:

1. Metoprolol is a cardioselective β-blocker that acts exclusively on the myocardial β1 receptors. Aspirin and clopidogrel are antiplatelet drugs. Atorvastatin is a lipid lowering agent.
2. Metoprolol is extremely useful as a prophylactic antianginal drug in post MI cases. Though it does not have any coronary vasodilator actions or improved coronary perfusion, it normalizes or stabilizes hemodynamic functions when they are altered as seen during MI. Particularly they stabilize any enhanced sympathomimetic effects often seen during or after MI. Thus it decreases heart rate, blood pressure and contractility, all leading to a decrease in myocardial oxygen requirements both at rest and during exercise. It improves exercise tolerance and reduces the frequency, severity and duration of angina.

   Aspirin and clopidogrel are antiplatelet drugs and inhibit platelet aggregation and useful to prevent possible thrombus formation and reinfarction and reduce morbidity and mortality.

   Atorvastatin is a HMG-coA inhibitor and inhibits cholesterol synthesis and lower LDL-C levels. As high serum lipid levels play an important role in endothelial plaque formation along with platelets and other thrombus forming elements, it is essential to use drugs that lower the lipid levels and prevent any future thrombus formation subsequent to MI.

Clinical Case Study-13

A male patient aged 56 years reported at the department of medicine (in the outpatient department) with a complaint of cough with productive sputum and fever for the past 4 days. A day before his visit tothe hospital he developed pain the right chest which intensified with inspiration. He had a past history of smoking for longer periods

On physical examination he was found to be weak and underweight and continuously coughing. His vital signs are – blood pressure 150/90 mmHg, apical heart rate 112/minute and regular, respiratory rate 24/minute and somewhat labored, body temperature 102° F. Both the lungs are resonant by percussion with locations of dullness in the right mid – anterior and right mid -lateral lung fields. Bronchial breath sounds of dullness in the lung fields. The heart functions were found to be normal.

Laboratory findings were – WBC 17,000/mm^3, neutrophils 70% lymphocytes 15%, eosinophils 8% basophils 7%. X- ray chest PA view revealed acute pneumonia in the right middle lobe (labor pneumonia) as evidenced by the presence of features of pneumonic consolidation. The diagnosis is confirmed by the presence of Gram-Positive diplococci in a gram stained sputum specimen and the diagnosis is further confirmed by identification of streptococcus pneumonia in sputum culture.

1. What are the types of Pneumonia?
2. From the clinical presentation how do you assess the type of pneumonia?
3. What are the possible microorganisms that can cause pneumonia?
4. What are the antibiotics of choice for the treatment of pneumonia?

Ans: There ae mainly two types of Pneumonia

1. One is community acquired and the other is nosocomial, or hospital acquired.
2. From the clinical presentation of the case the type of pneumonia is a community acquired as there is no history of the patient being admitted to a hospital and exposure to the surroundings and equipment. Nosocomial pneumonia otherwise known as hospital acquired pneumonia results from a person getting admitted to a hospital and who develops the features of pneumonia 48 hours after admission. It is commonly acquired from the hospital surroundings including the form other infected persons. It is also likely to be contacted through assisted ventilation (ventilator use) and admission in ICUs.
3. Community – acquired pneumonia is caused by streptococcus pneumoniae, Haemphilus influenzae, Moraxella catarrhalis, staphylococcus group, Group – A streptococci and a typical organisms like Legionella, Mycoplasma, Chlamydia Pneumonia and C.Psittaci.

   Nosocomial Pneumonia is usually caused by Pseudomonas aeruginosa, Escherichia Coli, Klabsiella Pneumoniae, Enterobacter species, Enterobacter species and Grama Positive Cocci.
4. A person without any underlying comorbidities, Azithromycin 500mg orally/day or Doxycycline 100mg orally twice a day is the usual approach to treat a patient. If the age of the patient is over65 years, and an alcoholic or with associated conditions like malignancy, asplenia, chronic heart/lung/liver/kidney disease, diabetes mellitus, moxifloxacin 400mg once a day given orally is the usual practice. The other drugs that can be used is these patients include cefuroxime 500mg once a day or Amoxacillin/ 0.5 gram PO 8th

hourly, Azithromycin 500mg PO once a day or Doxycycline 100mg PO 12th hourly. Ceftriaxone 1 gram IV/day, moxifloxacin 400mg IV/once a day can be given if the patient is admitted in ICU. If Pseudomonas infection is present in ICU admitted patients Cefepine 1g IV once a day along with azithromycin or moxa floxacillin given either orally or IV.

Clinical Case Study-14

A 73 year – old woman reports 8 months of substernal chest discomfort that occurs while she is walking moderate briskness and climbing stairs. The discomfort radiates to her jaws and is associated with dyspnea. It resolves at rest or administration of sublingual nitroglycerine and has not increased in frequency. The patient has a history of hypertension, dyslipidemia stage 3, chronic kidney disease, and an inferior myocardial infarction 9 years ago and 8 months of substernal pain. An exercise stress echogram performed 3 months ago showed changes indicative of ischemia when the patient reached 96% of her predicted maximum heart rate. Cardiac catheterization with coronary angiography revealed an occluded right coronary artery, with robust collateralization from left coronary artery. The occluded vessel is not suitable for percutaneous coronary revascularization. Clinical recordings showed BP in the normal range with a decrease of heart rate at 56 beats per minute.

She is currently taking aspirin 75mg/day, lisinopril 40mg/day. Her lipid levels showed – Total cholesterol 122mg/dL; LDL cholesterol 68mg/dL; HDL cholesterol 42mg/dL; triglycerides 80mg/dL

Which one of the following management options is most appropriate for the patient?

1. Replace carvedilol with extended release metoprolol 100mg/day
2. Replace atorvastatin with oral rosuvastatin 40mg/day
3. Initiate oral extended release isosorbide mononitrate 30mg/day
4. Initiate oral clopidogrel with a single 600mg dose, followed by 75mg/day

Ans: In a patient with chronic stable angina (i.e. typical anginal systoms precipitated by exertion and relieved with rest or sublingual nitroglycerine), optimization of the antianginal regimen is the mainstay of therapy, especially if coronary revascularization is difficult. The addition of oral isosorbide mononitrate 30mg/day is the best approach.

Clopidogrel is appropriate in a patient with an acute coronary syndrome, aspirin intolerance or previous coronary intervention, but it has not been shown to benefit patients with chronic stable angina. Switching to another beta – blocker instead of carvedilol is unlikely to improve symptoms in a patient who is already on optimal doses. Because, the patient is already on a high dose of atorvastatin, switching from it to rosuvastatin is unwarranted.

Clinical Case Study-15

A 16 – year – old boy is brought to the emergency department (ED) by police after witnesses reported him being disruptive near a local amusement center. An acquaintance of the patient reported that he might have ingested "some pills" several hours ago.

The patient's heart rate is 134 beats per minute, and his blood pressure is 156/100mm Hg. His pupils appear dilated. Although he is safely restrained on the stretcher, he appears nervous and showed belligerent gestures at the ED staff.

What is the most appropriate next step for this patient?.

1. Administer naloxone.
2. Administer haloperidol
3. Administer a benzodiazepine
4. Administer flumazenil

Ans: Administer a benzodiazepine

Reasoning: The patient's presentation is consistent with acute stimulant intoxication, which can cause physiological and psychiatric symptoms. Stimulants such as amphetamines, methylphenidate, 3 – 4 methylenedioxymethamphetamine (MDMA or **Ecstasy**) – act as sympathomimetics, and can cause tachycardia, hypertension, diaphoresis, and mydriasis. Increased availability of dopamine, norepinephrine, and serotonin can lead to psychiatric symptoms, such as visual and auditory hallucinations, paranoid delusions, agitation, and mania. Emergency management of these symptoms is necessary to prevent adverse consequences from the increased sympathetic drive, such as cardiac ischemia, stroke, pulmonary hypertension, acute heart failure, and renal failure. Treatment is also indicated in agitated patients who might harm themselves or others in their agitated state.

For agitation related to psychostimulant toxicity as present with this patient, benzodiazepines are strongly recommended. These agents will help alleviate the patient's elevated heart rate and blood pressure and also reduces his mental distress.

Naloxone is used to reverse an opioid overdose. This patient's presentation is not consistent with opioid overdose which manifests with miosis, sedation, and respiratory distress.

Antipsychotic drugs, such as haloperidol, should be used with greater caution in patients with a psychostimulant overdose because they can lower seizure threshold, precipitate cardiac arrhythmias, and impair heat loss.

Flumazenil, a benzodiazepine receptor antagonists, is used to treat benzodiazepine overdose. This patient does not present with symptoms of benzodiazepine intoxication, which would include altered mental status, sedation, and respiratory depression.

Clinical Case Study-16

A 52 year old man presented to the emergency department with severe right flank pain radiating to the right lower quadrant. The pain was insidious in onset, was constant, lasting 3 hours in duration and he had two episodes of emesis since its onset. He had no chest pain, dyspnoea, or bowel or bladder dysfunction. He had similar history two years back. His physical examination revealed no abnormality either abdominal or indigestion.

His blood pressure was 154/96, respiratory rate was 24/min, and body temperature at 99^0 F. A conventional radiograph (Kidney, ureter, bladder- KUB) revealed right ureteric calculus which was confirmed by enhanced CT scan.

1) What is the clinical presentation of the patient?
2) What are the drugs that can be used to provide relief from the acute severe pain?
3) What are the other drugs that could be useful and to supplement the analgesics used?
4) What are the other lines of treatment for recurrent episodes of urolithiasis?
5) What are the other causes of acute abdominal pain?

Ans:

1) It is a case of urolithiasis (calculus in renal tract). It occurs due to obstruction of the urinary flow by a kidney stone, increased pressure on the urinary tract wall, smooth muscle spasm of ureter, oedema, and inflammation near the stone. There would be sudden onset of severe loin pain (in the costovertebral angle, lateral to sacrospinous muscle, and beneath the 12th rib). Pain radiation or referred pain or migratory pain occurs due to passage of the stone along the ureter which may radiate to flank, groin, testis or labia majora.

   Tension in the renal pelvis leads to stimulation, synthesis of prostaglandins, which induce diuresis, and vasodilation which in turn increase intrarenal pressure. Release of prostaglandins cause ureteric smooth muscle spasm. The renal stones may be made up of urate, calcium, or cysteine crystals. Usually nausea and vomiting are present in an acute condition of renal colic.

2) The drugs that could provide relief from severe pain include Nonsteroidal anti-inflammatory drugs (NSAIDS) like diclofenac 75mg/3lL IM, Ketorolac 15-30 mg IV, acetaminophen 500mg/50 mL solution or ketoprofen 100 mg+ hyoscine butyl bromide 10 mg given as rectal suppository
3) The drugs that could be used to supplement the analgesics include morphine 0.1mg/kg IV or hydromorphone 0.02 mg/kg IV, Hyoscine butyl bromide (Buscopan) 20 mg as slow IV injection to relieve the spasm, and drotaverine (papavarine derivative) 40mgIV for the relief of spasm. Hyoscine and drotaverine can be used as antispasmodic drugs in hepatobiliary, GI colic conditions, irritable bowel syndrome, menstrual cramps and for shortening of duration of labor in primigravida whose labor is prolonged
4) The other lines of treatment for urolithiasis include extracorporeal shockwave lithotripsy
5) The other causes for acute abdomen include biliary colic, diverticulitis, appendicitis, pelvic inflammatory disease, ruptured ectopic pregnancy, ovarian disease, pepti ulcer disease, pancreatitis, diabetic ketoacidosis, gastroenteritis, splenic rupture, irritable bowel disease, and abdominal aortic aneurism (rupture)

1

Venous Thromboembolism (VTE)

-

Overview: Venous thromboembolism (VTE) encompasses deep vein thrombosis (DVT) and pulmonary embolism (PE). An embolus is any intravascular material that migrates from its original location to occlude a distal vessel. Although the embolus can be blood clot (thrombus), fat, air, amniotic fluid, or tumor, a PE is usually caused by a thrombus originating from the deep veins in the legs (deep vein thrombosis, DVT).

The coagulation cascade is an essential part of haemostasis. However, the same coagulation factors can give rise to clot formation in the circulation that is inappropriate (not for haemostasis). Thrombi can be formed in both the arteries and veins but they have different pathophysiology and lead to different outcomes. The following differences can be made out between arterial thrombosis and venous thrombosis.

	Arterial Thrombosis	**Venous thrombosis**
Mechanism	Typically from rupture of atherosclerotic plaque	Typically from combination offactors from Virchow's triad (endothelial damage, hypercoagulability, and statis)
Location	Left heart chambers, arteries	Venous sinusoids of muscle andvalves in veins
Diseases	Acute coronary syndrome (MI, unstable angina), Ischemic stroke, Limb claudication/ischemia	Deep vein thrombosis (DVT)Pulmonary embolism (PE)
Composition	Mainly platelets	Mainly fibrin
Treatment	Mainly antiplatelet drugs (ASA, clopidogrel and others)	Mainly anticoagulants (heparins,oral anticoagulants)

Etiology of Venous Thromboembolism

1) Endothelial damage (Surgery, caesarean section, catheter picc lines (peripherally inserted central catheter lines), trauma)
2) Endothelial dysfunction (smoking, hypertension)
3) Hypercoagulability
   (a) Hereditary (genetic origin due to mutations – Factor V Laden, prothrombin G20210A, Protein C and protein S)
   (b) Acquired – cancer, chemotherapy, oral contraceptives, and hormone replacement,pregnancy, obesity, and heparin induced thrombocytopenia
4) Stasis—Reduced mobility, polycythemia leading to endothelial injury

Some important risk factors for Deep vein thrombosis

1) **Reduced blood flow:** Immobility (Bed rest, general anesthesia, stroke, long flights)
2) **Increased venous pressure:** Mechanical compression or functional impairment leading to reduced blood flow in the veins (neoplasm, pregnancy, stenosis or congenital anomaly which increases outflow resistance)
3) **Mechanical injury to the vein:** Trauma, Surgery, IV drug abuse, Peripherally inserted catheters
4) **Increased blood viscosity:** Polycythemia rubra vera, thrombocytosis or dehydration

Clinical features of DVT

The clinical features of DVT may be due to venous obstruction and/or inflammation of the veins

Symptoms	Signs	Mechanism
Asymmetric Leg/ Calf swelling	Pitting edema onthe affected side	Swelling and pitting edema caused by venous obstruction. Normal difference between the two legs should be less than 1cm; greater than 3cm difference is considered significant
Pain, erythema	Localized tenderness along deep venous system	Pain, erythema, and tenderness are caused by vascular inflammation. Recruitment of inflammatory cells to thrombus, and venous stasis causes phlebitis
Dilated superficial veins (non – varicose)	Palpable cord	Dilated superficial veins are caused by obstruction of deep venous system. Palpable cord refers to superficial veins, which is a sign of superficial phlebitis

Clinical features of PE

Symptoms	Signs	Mechanism
Dyspnea	Tachypnea, decreased air entry,localized rales, wheezing	Hyperventilation to compensate for increases in dead space and in response to chemical mediators from platelets
	Parasternal heave,loud P2 and increased jugular venous pressure(JVP)	Increased pulmonary pressure (from vaso-constriction) causes right ventricular overload (loud P2) and right ventricular dilation (Parasternal heave), Right – sided heart failure causes increased JVP (jugular venous pressure) and eventually left - sided heart failure (tachycardia)
Palpitation	Tachycardia	As above
Pleuritic chestpain	Pleural friction rub,signs of plural effusion	Ischemia to the region, inflammation, increased vascular permeability
Hemoptysis and cough		PE causes damage to the pulmonary vasculature, which leads to bleeding into the airways. Cough is usually non-productive and may be triggered by irritation of the pleura or the airways

Treatment of venous thromboembolism

Anticoagulants: Anticoagulants are the first line drugs for the treatment of deep vein thrombosis.Typically, one of the parenteral agents are initiated for the early reversal of the symptoms followed by oral anticoagulants for the chronic use for a period of 3 months.

(I) Anticoagulants that can be used include

A) Unfractionated and low molecular weight heparins

B) Synthetic heparin derivative – Fondaparinux

C) Oral anticoagulants

1) Parenteral anticoagulants – Heparin, low molecular weight heparins like endoxapanin, dalteparin, tinzaparin, nadroparin

2) Oral anticoagulants:

a. Dabigatron (directly acting thrombin inhibitor)

b. Rivaroxabarin, Apixaban, Edoxaban, Betriaxaban (Factor Xa inhibitors)

3) Warfarin (Vitamin k antagonist) has been the mainstay of chronic VTE therapy for a long time. It has been replaced with newer oral anticoagulants like Rivaroxaban, apixaban and others because warfarin therapy requires regular monitoring of PT INR levels, apart from its drug interactions, bleeding risk and teratogenic effects when used in pregnancy.

(II) Thrombolytic agents like tissue plasminogen activator can also be used in an acute set up or early phase of venous thromboembolism.

2

Obesity, the Global Threat to Body Systems

Overview

Obesity is one of the most common preventable diseases. Obesity has a multifactoral etiology that includes genetic, environmental, socioeconomic, and behavioral or psychological influences. **Obesity is typically defined as a substantial accumulation of body fat for a given height and is associated with increased risk of numerous chronic diseases including type 2 diabetes (T^2D), hypertension, and cardiovascular disease (CVD)**. Body – mass index (BMI – weight in Kg/ height in **m^2**) is the most widely used formula to define overweight and obesity. For an individual, obesity is usually the result of an imbalance between calories consumed and calories expended. An increased consumption of high calorie foods, without an equal increase in physical activity leads to an increase of body weight.

Criteria for categorization of obesity and possible disease risk (relative to normal weight and waist circumference)

	Body mass index	Obesity class	Disease risk (relative to normal weight and waist circumference)	
			Men<40 inches (102 cm) Women<34 inches (88cm)	Men>40 inches Women>34 inches
Underweight	<18.5			
Normal	18.5 – 24.9			
Over weight	25.0 – 29.9		Increased	High
Obesity	30.0 – 34.9	1	High	Very high
	35 -39.4	2	Very High	Very high
Extreme obesity	>40.0	3	Extremely high	Extremely high

Obesity – Role in clinical conditions

Excessive body weight has a strong link to many disease conditions, particularly **cardiovascular diseases, type 2 diabetes mellitus**, **obstructive sleep apnea,** and **asthma, certain malignancies, osteoarthritis,** and thereby found to reduce life expectancy. Obesity is one of the leading preventable causes of death. It is also found that the mortality is lowest at a BMI of 20 – 24 Kg/**m^2** and less in non-smokers and 24-27 Kg/**m^2** in current smokers. On average, obesity reduces life – expectancy by six to seven years.

Morbidity

Obesity increases the risk of many physical and mental conditions. Obesity is associated with and the leading cause of metabolic syndrome, a combination of medical disorders which include TD2, high blood pressure, high cholesterol and high triglycerides levels. It has also been found that obese people are at a greater risk of developing extended COVID complications. Sedentary life style and obesity are strongly related toTD_2 and complications.

Health consequences of obesity

They fall into two categories – those attributable to increased fat mass such as osteoarthritis, obstructive sleep apnea and those due to increased number of adipocytes such as present in TD2 , malignancy, CV disease, non – alcoholic fatty liver disease, metabolic syndrome, and in conditions associated with proinflammatory and prothrombotic states.

The following table gives the obesity associated morbid conditions.

Medical Speciality	Condition
Cardiology	• **Coronary artery disease, angina, MI** • **Congestive heart failure** • **High blood pressure** • **High cholesterol** • **Deep vein thrombosis** • **Pulmonary embolism**
Endocrinology and reproductive medicine	• **Diabetes mellitus - Type 2** • **Polycystic ovarian syndrome** • **Menstrual disorders** • **Infertility** • **Complications during pregnancy** • **Birth defects** • **Intrauterine fetal death**
Neurology	• **Stroke** • **Migraine** • **Dementia** • **Multiple sclerosis** • **Carpal tunnel syndrome**
Respiratory	• **Obstructive sleep apnea** • **Asthma** • **Increased respiratory risk due to COVID**
Rheumatology and orthopedics	• **Gout** • **Osteoarthritis** • **Low back pain**
Urology and nephrology	• **Erectile dysfunction** • **Urinary incontinence** • **Chronic renal failure** • **Hypogonadism**
Gastroenterology	**GERD** • **Fatty liver disease** • **Cholelithiasis**

Table *Contd...*

Medical Speciality	Condition
Oncology (Malignancies)	• **Esophageal** • **Colorectal** • **Pancreatic** • **Gall Bladder** • **Endometrial** • **Hepatocellular** • **Renal**

Pathophysiology of obesity

Body weight is mainly influenced by the appetite of a person (the desire to eat) and satiety (the sensation of fullness). Many signaling molecules and hormones control appetite and satiety in the cellular, peripheral and central nervous systems. There is a genetic component in the causation of obesity. Body weight is determined by energy balance, that is the balance regulated by energy intake and the energy expenditure. If the intake and expenditure are balanced the body weight remains at the desired levels. If the intake overtakes than the expenditure, weight increases accordingly. Hypothalamus is the master regulator of energy homeostasis. Hypothalamus contains hormone-and nutrient-sensing nuclei that organize central and peripheral responses for maintaining normal body weight, food intake, energy expenditure, and nutrient partitioning.

Hunger and satiety signals that regulate eating behavior in the human body

Peripheral signals are generated by peripheral systems such as gut, fat tissue, the liver and the pancreas. These signals are relayed to the CNS through the peripheral nervous system to stimulate or suppress the **hunger center or satiety center in the hypothalamus**. There are two signals episodic and tonic as shown below

	Peripheral system		**Central nervous system**
Types	**Episodic (*meal to meal*)**	**Tonic (Days and weeks)**	
Hunger signals	**Ghrelin** Stimulates appetite, Increase body weight	Progesterone	AgRP, NeuropeptideY, MCH, orexins, Endocannabinoids, β – endorphin, Dynorphin, galanin
Satiety signals	Cholecystokinin, **GLP – 1** PYY, amylin, obestatin, enterostatin	Leptin, estrogens	Melanocortins, Serotonin (5 – HT), Norepinephrine, Dopamine

AgRP- Agouti-related peptide/protein synthesized in Neuropeptide-Y increases appetite and decreases energy

MCH- Melanin concentrating hormone regulates feeding behavior

Obesity and inflammatory markers

Obesity is also referred to as chronic – low grade inflammation or "metabolic inflammation" which is often the focus in the pathogenesis of several diseases such as coronary artery disease, atherosclerosis, and insulin resistance. Obesity is strongly associated with increased adiposity and increases storage of adipocytes at many areas in the body particularly visceral areas (***Visceral adiposity***). Adiposites produce and secrete several proteins called *adipokines which play important role in inflammation.* These adipokines include TNFα , leption, resistin, visfanin, IL – 6, and adiponectin. There are anti – inflammatory adipokines which include transforming growth factor – beta (TGF), IL – 4, IL - 10, IL – 13, IL – 1 receptor antagonist (IL – 1Rα). An imbalance between inflammatory and anti-inflammatory adipokines results in increased accumulation of adipocytes and fat accumulation.

The pathogenesis of obesity can be explained by the following flow chart.

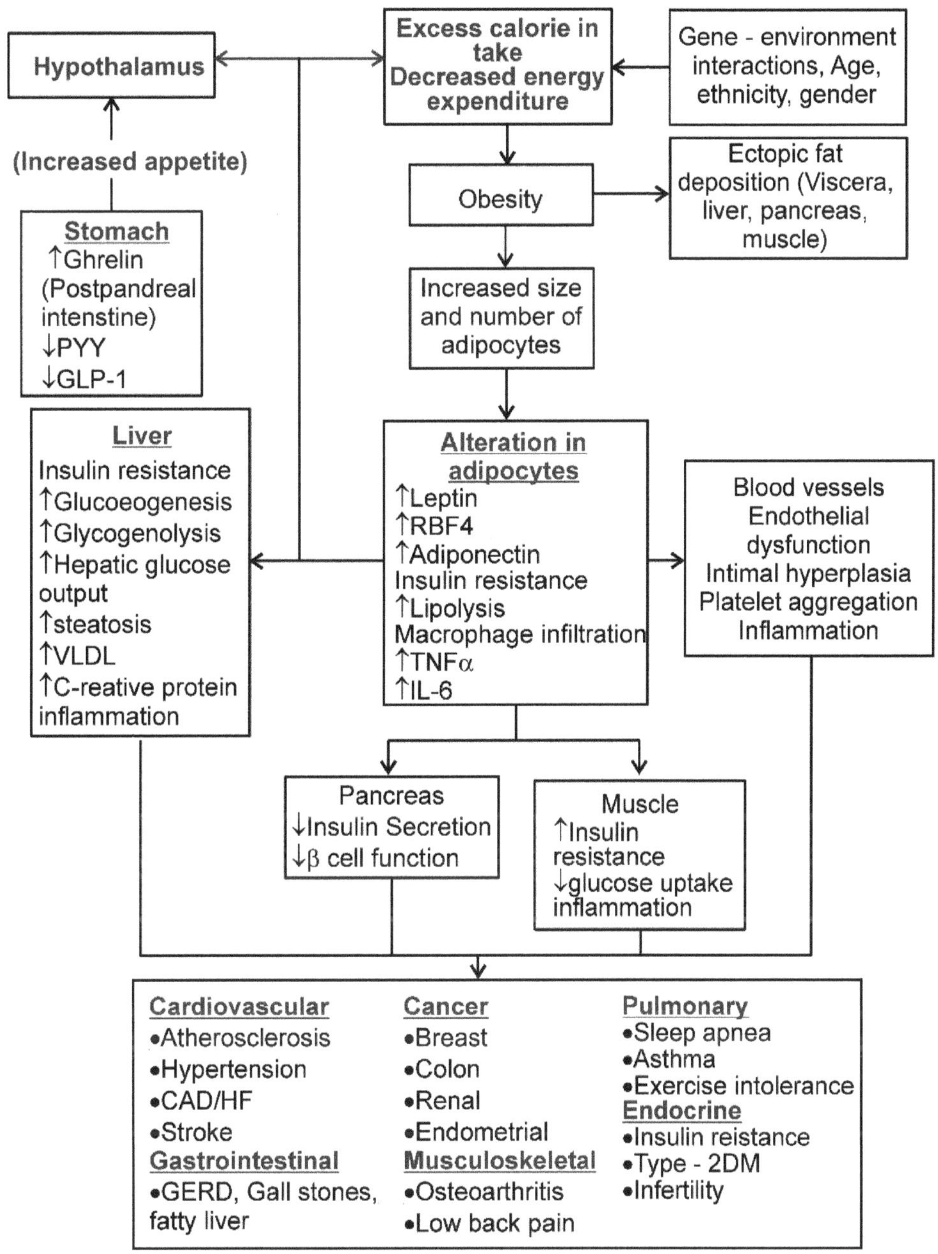

Management and treatment guidelines of obesity

Weight loss should be recommended for all patients with obesity and also for overweight patients with comorbid conditions such as prediabetes, diabetes, hypertension, and dyslipidemia. For most patients who need to lose weight for medical reasons, the initial goal should be 5% - 10% weight loss over the first six months. A common theme of various professional guidelines developed in many countries is the emphasis on a **multimodal lifestyle intervention that includes dietary changes, increase in physical activity, and behavioral modification**. Pharmacotherapy, medical devices and bariatric surgery are other treatment options for patients needing additional interventions particularly as there is likely worsening of the comorbid conditions related to obesity over a period. **At present the overweight or obesity are diagnosed more on the basis of BMI and waist circumference, but not based on any biomarker that is specific to the condition.**

Lifestyle interventions

To successfully achieve clinically meaningful weight loss of 5 – 10%, a comprehensive intense lifestyle intervention is needed that includes at least 14 – in – person sessions within 6 months. Effective weight loss interventions, which include dietary modification with the help of prescription of a calorie – reduced diet, increased exercise or physical activity, and behavioral strategies to foster adherence to dietary and physical activity recommendations, can be delivered by motivational guidance from individuals or through group sessions. This approach is needed for both immediate and long term goals. Weight loss of 5 – 10% results in improvement in cardiometabolic risk factors and also the needs for any modification in the treatment strategies to treat cardiovascular and metabolic disease conditions.

Mediterranean diets have been found to protect against CV disease. Mediterranean diet includes plenty of fruits, vegetables, nuts, legumes, whole grains, fish (salmon, sardine, shrimp, mackerel), yogurt, milk, eggs, olive oil, avocados and avocado oil. The foods that need to be curtailed include red meat, trans fats, refined oils, fast food, added sugar in beverages and soft drinks.

Pharmacotherapy

Pharmacotherapy should be considered for patients with a BMI of ≥ 30 kg/m^2 and ≥27 kg/m^2 with weight – related comorbidities such as T2D and those who failed to respond to lifestyle modifications and dietary control.

The following drugs approved for the use in the pharmacotherapy of obesity

1. Lorcaserin is a serotonergic drug with selective antagonism for 5-HT2**c** receptors. It has produced onlyless than 5% weight loss over a period of 12 weeks. Though it is well tolerated, it has low efficacy.
2. Phentermine + Topiramate Of all the anti-obesity drugs, this combination of drugs has yielded a weight loss of 8.6% at the end of one year treatment. Combination consists of 15mg of phentermine and 92mg of topiramate. Paresthesia is the most common adverse effect produced by the drug combination. As topiramate is a teratogenic drug, it is contraindicated during pregnancy.
3. Naltrexone + Bupropion it is combination drug of naltrexone (32mg) and buproprion (360mg) and given orally once daily. It has yielded a weight loss of 3.3% - 4.8%.
4. Diethylpropion is a CNS stimulant similar to amphetamine. It causes appetite suppression and is used together with diet restriction and exercise to treat obesity in those who have a BMI of at least 30Kg/m^{2}and given after diet and exercise have been tried without success. It is indicated for monotherapy only and treatment should be continued only if the patient has satisfactory weight loss within the first 4 weeks of treatment, (a weight loss of least 2.5kg.) It is used in the management of exogenous obesity as a short – term adjuvant (a few weeks) on a regimen of weight reduction based on diet restriction and physical exercise. The immediate release preparation is available as 25 mg tablet taken 3 times a day 1 hour before meals.

   The controlled release 75 mg tablet is taken once a day. It is likely to produce many CNS stimulant effects similar to amphetamine.
5. Liraglutide is a glucagon – like peptide 1 receptor agonist which is in use to treat diabetes mellitus for some years and is also found to be effective to reduce body weight and being prescribed for obesity. It is recommended for use in patients of obesity with BMI of 30kg/m^2 or more or 27kg/m^2 or higher who have at least one weight related comorbid condition like hypertension, dyslipidemia, insulin resistance, type – 2 DM. The dose of liraglutide for obesity is 3mg/day given subcutaneously (SC) in contrast to 1.2 – 1.8mg given for T2DM.

6. Semaglutide is also a GLP – 1 receptor agonist and approved for the treatment of chronic weight management in adults. As with liraglutide it is recommended for use in patients of BMI of 30 kg/m^2 or more or 27kg/m^2 or higher in persons of obesity with associated comorbid conditions. It is given as a once weekly SC injection in a dose of 0.25mg to begin with and increased up to 2.4mg once weekly over 16 weeks. It is better tolerated with few GI side effects like nausea, vomiting and diarrhea.
7. Tirzepatide is a dual glucose – dependent insulotropic polypeptide (*GIP)* and glucagon – like peptidel *(GLP – 1*) agonist. It is a promising weight loss drug effective to treat obesity regardless of BMI, age, and of obesity – related complications. It is given subcutaneously in gradual incremental doses of 5mg, 10mg and 15mg once weekly. It is an effective weight loss medication independent of associated T2DM.

3

Calcium Channel Blockers- Some Perspectives

Overview

Calcium channel blockers are a group of drugs that are used in a wide variety of clinical conditions like hypertension, cardiac arrhythmias, peripheral vascular disorders, prophylaxis of migraine, vestibular disturbances and preterm labor. Their efficacy as far as the use in cardiovascular conditions is concerned is more or less similar to β- adrenergic blockers, though they act by different mechanisms.

Calcium channels and their location

A calcium channel is an ion channel which shows selective permeability to calcium ions. Calcium channels are predominantly voltage-gated channels though there are ligand-gated channels (with formation of second messenger **IP3**) and receptor-operated calcium channels which facilitate Ca^{2+} entry intracellularly.

Voltage-gated calcium channels

Type	Voltage	Location
L – Type	High voltage – activated	Cardiac myocytes, pacemaker, vascular smooth muscle
T – Type	Low voltage – activated	Thalamic relay neurons, cells that have pacemaker activity in the central neurons system
N – Type	High voltage – activated	Throughout the brain and peripheral neurons system
R – Type (Residual)	Intermediate voltage-gated	Cerebellum
P – Type	High voltage-gated	Cerebellum

Ligand-gated calcium channels

Type	Gated by	Function
IP3 receptor	IP3	Releases calcium from endoplasmic/ sarcoplasmic reticulum in response to IP3
Ranodinereceptor	Gated by dihydropyridine receptors in T – tubules and increased intracellular Ca^{+}	Release of calcium from the endo-plasmic/sarcoplasmic endothelium

Classification of calcium channel blockers

Chemical classification

1	Dihydropyridines	Nifedipine, Nimodipine, Amlodipine, Felodipine, Nicardipine, Nitrendipine,Isradipine, Lercandipine, Clevidipine, Clinidipine, Lacidipine, Cilnidipine.
2	Benzothiazepines	Diltiazem
3	Phenyl alkylamines	Verapamil
4	Diaryl aminopropylamine ether	Bepridil
5	Benzimidazole – substituted tetralines	Mibefradil

Classification of Calcium channel blockers according to duration of action

1. **Dihydropyridines**

i	Short acting	Nifedipine, Nicardipine, Nimodipine, Nicardipine(IV)
ii	Intermediate acting	Nisoldipine, Nitrendipine, Isradipine, Clinidipine
iii	Long acting (up to 24 hrs)	Amlodipine, Clevidipine, Lercandipine, Nicardipine ER;(twice daily doses) Nifedipine – gastrointestinal therapeutic system (GITS), Nifedipine-ER, Azelnidipine, lacidipine, levoamlodipine, cilnipidine,

2. **Non Dihydropyridines**

   Verapamil – IR, ER, SR

   Diltiazem – ER, SR

   Bepridil – Long acting

   IR – Immediate release;

   ER – Extended release;

   SR – Sustained release

Mechanism of action of calcium channel blockers

Calcium channel blockers (CCBs) inhibit the voltage-gated L-type of calcium channels (which require larger depolarizations) on cardiac myocytes, vascular smooth muscle cells and cells within SA and AV nodes preventing influx of extracellular calcium. CCBs act by either deforming the channels, inhibiting ion-control gating mechanisms, end/or interfering with the release of calcium from the sarcoplasmic / endoplasmic reticulum. Calcium flux via these channels serves for excitation – contraction coupling and the mobilized calcium combines with calmodulin, which in turn activates myosin light chain kinase that is followed by interaction between actin and myosin and formation of actomyosin which causes contraction of vascular smooth muscle. These cellular responses are blocked by calcium channel blockers. The overall response is relaxation of coronary and peripheral vasculature and also the inhibitory actions on cardiac myocytes and pace maker cells.

The calcium channel has three receptor binding sites. Verapamil blocks the phenyl alkylamine site and diltiazem, the benzothiazepine site and dihydropyridines bind to 1, 4 dihydropyridine site.

Classification of Calcium channel blockers according to their development

First generation: Verapamil, diltiazem, nifedipine

Second generation: Amlodipine, felodipine, isradipine, nicardipine, nimodipine and others)

Third generation: Clevidipine and lecardipine.

Fourth generation: Clinidipine

Each group shows predominant individual actions, though they share common properties. Thus, the actions of dihydropyridines are more on the smooth muscle vasculature, while diltiazem and verapamil have more actions on the cardiac pacemaker activity though they also have action on smooth muscle vasculature which is not prominent compared to dihydropyridines.

Pharmacological responses

Actions on the Cardiac cell and Pacemaker tissue

Calcium channel blockers (CCBs) prevent the entry of calcium into the cardiac pacemakers (SA node and AV node) and cardiac myosites there by causing decreased contractility of the heart that results in negative inotropic and chronotropic effects. There is further a decrease of conduction velocity which explains their use in cardiac arrhythmias. Dihydropyridines produce reflex sympathetic activity which is likely to nullify the negative inotropic effects that they cause, and also produce peripheral edema. In the cardiac muscle, CCBs account for the shortening of phase 2 (plateau) of the cardiac action potential.

In cardiac pacemaker tissue, CCBs are responsible for shortening /slowing of phase 0 of the pacemaker potential decreasing the pacemaker activity (SA and AV nodal activity).

Selectivity of calcium channel blockers for cardiovascular effects

a. Dihydropyridines have greater effects on the vascular smooth muscle compared to their effects on cardiac effects

b. All the dihydropyridines (DHPs) have the common mechanism of action with regard to a decrease of vascular resistance and causing fall of blood pressure. They also cause coronary vasodilatation increasing coronary blood flow and stand a better chance for treating angina than diltiazem or verapamil. DHPs are a better choice for treating hypertension and other vasculature related clinical conditions. Lacidipine, levoamlodipine, cilnipidine, clevidipine have high degree of selectivity of vascular smooth muscle and long acting with a half-life of 13-19 hours and given once daily doses

c. Nicardipine has selective action on the coronary blood vassals

d. Nimodipine has selective action on the cerebral blood vassals

e. Amlodipine produces lesser reflex sympathomimetic affects compared to other agents of the same class. Lacidipine does not produce reflex tachycardia

f. Diltiazem, verapamil have more selectivity for the cardiac muscle and hence produce negative inotropic, chronotropic and dromotropic (conduction velocity) effects more prominently than dihydropyridines. Hence they have become the drugs of choice for the treatment of cardiac arrhythmias. Their vascular selectivity is muchless than that of dihydropyridines.

General pharmacokinetic properties of calcium channel blockers

1. All the calcium channel blockers (CCBs) are given orally except clevidipine which is given IV. They are all well absorbed when given orally.
2. They have a relatively large volume of distribution and are highly proteinfound.
3. All the CCBs are highly lipid-soluble without exception
4. They undergo extensive hepatic metabolism, except clevidipine which is hydrolyzed by plasma esterases, giving it an extremely short half life (1-2 minutes)and hence given IV.

Clinical uses of Calcium channel blockers

1. **Hypertension:** Calcium channel blockers are the first line drugs for treating moderate to severe hypertension either alone or in combination with diuretics and β-blockers. In severe persistent hypertension, they can be combined with ACE inhibitors or angiotensin ii receptor blockers. Clevidipine is an injectable short acting dihydropyridine used in patients with hypertension, including perioperative hypertension, hypertensive emergencies or in situations where oral therapy is not feasible or desired. It is administered via continuous IV infusion and has a very quick onset of action and also a short duration of action allowing rapid dose titration.
2. **Variant angina / Prinzmetal angina / vasospastic angina:** Calcium channel blockers by virtue of their coronary vasodilatory action relieve the coronary spasm associated with this type of angina. Nicardipine, isradipine, are the drugs of choice in this category
3. **Exertional angina / post MI angina:** Calcium channel blockers by virtue of their antihypertensive effect, negative inotropic and chronotropic effects reduce myocardial oxygen demand and hence useful in the treatment of exertional angina. However there is a possibility of aggravation of angina due to reflex sympathetic activity by dihydropyridines. This is better managed by the co administration of β-blockers which antagonize the reflex sympathetic activities. However, diltiazem has become popular for the management of post myocardial infarction angina because of absence of reflex sympathetic activity with its use in non-Q wave myocardial infarction.
4. **Cardiac arrhythmias:** Verapamil and diltiazem are the drugs of choice in the control of supraventricular tachycardia and also to decrease ventricular responses in atrial fibrillation or flutter. This action is due to their action on SA and AV nodes resulting in the decrease of conduction velocity and other actions on pacemaker activity.
5. **Peripheral vascular disease / Raynaund's and Burger's diseases:** By causing peripheral vasodilatation calcium channel blockers are useful in peripheral vascular disorders like Raynaud's and Burger's diseases.
6. **Subarachnoid hemorrhages:** By producing cerebral vasodilatation, calcium channel blockers reduce cerebral congestion secondary to subarachnoid hemorrhage. Nimodipine is the drug of choice in this condition.
7. **Preterm labor:** Calcium channel blockers are useful in the treatment of preterm labor by virtue of their relaxant effect on the gravid uterus. Nifedipine is more specific for uterine relaxant effects than the rest.
8. **Prophylaxis of Migraine:** Calcium channel blockers are found to be as effective as β-blockers or clonidine in providing prophylaxis to abort possible attacks of migraine
9. **Vestibular disturbances:** Calcium channel blockers such as cinnarizine, flunarizine, verapamil, and nimodipine are useful in treating vestibular disturbances like vertigo and Menier's desease.
10. **Renal disorders:** Blood pressure control is effective in preventing the complications that are likely to occur or associated with cardiovascular disease and chronic kidney disease (CKD). Furthermore, lowering BP can slow the rate of renal disease progression. The GFR reduction rate slows down by a good BP control. Hence effective management of hypertension is essential for the management of CKD. Calcium channel blockers are frequently used in combination with RAAS inhibitors and diuretics for better therapeutic outcomes in patients with hypertension and CKD.

Some commonly used calcium channel blockers and their doses, indications and adverse effects

Verapamil	Arrhythmia (supraventricular), Atrial fibrillation, migraine, hypertension, angina	75–150 μg/kg/IV or 80–160 mg orally every 8 h	Hypotension, flushing, dizziness, bradycardia, and constipation
Diltiazem	Supraventricular tachycardia, sinus tachycardia, atrial tachycardia including atrial fibrillation	75–150 μg/kg/IV or 30–80 mg orally every 6–8 h	Bradycardia, hypotension, AV nodalconduction defects in the presence of β-adrenergic blockers
Nifedipine	Angina, hypertension, Raynaud's disease	3–10 μg/kg/IV or 20–40 mg orally every 8 h	Tachycardia, flushing, nausea, dizziness, ankle edema, hypotension
Nicardipine	Angina, hypertension, CCF	20–40 mg orally every 8 h	Edema, dizziness, flushing and fatigue
Isradipine	Hypertension	2.5–10 mg orally twice daily	Headache and fatigue
Felodipine	Hypertension, Raynaud's phenomenon, CCF	5–10 mg orally once daily	Headache and dizziness
Amlodipine	Hypertension, angina	5–10 mg orally once daily	Headache and edema
Nimodipine	Subarachnoid hemorrhage, migraine	40 mg orally every 4–6 h	Headache and diarrhea
Nisoldipine	Hypertension	20–40 mg orally once daily	Hypotension and dizziness
Nitrendipine	Investigational for angina, hypertension	20 mg orally once daily	Hypotension and dizziness
Bepridil	Angina, hypertension	5–10 mg orally once daily	Hypotension, dizziness and ankle edema
Mibefradil	Angina, hypertension	50 mg orally once daily	Hypotension, headache, dizziness, ankle edema and tachycardia
Lacidipine	Hypertension	2- 6 mg orally/day as single dose	Flushing, fatigue, ankle edema Flushing, dizziness, fatigue, headache,
Levoamlodipine	Hypertension	2.5- mg/ orally/day as single dose	Headache, palpitation, fatigue, ankle edema
Cilnipidine	Hypertension	5 mg once daily given orally	Hypotension, headache, ankle edema,

Contraindications of calcium channel blockers

Non- dihydropyridines are contraindicated in those with heart failure with reduced ejection fraction, second or third degree AV blockade, and sick sinus syndrome because they cause bradycardia, worsening of cardiac output, acute MI, and pulmonary congestion.

4

Menopausal Syndrome and Role of Hormone Replacement Therapy (HRT) and other Treatment Guidelines

Overview

Menopause by definition is the final menstrual period in a woman's reproductive life. It is a universal and irreversible part of the overall aging process as it involves a women's reproductive system. Menopause is diagnosed after 12 months of amenorrhea and is characterized by a myriad of symptoms. Hormonal changes and clinical symptoms occur over a period leading up to and immediately following menopause. This period is frequently termed the **climacteric or perimenopause (**transition phase before menopause**)** and the symptoms begin years before menopause. The average age of occurrence of menopause is 50 – 52 years. The symptoms can be hastened because of oophorectomy, hysterectomy, autoimmune disorders, use of chemotherapy and radiation therapy.

Clinical Findings

During the menopausal transition, physiological changes in responsiveness to gonadotropins and their secretions occur, with wide variations in hormone levels. Women often experience the following symptoms.

Hot flashes, night sweats, insomnia, weight gain and floating mood changes, irregular menstruation, depression, anxiety states, headache, feelings of tiredness, irritability, feelings of sadness, breast tenderness, vaginal dryness, reduced sex drive, dyspareunia, and physical changes like build-up of fat around waist, weight gain and changes in skin color occur.

Osteoporosis due to increased bone loss occurs in the late menopausal transition and continues for the first few years after menopause with a possibility of fractures of the bones which become fragile. There is an accelerated rise in plasma cholesterol, LDL cholesterol and triglycerides levels.

Menopausal Hormonal Therapy (MHT)

MHT is indicated in menopausal women when the expected benefits of treatment are anticipated to be greater than any possible adverse effects. MHT includes the use of conjugated equine estrogens, bazedoxifene (selective estrogen receptor modulator – SERM) and tibolone (an estrogen preparation having estrogenic, progestational and androgenic effects). MHT is the most effective treatment for vasomotor symptoms associated with menopause – related complaints such as joint and muscle pains, mood changes, sleep disturbances, CV risk, genitourinary complaints, irregular menstrual cycles, and bone loss.

Possible Mechanism of Action of MHT for the Relief of Vasomotor Symptoms

Recent research had showed that a chemical pathway involving Neurokinin- B and Neurokinin – 3 receptors involved in the development of hot flashes, where it interacts with the temperature controlling mechanisms in the brain. Neurokinin-B binds to the neurokinin B receptor to stimulate its effects. In postmenopausal women, estrogen deficiency increases neurokinin B, so that the pathway is overstimulated, leading to hot flashes and nocturnal sweats. Estrogen therapy prevents or reverses overstimulation of the pathway and thus prevents the vasomotor symptoms.

Reversal of Genitourinary Changes and Symptoms

MHT is effective in the treatment of vulvovaginal atrophy (VVA), now considered as a component part of genitourinary syndrome of menopause (GSM). Local low dose of estrogen therapy is preferred for women whose symptoms are limited to vaginal dryness or associated discomfort with intercourse or for the prevention of recurrent urinary tract infections. The hormone therapy (MHT) reverts vaginal tissue back to the premenopausal state.

Role of MHT in the Changes in the Bone and CV Risk

In terms of bones, the hormone therapy has been shown to significantly lower the risk of vertebral or other osteoporosis – related fractures in postmenopausal women. Estrogens inhibit bone resorption by a mechanism of decrease of interleukins that activate and promote survival of osteoclasts. But, hormone therapy alone by itself does not confer any benefit for the prevention and treatment of osteoporosis in postmenopausal women who require bisphonates, calcium preparations and Vitamin D to ensure a better treatment choice.

In terms of CV benefits it is known that in estrogen alone dosages, MHT may decrease the risk of MI and all – cause mortality when initiated early. These positive CV benefits are not evident in the estrogen – progesterone combination therapy. It works by lowering LDL levels, triglycerides and an increase of HDL levels. Estrogen replacement has a better beneficial effect in women with premature menopause.

Other Beneficial Effects

In body composition, MHT prevents accumulation of central and visceral adiposity. It improves glucose tolerance, lowers the risk of metabolic syndrome, and reduces the blood pressure. It significantly reduces the progression of subclinical atherosclerosis if started early in the menopause. MHT also improves cognition and mood changes associated with menopause.

Drugs used in Hormone Therapy (MHT)

1) Conjugated equine estrogen (CEE) Premarin 0.625 – 1.25mg/day or ethinyl estradiol 0.01 – 0.02mg/day is given for shorter periods if vasomotor symptoms like hot flashes and sleep disturbances are the main indications for replacement therapy. For women who have undergone hysterectomy, estrogen alone can be given 5 days per week or continuously, as progestins are not required to reduce the risk of endometrial hyperplasia and cancer. In women with intact uterus a combination of estrogen and progesterone is given when there is a risk of endometrial cancer or hyperplasia seen in early screening.
2) For long term control of features like osteoporosis, vaginal atrophy, and urogenital atrophy the replacement therapy is indicated. It consists of a fixed combination of 1mg estradiol and 5mg of dihydrogestirone given once daily. Addition of progestin to estrogen in long term therapy decreases the risk of endometrial hyperplasia and endometrial carcinoma which are the adverse effects of estrogens. The cyclic therapy consists of giving estrogen alone for the fifteen days followed by progesterone for the next 10 days. This combination is continued for 2 months followed by continuous therapy for further periods. This can reduce breakthrough bleeding.

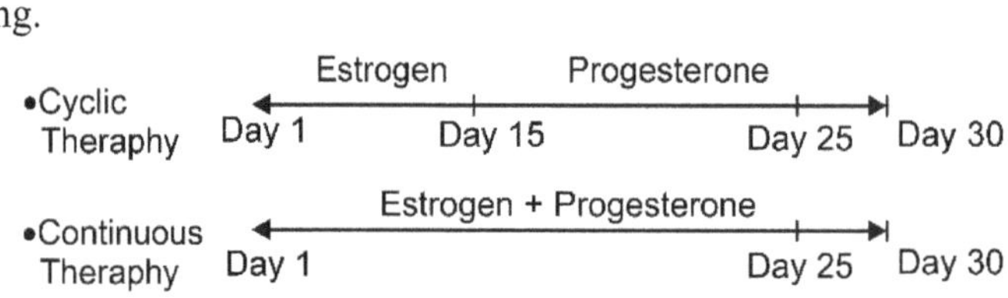

3) For the better control of symptoms on continuous basis addition of bazedoxifene 20mg/day is needed to the combination of estrogen and progesterone. **Bazedoxifene** is a 3rd generation selective estrogen receptor modulator (SERM) that increases bone mineral density and is approved for use in the prevention and treatment of osteoporosis in postmenopausal women. It prevents vertebral, hip, and long bone fractures. **Lasoxifene** 0.25 to 0.5mg/day and **arzoxifene** (20mg/day) are still the better SERMS which have a better choice since they reduce the incidence of breast cancer, and vertebral fractures in postmenopausal compared to bazedoxifene.

Tibolone

It is an estrogen preparation and found to be specifically effective in treating symptoms of menopause. ***It has estrogenic, progestational and androgenic effects*** beneficial to patients suffering from postmenopausal symptoms. It relieves estrogen withdrawal symptoms (vasomotor symptoms) such as hot flashes, sweating, insomnia, mood disturbances, headache, stress, impaired cognitive function, and vaginal dryness. Its positive progesterone effects include a reduction of endometrial thickening and subsequent bleeding. It obviates the necessity of using progesterone in post hysterectomy women for the control of postmenopausal symptoms. By virtue of its androgenic effects, it causes a sense of sexual wellbeing, elevated mood, and improves dyspareunia and libido. Tibolone also prevents bone loss and possibly **the combination therapy (estrogen and bazedoxifene + tibolone) is considered to be one of the best choices for the management of symptoms of menopause.**

Other Routes of Administration of Estrogens:

Estrogens can also be given as transdermal patches (estradiol) 0.075mg, 0.05mg or through vaginal route as 0.01% cream or 10mcg vaginal tablet insert in those who cannot tolerate oral administration. Through these two routes of administration, estrogens bypass the first pass metabolism thus offering increased bioavailability and reduced peripheral effects.

Adverse effects of Estrogens

The adverse effects of estrogens can be noted as early and delayed manifestations and vary according to the dose administered and duration of therapy.

Gastrointestinal symptoms include anorexia, nausea and vomiting, increased risk of cholesterol gall stones producing cholestatic jaundice.

Cardiovascular effects include thrombophlebitis and thromboembolism producing deep vein thrombosis (DVT), pulmonary embolism, venous thromboembolism (VTE). Increased risk of coronary heart disease is more evident in postmenopausal women in the age group of 60 years and above.

Uterine hyperplasia and uterine bleeding: Estrogens can produce endometrial hyperplasia with attendant enhanced risk of endometrial carcinoma. Uterine bleeding is the common manifestation of uterine hyperplasia which is usually regulated or prevented by the combination of estrogen with progesterone.

Salt and water retention can occur with the use of estrogens causing edema, increased premenstrual tension, and can aggravate migraine attacks.

Contraindications of Estrogens and Menopausal Hormone Replacement Therapy

Hormonal replacement therapy is contraindicated in women with underlying cardiovascular disease, history of earlier episodes of thromboembolism, hypercholesterolemia, stroke, gall bladder disease, breast cancer.

5

Septic Shock and Management Strategies

Overview

Septic shock is the severe form of sepsis occurring or originating from anywhere in the body which carries a high morbidity and mortality rates. In response to the inciting agent – a microorganism, the pro and antiinflammatory arms of immunity areactivated in concert with the activation of monocytes, macrophages and neutrophils that interact with the endothelium through pathogen recognition receptors to release cytokines, proteases, kinins, reactive oxygen species and nitric oxide. This leads to damage of the endothelium (**microvascular injury**) and also activates coagulation and complement cascades which further increase vascular injury, leading to capillary leak and capillary permeability that further lead to a decrease of peripheral vascular resistance and hypotension.

This cascade of events is responsible for the clinical signs and symptom of sepsis andprogression from sepsis to shock. It is the degree of responses shown by the proinflammatory cascade and the antiinflammatory signals set to control the overall inflammatory cascade that determines the progression of the condition with the resultant end effect. **Functionally, septic shock is defined by persistent hyportension despite fluid replacement.** A prompt and effective antimicrobial therapy provides better outcomes with reduced morbidity and mortality.

Etiology

Both the Gram positive and Gram-negative organisms (63%) are the responsive agents for the sepsis followed by septic shock. The most common organisms involved in the septic shock include ***Staphylococcus, Pseudomonas and Escherichia Coli.***

The source of the causative organism may be through a nosocomial infection or due to performance of more invasive procedures. The common sites of infection includerespiratory, bloodstream and genitourinary systems. Sepsis can also be caused by rupture of an intraabdominal or intrapelvic abscess, meningitis, head and neck infections, deep neck space infections, pyelonephritis, renal abscess, acute prostatitis/prostatic abscess, severe skin or skin structure infections, post-surgical infections or any systemic infections. Sepsis syndromes caused by multidrug – resistant bacterial strains (methicillin – resistant Staphylococcus – MRSA), vancomycin – resistant enterococci (VRE) are on the rise in the studies made (European prevalence of infection in intensive care (EPIC II study, 2009).

Risk factors that predispose to sepsis include diabetes, malignancy, chronic kidney disease, and liver disease; use of corticosteroids, immunodeficiency clinical conditions, burns, major surgery, trauma, long presence of indwelling catheters, prolonged hospitalization particularly in ICU, hemodialysis, and advanced age.

Clinical features and progression: The origin of the condition is one of generalised systemic inflammatory responses (SIRS) and ending in multiorgan failure before the fatality occurs.

The Earliest Signs of Inflammation Include

1. Fever (temperature higher than 38^0C) or hypothermia (less than 36^0C)
2. Tachycardia (heart rate more than 90 beats/minute)
3. Tachypnea (respiratory rate more than 20 breaths/min)
4. Leukocytosis and other laboratory findings of a typical septicemic shock (culture and sensitivity of the organism sourced from body fluids suspected to be the origin of the infection)

Complications

End organ failure is a major contributor to mortality in sepsis and septic shock. The complications with the greatest adverse effect on survival are acute respiratory distress syndrome (ARDS), acute kidney injury (renal failure) and disseminated intravascular coagulation (DIC).

Management

The initial lines of treatment of septic shock include initiation of empirical antimicrobial therapy until culture reports become available at which more specific antimicrobial agents could be used. In addition, supportive therapy is given aimed at maintaining organ perfusion and to provide respiratory support when necessary.

1. **Fluid replacement:** The landmark of septic shock is systemic vasodilatation with different levels of hypovolemia. Fluid replacement is the first line intervention to restore the hemodynamics and increase oxygen delivery to match oxygen demand in septic patients. In those patients an initial fluid load of 20-30 ml/Kg body weight (1.5-3 liters) is required which is mostly in the form of crystalloids (isotonic 0.9% sodium chloride, lactated Ringer's solution, 5% dextrose in water) and Ringer's solution. The reason behind administration of fluids to septic shock patients is based on the presence of vascular changes, namely vasodilatation resulting in hypovolemia attributable to the release of inflammatory mediators in the vascular endothelium. Fluid administration maintains perfusion pressure and blood flow to the tissues. Early fluid resuscitation can prevent or restore tissue hypoxemia and minimize the progression to cell and mitochondrial dysfunction and the establishment of multiple organ failure secondary to systemic inflammation and tissue hypoperfusion.
2. **Vasopressors:** Vasopressors should be initiated in patients of septicemia who do not respond to fluid resuscitation and while the status of sepsis continues. Vasopressors can be initiated and continued simultaneously with fluid resuscitation, especially in patientswith severe hypotension.

The aim of initiation of vasopressor use is to maintain a mean arterial pressure of 65mmof Hg.

a) **Noradrenaline:** Should be provided as the first-line vasopressor. Noradrenaline increases mean arterial pressure through vasoconstriction with little effect on heart rate, stroke volume, and cardiac output. The dosage may range from 0.2 to 1.5 mcg/Kg/min which can go up to 3.3mcg/Kg/min because of the down regulation of α-receptors in septicemic shock.

b) **Vasopressin**: Vasopressin induces vasoconstriction by acting on peripheral **(V_1)** receptors in the blood vessels. Additionally it inhibits the inflammatory cytokine interleukin which is released in response to trauma or infection and that produces vasodilatation due to release of endothelial nitric oxide. Vasopressin decreases nitric oxide-mediated vasodilatation, commonly present in septic shock. Very low doses of vasopressin (from 0.01 to 0.05 units/min) have been shown to improve mean arterial pressure.

c) **Terlipressin**: A long acting vasopressin **(V_1)** agonist is being used in doses of 1-2mg every 4-6 hours. This is indicated in common settings of septic shock refractory to catecholamine (noradrenaline) inducted vasoconstriction and a failure of reaching a target mean arterial pressure (65 mm Hg). Traditionally, terlipressin has been used as a drug of last choice.

Other vasopressors like adrenaline, dopamine, phenylephrine are not commonly used in septic shock as they are likely to produce tachycardia and arrhythmias.

1. **Antibiotics used in septic shock:**

   One of the foremost initial therapies is antibiotic coverage in a case of septic shock. Empiric therapy which is immediately provided should be comprehensive and should cover all the likely pathogens in the context of the clinical setting.

   1. The first choice of antibiotic coverage includes a **3rd or 4th generation cephalosporin** such as **cefotaxime** 1 to 2 g given IV/IM or **cefepime** 1g IV 6th hourly in combination with **vancomycin** 500mg IV every 12hours
   2. The second choice would be **vancomycin + ticarcillin/tazobactam** 3g 6th hourly IV
   3. The other combinations include
      a) **Cefepime + Metronidazole** (500mg IV – 6th hourly)
      b) **Ceftriaxone** (1g IV – 12th hourly) + **Clindamycin** (600-1200mg/day)
      c) **Imipenem – Cilastatin** is used for treatment for multiple organism infections in which other agents do not have wide – spectrum coverage or contraindicated because of their toxicity.

   Ultimately the choice of selection of a suitable antibiotic in septic shock depends on the probable site of infection responsible for sepsis apart from the likely organisms responsible for the cause of the same after the confirmation by laboratory tests

Conclusion

Septic shock is an emergency clinical condition that needs medical attention without delay. Prompt diagnosis and assessment is vital to proceed with the management which should restore the vital functions as early as possible and before the end organ failure sets in which may cause fatality.

6

Phosphodiesterase Inhibitors

Overview

Phosphodiesterases are a diverse family of enzymes that play a key role in regulating cell functions by directly increasing the intracellular levels of cyclic adenosine monophosphate (c-AMP) and cyclic guanine monophosphate (c-GMP), both of which are "**second messengers**" that regulate the primary effects of hormones and neurotransmitters.

Phosphodiesterase inhibitors are a class of medicines used in the management and treatment of pulmonary arterial hypertension (PAH), benign prostatic hyperplasia (BPH), chronic pulmonary obstructive disease (COPD), erectile dysfunction (ED), acute decompensated heart failure (HF), psoriatic arthritis (PA), atopic dermatitis (AD) and neonatal apnea. Phosphodiesterase inhibitors owe their activity due to prevention of breakdown of cAMP and /or cMP followed by relaxation of the smooth muscle, and vasodilatoty and bronchodilatory effects.

Subtypes of phosphodiesterase

The super family of PDE enzymes is classified into 11 families, namely PDE 1 to PDE 11, the classification of which is mainly based on tissue distribution, pharmacological properties and substrate specificities. PDEs have different substrate specificities. Some are c-AMP selective hydrolases (PDE4 and 8); others are c-GMP – selective (PDE 5, 6 and 9). Others which hydrolyze both c-AMP and c-GMP (PDE1,2,3,10 and 11).

Mechanism of action

Phosphodiesterase inhibitors exert their effects on their targeted enzymes (PDE 3, PDE 4, PDE 5, and PDE 9) preventing degradation of c-AMP or c-GMP further increasing their levels in smooth muscle cells, causing relaxation and vasodilatory effect in the target tissue.

Class selectivity of PDE inhibitors and the resultant pharmacological effects:

1. **PDE3 – inhibitors** (cilostazol, dipyridamole, milrinone, amrinone, vesnarinone, enoximone) exert their effects by increasing c-AMP and c-GMP levels in myocardium, peripheral vasculature and platelets. This further causes positive inotropic effects in the myocardium by increasing the inward flux of calcium and also intracellular mobilization of Ca^{2+} from the sarcoplasmic reticulam. An increase of c-AMP and c-GMP cause relaxation of peripheral vasculature and increase the peripheral circulation and hence used in **peripheral arterial disease (PAD)(cilostazol).** In platelets, an increase of concentration of c-AMP leads to a decrease of platelet aggregation. Dipyridamole is an inhibitor of platelet phosphodiesterase increasing the formation of platelet c-AMP and thus **decreasing platelet aggregation**.
2. **PDE4 inhibitors** (Xanthines – Caffeine, theophylline, aprimilast, roflumilast, crisaborole) The c-AMP – specific PDE4 is highly expressed in the brain, cardiovascular tissues,smooth muscles, keratinocytes and immunocytes (including T cells, monocytes,macrophages, neutrophils, dendritic cells, eosinophils). The inhibition of PDE4 elevates intracellular level of c-AMP and subsequently modulate the inflammatory

responses and maintain immune balance. Hence PDE4 inhibitors find a place in the treatment of various inflammatory conditions such as **bronchial asthma, COPD, atopic dermatitis,inflammatory bowel disease, rheumatic arthritis, lupus, and neuro inflammation**.

3. **PDE 5 inhibitors:** (Sildenafil, vardenafil, avanafil, tadalafil)

   They block the breakdown of PDE5 and increase c-GMP levels in corpus cavernosum of penis and vasculature of the lung and are the drugs of choice to treat **erectile dysfunction and pulmonary hypertension.**

Clinical uses of phosphodiesterase inhibitors

1. **Erectile dysfunction** – Sildenafil, vardenafil, avanafil and tadalafil
2. **Benign prostatic hyperplasia** – Tadalafil
3. **Pulmonary artery hypertension** – Sildenafil, tadalafil
4. **Platelet aggregation** – Dipyridamole to prevent thrombosis in CVS diseases- Angina, post MI
5. **Intermittent claudication** in peripheral arterial disease – Cilostazol,pentoxyphylline
6. **Congestive heart failure** – Milrinone, Inamrinone, Vesnarinone, enoximone are used for short term treatment of decompensated congestive heart failure.
7. **COPD, bronchial asthma** – Caffeine, theophylline and its derivatives, Roflumilast, Ibudilast. Ibudilast exerts their actions by non-selective PDE inhibition of PDE3, PDE4, PDE10 and PDE11, decreasing nitric oxide production, and pro-inflammatory cytokine LTB_4. Caffeine exerts its effects on PDEs by non-selective inhibition of PDE1, PDE4 and PDE5, promoting c-AMP accumulation. Caffeine also inhibits adenosine and GABA receptors and enhances intracellular calcium release, improving and enhancing cognition, memory, energy fatigue and drowsiness.
8. **Thrombocytopenia** – Anagrelide is PDE3 inhibitor which decreases platelet count and platelet aggregation further preventing thrombotic complications in myeloproliferative disorder such as essential thrombocytopenia, polycythemia vera and chronic myeloid leukemia.
9. **Inflammatory diseases** – Roflumilast a PDE4 inhibitor has been in use to treat COPD and asthma. It is also approved for use to treat ulcerative colitis and other inflammatory bowel diseases (Crohn's disease). Apremilast has been approved for the treatment of psoriasis, psoriatic arthritis. Similarly Crisaborole has been approved for the treatment of atopic dermatitis. Rivamilast is being tried for the treatment of rheumatic arthritis, asthma, psoriasis and other inflammatory disorders.

Administration details of some PDE inhibitors in clinical conditions

1. Erectile dysfunction
   a) Sildenafil – 25-100mg/day orally (available as 25, 50, 100mg tablets)
   b) Vardenafil – 5-10mg/day orally (available as 2.5, 5, 10mg tablets)
   c) Tadalafil – 5-20mg/day orally (available as 2.5, 5, 10, 20mg tablets)
   d) Avanafil – 50mg to 200mg (available as 50, 100, 200mg tablets)
2. Benign prostatic hyperplasia (BPH) – Tadalafil – 5mg/day orally

   (available as 2.5, 5, 10mg tablets)
3. Pulmonary arterial hypertension (PAH) – Sildenafil – 20mg 3 times per day

   Tadalafil – 40mg/day

   Sildenafil is also available for IV

4. Psoriatic arthritis – Apremilast (oral tablets)

   Day 1 – 10mg/day; Day 2 – 10mg twice/day; Day 3 – 10mg twice/day;

   Day 4 – 20mg twice/day; Day 5 – 20mg in the morning and 30mg twice/day;Day 6 – 30mg twice/day.

5. Asthma and COPD — Aminophylline, an ethylenediamine derivative of theophylline is indicated for treatment of severe acute asthma not responding to treatment with bronchodilators, steroids, and magnesium. It can also be given for a case of COPD exacerbation with inadequate response to nebulizer therapy. The usual dose in either condition is 5mg/Kg given IV over a period of 20 minutes. A maintenance dose of 0.3 mg/Kg/ hour may be needed till the symptoms subside. But with the advent of powerful β2 agonists and anticholinergics the use of aminophylline is considered for severe acute cases only. Roflumilast – It is a long acting PDE-4 inhibitor that reduces inflammation produced by eosinophils, and neutrophils, airway remodeling and bronchoconstriction and useful to treat bronchial asthma and acute exacerbation of COPD associated with cough and sputum. It is given orally in a single dose of 500mcg/day

6. Peripheral artery disease

   Cilostazol – 100mg/day orally

   Pentoxyphylline – 400mg 3 times a day taken orally

7. Decompensated heart failure

   Milrinone – 50mcg/kg IV as bolus and 0.25 – 1mcg/kg/min as infusion Amrinone – 0.75mg/kg IV as bolus over 2-3 minutes followed by 5-10mcg/kg/min as infusion

   Vesnarinone – 60mg given orally once daily

8. Atopic dermatitis – Crisaborole 2% topical ointment

9. Premature apnea (Neonatal apena) – Caffeine citrate 10mg/ml to 20mg/mlgiven IV or orally (as solution) once a day.

10. Post-operative thromboembolic prophylaxis or post MI

    Preventing thrombosis – Dipyridamole – 75 to 100mg 4 times given orally a day.

11. Thrombocytopenia – Anagrelide 0.5 mg 4 times a day or 1 mg twice a day given orally.

7

Osteoporosis and some New Treatment Choices

Osteoporosis is defined by World Health organization (WHO) as a bone mineral density of 2.5 standard deviations or more below the peak bone mass (average of young, healthy adults) as measured by **dual – energy X – ray absorptiometry**. The term "**established osteoporosis**" includes the presence of a fragility fracture.

There are two forms of osteoporosis

1. Primary osteoporosis
   a. Type I – It is called as postmenopausal osteoporosis
   b. Type II – It is known as senile osteoporosis that occurs after the age of 75 years and is found in both men and women.
2. Secondary osteoporosis – This may arise at any age and can affect men and women equally. This results from chronic predisposing medical conditions or diseases or prolonged use of steroids for different clinical conditions such as rheumatoid arthritis, bronchial asthma, COPD, and men receiving androgen – deprivation therapy for prostate cancer. Malabsorption of calcium plays an important role in the cause of osteoporosis.

Normal bone structure

Histologically, the disorder is characterized by a decrease of cortical thickness and in the number and size of the trabeculae of the cancellous bone. Trabeculae are perforated and may be fractured, and trabecular connectivity reduced. Bones consist of a matrix of firm, resistant connective tissue containing mineral salts (hydroxyapatite crystals and amorphous calcium phosphate) and cells. The outer cortical area (80% of skeletal mass) referred to as compact bone, is dense and solid and covered by periosteum. It predominates in the vertebrae, epiphyses of long bones and the iliac crest. Trabecular bone (20% of skeletal mass) has a large surface area and is metabolically more active and more affected by factors that lead to bone loss. It predominates in vertebrae, epiphysis of long bones and in iliac crest.

Inside the trabecular bone lies the marrow cavity, the site of haematopoiesis. Bones possess a degree of elasticity and deformability. Osteoblastic activity causes bone formation and osteoclastic activity causes bone resorption and bone loss.

Clinical course

Osteoporosis means loss of bone per unit volume. The micro – architecture is increasingly destroyed, and bone becomes more porous and is less able to withstand stresses which may result in fractures. Bone atrophy can occur in all the bones but is more likely within the vertebrae, neck of the femur, wrist joint, and metatarsophalangeal joints. The vertebrae become flat, compressed and break which may result in kyphosis which makes the upper part of the body to bend forward.

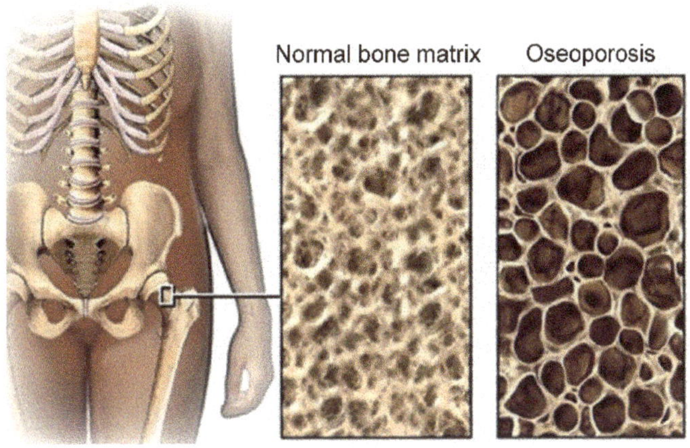

Pathogenesis -Bone remodelling

Bone morphogenesis and remodeling depend on the combined activities of osteoblast–mediated bone formation and osteoclast –mediated bone resorption.

The process is a dynamic one that occurs throughout the life of an individual. This mechanism not only protects the integrity of bones, but also makes the bones an adequate reservoir of calcium and phosphorous.

Three process of osteoblastic and osteoclastic activities results in bone remodeling

1. Initial stage of differentiation of osteoclastic precursor cells, activation of osteoclasts and bone resorption.
2. Osteoclast apoptosis occurs in the intermediate stage, and in the meantime, osteoblasts accumulate and differentiate to form new bone in the bone lacuna.
3. During the final stage, bone resorption overtakes the bone formation resulting in bone remodeling. An interplay between the bone resorption and bone formation is the ultimate cause of bone remodeling. The control and regulation of osteoclast activation and differentiation is achieved by a family of TNF receptor / TNF – like proteins – osteoprotegerin (OPG), the receptor activator NF – KB (RANK) and RANK ligand (RANKL). The activation of TNF receptor/TNF like proteins and NF – KB pathway leads to the expression of multiple inflammatory and innate genes. TNF – α activates NF – KB.

Risk factors: Risk factors for osteoporosis include nutritional deficiencies due to inadequate intake of calcium and vitamin D, genetic predisposition, chronic illness, and environmental factors that contribute to the changes in bone architecture and subsequent developments.

Women for example, have a greater genetic predisposition to develop osteoporosis as their bones are less dense even at the age of 20 or 30 years. Age related bone loss is more rapid in women, because bone mass is closely associated with hormone balance. The risk is high in postmenopausal women when estrogen protection is lost. Estrogens minimize or decrease bone resorption.

The other factors which can cause osteoporosis include alcoholism, chronic hepatic, or renal disease. Excessive acid intake in the form of high – protein diets may contribute to dissolution of bone. Acidosis directly increases osteoclastic activity. Prolonged use of heparin also potentiates bone loss. Immobilization for longer periods also contributes for bone loss. The conditions in which osteoporosis is a common feature are hypogonadism, hyperadrenocorticism, chronic glucocorticoid administration, hyperparathymidism, thyrotoxicosis, malabsorption, calcium deficiency and scurvy. Osteoclasts dissolve the minerals out of bony tissue and dissolve the connective tissue by enzymes, thus causing resorption. Osteoblasts replace the minerals and the connective tissue and facilitate bone formation.

Screening and diagnosis

The gold standard for diagnosing osteoporosis utilizes bone mineral density (BMD) measurements,especially in the hip and lumbar spine, the most common areas of osteoporosis with **dual – energy X – ray absorptiometry (DXA)** device or the occurrence of non-traumatic hip or vertebral fractures. Resulting T scores are used to interpret BMD and to correlate results with fracture risk.

T -Scores and WHO Diagnostic criteria for osteoporosis	
Normal	-1.0 or higher
Osteopenia	-1.0 to -2.5
Osteoporosis	-2.5 and lower
Severe osteoporosis	-2.5 and lower with one or more fragility fractures

Treatment of osteoporosis

The classes of drugs that can be used to treat osteoporosis include

1. Bisphosphonates - Alenronate, ibandronate, etidronate, zolendronic acid, pamidronate,tiludronate
2. Selective estrogen receptor modulators (Estorgen Agonists/Antagonists) - Raloxifene (**2nd** generation), ormeloxifene, toremifene, lasoxifene, arzoxifene, bazedoxifene (3rd generation)
3. Parathyroid analogues – Teriparatide, Abaloparatide, ostabolin
4. Calcitonin – calcitonin – salman nasal spray
5. Monoclonal antibodies – Denosumab, Romosuzamab

1. **Bisphosphonates:** Bisphosphonates bind with high affinity to hydroxyapatite crystals and inhibit osteoclast mediated bone resorption, leading to a decrease in bone turnover and a net gain in bone mass. They increase the bone mineral density and decrease the risk of fractures.

   For maximum gut absorption, all oral bisphosphonates should be taken with plenty of water in a sitting or standing posture because of their propensity to cause severe esophageal problems and to prevent oesophageal regurgitation. They are taken on empty stomach or at least 2 hours before or after meals as food retards their absorption (only 10% and further reduced in the presence of food).

   Bisphosphonates are available in multiple formulations. Alendronate, risedronate, and ibandronate are available as oral tablets. Zolendronic acid and ibandronate are available as IV preparations. The following table gives the preparations available, prophylactic dose, treatment doses of some commonly available bisphosphonates.

Bisphosphonate	Prophylactic dose	Therapeutic dose
Alendronate	5mg PO/dayOr 35mg PO once weekly	10mg PO/dayOr 70mg once weekly
Risedronate	5mg PO/dayOr 35mg once weekly	5mg PO/dayOr 35mg once weekly
Ibandronate	2.5mg PO/dayOr 150mg once weekly	2.5mg PO/dayOr 150mg once monthly or 3mg IV every 3 months
Zolendronic acid	5mg IV every2 years	5mg IV once yearly
Pamidronate	-	20mg IV/day given for 3 days

Adverse effects of bisphosphonates – GI disturbances including peptic ulcers, esophagitis (sometimes with erosions and strictures), osteonecrosis (zolendronic acid) of jaw, especially in patients with malignant disease.

Contraindications of bisphosphonates: Decreased renal function (creatinine clearance should be considered before administration), esophageal motility disorder and peptic ulcer disease being the main contraindications of bisphosphonates. The GI adverse effects can be overcome by the IV administration of pamidronate, zolendronate (zolendroic acid) and ibandronate.

2. **Selective estrogen receptor modulators**

   Raloxifene exhibits dual agonist and antagonistic properties in estrogen pathways. Being highly selective, raloxifene produces the desired estrogenic effects on bone and plasma lipids and without any major adverse effects on breast and uterus. Raloxifene increases bone mineral density (BMD) and prevents vertebral and long bone fractures. It is given orally in daily dose of 60mg.

   Bazedoxifene (20mg) and conjugated estrogens (0.45 mg) are given orally as combination therapy once daily for prevention of osteoporosis with an additional indication of treating vasomotor symptoms.

   Lasoxifene given orally in daily doses of 0.5mg for extended periods prevents the occurrence of fractures of femoral neck and spine and also found to be with reduced risk of developing breast cancer, coronary heart disease, and stroke.

3. **Parathyroid Analogues (PTH and fragments of PTH)**

   PTH and fragments of PTH given in small doses stimulate osteoblast activity and enhance bone formation and can be used selectively to treat osteoporosis in both males and females. **Teriparatide** is the main drug used for the purpose, particularly for the initial treatment of postmenopausal osteoporosis in those with prior fragility fractures or with high fracture risk and for those who are unable to take oral therapy. It is given in doses of 20mcg subcutaneously once daily. **Abaloparatide** is the second recombinant human PTA analogue indicated in women postmenopausal osteoporosis at high risk for fractures and given in doses of 80 mcg subcutaneously once daily into the periumbilical region of abdomen. The duration of therapy is for 2 years. **Ostabolin,** another peptide analogue, is also useful in osteoporosis and it increase bone mass with less effect on bone resorption than PTH or teriparatide and given both subcutaneously (50mg) or by inhalation(1.2mg) route.

4. **Calcitonin**

   The effects of calcitonin on normal human bone physiology are unclear; however calcitonin receptors have been discovered on osteoclasts and has antiresoptive effects in bones thereby inhibiting bone resorption and an increase in serum calcium levels. It inhibits renal tubular reabsorption of calcium and phosphorus.. However, this is a minor effect with no physiological significance. It is a short- lived effect because kidneys become resistant to calcitonin. Calcitonin is given for the treatmentof osteoporosis in women who have been in postmenopausal period for more than 5 years and when alternative treatments are not feasible. When given in doses of 200IU intra-nasally once daily reduced the risk of new vertebral fractures by 33%. It has not been found to be effective in non-vertebral fractures unlike bisphosphonates and denosumab.

5. **Monoclonal antibodies (RANKL – Targetted therapies)**

   Denosumab is a fully human monoclonal antibody that binds and inhibits RANKL and reduces bone resorption and found to be useful to treat osteoporosis in postmenopausal women. RANKL is a transmembrane protein required for the formation, function and survival of osteoclasts. Denosumab is available as an injectable formulation in either a prefilled syringe or a single – use vial.It is given in a dose of 60 mg subcutaneously every six months.

Denosumab can cause hypocalcemia, hence calcium levels should be corrected prior to treatment initiation. It is found to be safe in CKD up to stage 3, but not recommended in patients on dialysis or with stage 5 CKD. It is safe for administration in patients with hepatic impairment.

Nonpharmacological treatment of osteoporosis: It includes adequate intake of calcium and Vitamin D, weight – bearing exercise, smoking cessation, limitation of alcohol/caffeine consumption and fall – prevention techniques. The calcium requirement in a male patient is 1000mg/day between the age group of 50-70 years and up to 1200mg in women between the same age group. Vitamin D requirement is 600 IU/day for men and 800IU for women inthe same age group (50 – 70 years) Vitamin D3 supplements that are given usually include Cholecalciferol (Vitamin D3) 6 lakh IU once weekly orally or given once as a single dose. Ergocalciferol (Vitamin D2) can also be given in doses of 1.25 mg equivalent to 50, 000 units per day.

Postmenopausal osteoporosis: American college of endocrinology (ACE) provides evidence – based information for management of postmenopausal osteoporosis(PMO). In those with no prior fragility fractures or with moderate fracture risk, alendronate, risedronate, zolendronic acid or denosumab are appropriate as first – line options, while ibandronate and raloxifene are considered as alternatives. In those with prior fragility fractures or indicators of high fracture risk, denosumab, teriparatide and zolendronic acid are preferred as first line drugs.

Conclusion

Osteoporosis is an age – related metabolic bone disease characterized by low bone density and deterioration of bone architecture that increases the risk of fractures. Osteoporosis- related fractures can increase pain, disability, nursing homecare, total health care costs, and mortality. Elderly (60 years above) should take all care in attending to daily chores in order to prevent a possible fall, sustaining injury and likely fracture of a bone.

Age, assessment of risk factors, dietary habits, underlying disease conditions (comorbidities), physical activity and other lifestyle changes play an important role in the diagnosis and managementof osteoporosis.

Osteoporosis can be effectively prevented and treated with the medications, reduce hospitalizations and reduce morbidity and mortality and improve the quality of life.

8

Dyslipidemia - Retrospect and the Prospect

Overview

Coronary artery disease **(CAD)** is a growing public health problem and is responsible for an increase in morbidity and mortality worldwide. It is the single most important cause of premature deaths in many advanced and developing countries alike. One of the contributing factors and also the foremost one of CAD being atherosclerosis that results in atheroma and thrombosis. Hyperlipidemia is a major cause of atherosclerosis in coronary arteries, cerebral blood vessels and peripheral blood vessels resulting in ischemic heart disease, congestive heart failure, stroke and claudication. Dyslipidemia denotes not only hypercholesterolemia but also reduced levels of high-density lipoprotein cholesterol (HDL-C). Apart from dyslipidemia the other comorbid conditions that promote CAD include smoking, consumption of alcohol, diabetes mellitus, hypertension and a family history of premature coronary heart disease. Hence it is important to target blood cholesterol levels thereby reduce the incidence of atherosclerosis and its further complications. This helps not only to arrest the progression of vascular atherosclerotic changes but also reverse the progression to a greater extent.

Multiple evidence – based guidelines exist throughout the world to link the atherosclerosis and cardio vascular diseases(ASCVD), the main common theme however being the targeted therapy for lowering low – density lipoprotein cholesterol (LDL – C). It is strongly emphasized in all of the guidelines.

Pathogenesis of Atherosclerosis: Atherosclerosis is primarily an inflammatory response to a blood vessel injury. It arises from chronic or repetitive injury to the vessel wall (endothelial lining) which triggers a hyperplastic response by prominent inflammatory components. Initially there is a congregation of monocyte – derived macrophages and platelets. This is followed by active and passive transport of lipid particles(LDL particles) into the subendothelial space. Endothelial cells and monocyte/ macrophages generate free radicals that oxidize LDL resulting in lipid peroxidation. The monocytes are converted to macrophages. Phagocytes (macrophages) scavenge (Phagocytize) oxidized lipoprotein complexes and become "foam cells". These changes contribute to the lipid component of the fatty streak marking the beginning of atherosclerosis, that is the formation of **subendothelial fibrous plaque**.

Before the phagocytes perish, they secrete multiple growth factors that serve as the principal mitogens for connective tissue cells such as fibroblasts and smooth muscle cells (SMC). Collagen is another principal contributor to atherosclerotic plaque formation and its production leads to the formation of hardfibrous plaques. In response to increased plaque volume, negative arterial remodeling takes place that results in the narrowing of the lumen of the blood vessel. Rupture of the atheromatous plaque leads to the development of atheroma which results in thrombus formation and occlusion of the blood vessel. Normally any temporary occlusion of the coronary blood vessels can dilate in response to ischemia due to the action of nitric oxide (NO), the endogenous vasodilator. But in the presence of lipoprotein plaque, this function of arterial dilatation is impaired. Whereas chronic vascular injury is tolerated and efficiently repaired in young individuals, repair is less efficient in older individuals who are most probably associated with comorbidities like hypertension, diabetes mellitus, and those habituated to smoking, or with low immunity and active bacterial and viral infections. The risk factors and complications that could be associated with the atherosclerosis can be explained as follows.

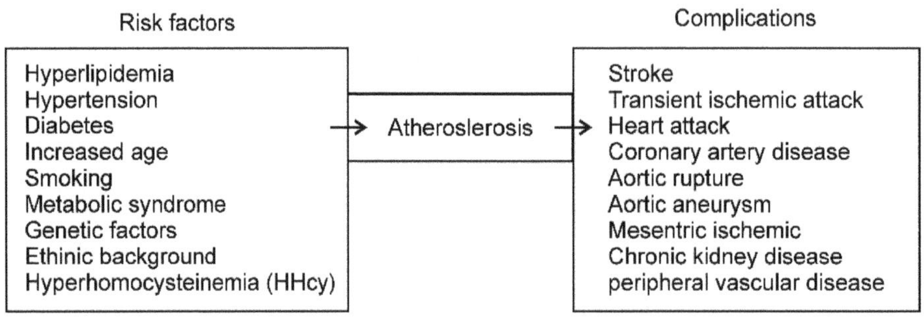

In these individuals there is accumulation of repair cells, excess extracellular matrix, inefficient removal of cholesterol–rich debris, negative remodeling (contraction) of the artery and persistent inflammation. **Plaques located near the lumen and contained only by the fibrous caps can easily rupture and release cholesterol and procoagulant–rich debris, leading to life threatening complications including thrombosis, MI and stroke.**

Reducing the levels of atherogenic lipoproteins and inhibiting their oxidation restores endothelial function, reduces coronary events, strokes, and peripheral arterial embolic episodes and also arrest the new plaque formation. It further reduces the rate of progression of atherosclerosis and even induces regression with aggressive lipid lowering therapy. Though the reduction of LDL and triglyceride levels is paramount in preventing atheromatous changes, it is an increase of HDL levels that contributes to the ultimate benefit of enhancing the endothelial function and removing cholesterol from the cells and lipid pools. However also, evidence from many genetic, epidemiological, and Mendelian randomization studies and from different kinds of therapies, it is shown a consistent dose-dependant log-linear association between LDL-C and ASCVD risk. There is proportionate risk reduction parallel to lower LDL-C levels.

Hyperlipidemia or Hypercholesterolemia: It is the term used to denote raised serum levels of one or more of total cholesterol, LDL cholesterol, and triglycerides or both total cholesterol and triglycerides (Combined hyperlipidemia). Dyslipidemia is a wider term that also includes low levels HDL cholesterol. The normal range of lipids for adults is as follows (mg %).

Lipid	Good	Borderline	High
Total Cholesterol	Less than 200, the lower the better	200 – 239	240 and more
LDL cholesterol	Less the 100; below 70 if coronary artery disease is present	130 – 159	160 or higher; 190 is considered very high.
Triglycerides	<120	120 – 199	200 – 399 ≥ 500 (Very high)
HDL cholesterol	60mg and higher	40 – 59	Less than 40 (Risk factor forCAD)

A low total cholesterol (<200mg %) and a normal or high HDL (≥ 45 mg% for men and 55mg % for women) in the absence of other risk factors or a family history of atherosclerosis generally infers a low risk for CAD. For a person with CAD or other risk factors, it is desirable to have a periodical assessment of lipid profile. The following equations may be taken into consideration for assessing the cholesterol levels in the body.

Total cholesterol = HDL + LDL + (Triglycerides/5)

LDL cholesterol = Total cholesterol - HDL cholesterol – triglycerides/5

Very low-density lipoproteins (VLDL), intermediate – density lipoprotein (IDL) and LDL particles (LDLP) are all components of apolipoprotein B(apoB) which itself is a risk factor for atherosclerotic vascular disease (ASCVD).

Lipoprotein a (LPa) is an independent risk factor for ASCVD, and is a link for atherosclerosis, stroke, MI, aortic valve disease, peripheral artery disease and heart failure. LPa has proiflammatory, proatherogenic, and prothrombotic properties. It is also linked to be associated with chronic kidney disease (CKD) as evidenced by lower GFR levels and high urinary albumin: creatinine ratio(UACR). Usually a reading of LPa of more than 40mg/dL is considered to be pathognomonic. Apart from the estimation of the plasma lipids as mentioned above, the estimation of LPa assumes significance in the diagnosis of premature cardiovascular disease,a family history of elevated LPa levels, familial hypercholesterolemia and those with recurrent CV disease despite optimal medical treatment.

Treatment guidelines

2019 European society of cardiology/ European Atherosclerosis society (ESC/EAS) guideline which are being adopted in majority of Indian hospitals also since then are the basis for the management of dyslipidemias and their role in many CV diseases(ASCVDs). Any patient with documented ASCVD (eg. Previous ACS, stable angina, coronary revascularization, stroke, transient ischemic attacks or peripheral artery disease) is considered to be at very high risk and those patients with LDL > 55mg/dL and LPa levels more than 50mg/dL and associated with comorbidities of diabetes mellitus, CKD, hypertension, current smoker, a family history of CV episodes are also considered to be at high risk.

Although fibrates (Gemfibrogil, bezafibrate, ciprofibrate), bile acid sequestrants (Cholestyramine, colestipol, colesevelam) are also effective in lowering LDL-C levels acting by different mechanisms, the following groups of drugs are chosen because they provide a sustained, reliable, consistent and therapeutically beneficial effects in lowering LDL-C levels and preventing the development of ASCVDs. Some of them also exhibit novel mechanisms of action making them more effective in treating both primary hyperlipoproteinemia also known as familial hyperlipoproteinemia and secondary hyperlipoproteinemia usually associated with diabetes mellitus, hypothyroidism, nephritic syndrome, primary biliary cirrhosis, chronic alcoholism, uremia, and prolonged use of oral contraceptives.

Statins: By all considerations statins are taken as the choice as the first – line drugs for the treatment of cardiovascular events as mentioned earlier. Statins block HMG-COA reductase enzyme which isresponsible for the production of cholesterol in the liver followed by a reduction of circulating LDL – C levels. In addition statins have pleotropic effects like improvement of endothelial functions, increased nitric oxide bioavailability, antioxidant properties, inhibition of inflammatory responses and stabilization of atherosclerotic plaques. They may also lower triglycerides. Medications in this class include the **moderate intensity statins** lovastatin (20-80 mg), fluvastatin(10-40 mg), pitavastatin (2mg), pravastatin (20 – 40mg) and simvastatin (20 – 80mg) and the **high – intensity statins** atorvastatin (20 – 80mg) and rosuvastatin (10 – 20mg). The doses of statins depends upon the level of the ASCVD and the associated risk factors and the levels of LDL-C .Moderate intensity statins cause a reduction of 30% LDL reduction, while high – intensity statins cause a reduction of 50% LDL – C. Both the patient and the attending medical practitioner should be wary of the possible adverse effects of statins particularly while using high – intensity statins.

Niacin: Niacin decreases LDL-C and triglyceride levels with an increase of HDL-C concentration, the appreciable action being an increase of HDL-C levels. Like statins, niacin also elicits favorable effects for prevention and control of atherosclerotic changes in coronary arteries, thus preventing coronary events. It inhibits lipolysis of triglycerides through hormone sensitive lipase activity, leading to reduced triglyceride breakdown which consequently leads to reduced availability of fatty acids. This leads to reduced synthesis of VLDL, triglycerides and further to reduced LDL-C . An increase of plasma Apo-A-1 increases HDL-C levels. It is mainly indicated in familial combined hyperlipidemia usually in combination with statins.

Ezetimibe: It is a selective cholesterol absorption inhibitor that lowers LDL – C blocking absorption of cholesterol in the intestines. It decreases cholesterol transport from micelles into enterocytes by selectively inhibiting cholesterol uptake through brush border protein named NPCIL-1 (transport protein). By the addition of this drug to statins increases the magnitude of LDL – C lowering by 20% to 25%. Thus either moderate – intensity or high intensity statin can be added with ezetimibe for a sustained and effective lowering of cholesterol levels in high risk patients.

Clinicians should obtain baseline liver function tests before starting ezetimibe. When the combination is being given liver function tests should be carried out and the liver function monitored periodically. If any change in the liver function noticed, ezetimibe should be discontinued. Ezetimibe is contraindicated during pregnancy and lactation, and patients with existing liver disorder. The normal dose of azetimibe is 10mg once daily.

PCSK9 inhibitors: When patients do not achieve adequate LDL – C lowering using statins and ezetimibe, PCSK9 inhibitors may be useful. These agents are monoclonal antibodies that bind to the PCSK9 (Proprotein convertase subtilin/ kexin type 9) protein. Normally LDL receptors (LDL–R) present on the surface of the hepatocytes bind to LDL particles and remove them from circulation. LDL-Rs return to thecell surface cyclically to continue the process of removal of LDL particles and thus recycling of LDL receptor takes place for effective removal of LDL particles. PSCK9 is a serine protease secreted in hepatocytes and after secretion binds to LDL-R and prevents their recycling thus inhibiting removal of LDL particles. By blocking PCSK9 by drugs like **alirocumab**, **evolocumab, evinacumab** the availability of LDL-R is increased (by an increase of recycling of LDL-R) for effective removal of LDL particles, followed by a decrease in blood LDL – C levels. PCSK9 inhibitors can lower LDL – C by 55% to 72%. They can also cause a modest increase of HDL – C and a decrease of triglycerides. They are indicated in adult patients with established CVD and as an adjunct to diet as monotherapy or in combination with other lipid – lowering agents in conditions like primary hyperlipidemia or heterozygous familial hypercholesterolemia to reduce LDL – C. The starting dose of arilocuomab is 75mg given subcutaneously every 2 weeks. LDL – C levels should be monitored every 4 to 8 weeks and the dose adjusted accordingly.

Inclisiran is a first in–class cholesterol–lowering small interfering RNA–based drug. It inhibits the expression of PCSK9 gene and has extraordinary biology. It gets targeted to the liver with N – acetylgalactosamine and produces the same favorable lipid levels as statins or PCSK9 inhibitors. It can be used at a lower dose and can be given every six months. A single injection given for a period of six months has decreased LDL – C to the extent of 50%. It has every good safety profile as far as the adverse effects on the muscle and liver are concerned. It is given as a first dose of 284mg subcutaneously, followed by similar dose on day 90 (3 months) and later 180mg every six months. It acts in LDL-R pathways similar to PCSK9 inhibitors.

Pelacarsen is a hepatocyte directed antisense oligonucleotide targeting **LPa** gene mRNA and lowers **LPa** significantly and is considered to be one of the choices to be used for prophylaxis of MI in such patients who have high values of LPa of more than 40 mg/dL. It has reduced LPa levels in a dose dependant manner 35% at a dose of 20 mg every 4 weeks, 56% at a dose of 40 mg every 4 weeks, 58% at a dose of 20 mg every 2 weeks, 72% at a dose of 60 mg every 4 weeks and 80% at a dose of 20 mg every week.

Bempidoic acide (BA): It inhibits cholesterol synthesis in the same pathway that statins work on. Bempedoic acid is converted to conjugate of bempidotic acid, the active form in the liver by an isoenzyme ACSVL-1 which is present only in the liver, not in the skeletal muscle thus sparing any adverse effects on the skeletal muscles. It targets ATP – Citrate lyase (ACL) an enzyme upstream of HMG – COA reductase, thereby inhibiting the lower pathway in the synthesis of cholesterol. It up-regulates LDL receptors and lowers LDL – C levels. It is usedin primary hypercholesterolemia (familial and non-familial) and mixed dyslipidemia usually in a fixed dose combination with ezetimibe. (180 mg bempidotic acid + 10 mg ezetimibe)

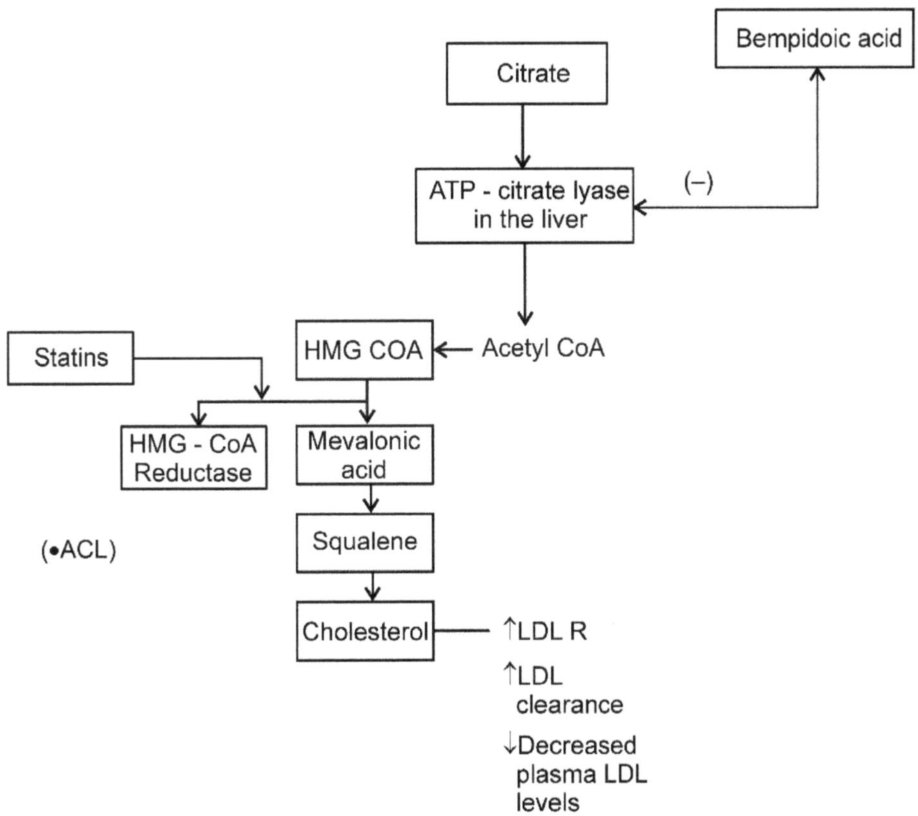
Bempidoic acid
Citrate
(–)
ATP - citrate lyase in the liver
Statins
HMG COA
Acetyl CoA
HMG - CoA Reductase
Mevalonic acid
Squalene
(•ACL)
Cholesterol
↑LDL R
↑LDL clearance
↓Decreased plasma LDL levels

9

Standard and Approved Guidelines for Antibiotic use

Overview

Infections caused by microorganisms have threatened human life from time immortal. During the Pre- antibiotic era, these have been a major concern for high morbidity and mortality in humans. Some of the virulent organisms with the potential to spread infection from one infected person to another at a very rapid rate may cause worldwide pandemics, epidemics or outbreaks as we have seen recently with SARS COVID – 19 viral infection which had taken a total mortality of 50 lakh lives worldwide with many people left with recoverable or non – recoverable post COVID complications causing a heavy burden on the human resources and strained economics. With the introduction or commencement of use of antimicrobial therapy over the years with the discovery of penicillin in 1943, a rapid and effective treatment choices could reduce the morbidity and mortality rates. The discovery of new antibiotics had become necessary and imperative because of bacterial resistance due to various causes that include irrational use, self-medication and misuse of drugs. This apart from antimicrobial resistance due to several mechanisms related to the microbial organisms like inactivation by the enzymes like beta lactamases, impermeability of the outer membrane to the accessibility of the antibiotic, mutations in the target site of action and due to efflux mechanism.

In view of the possible resistance due to improper selection, improper clinical application, improper dosage, improper route or administration and drug interactions it has become necessary to select the right antibiotic, for the right purpose with the right dose and route of administration, and also the knowledge the possible organisms that are likely to cause the clinical condition, the National centre for Disease Control (NCDC) Government of India had brought out guide lines for presumptive therapy for adult patients suspected of infection. These guide lines are adopted in most of the health care facilities in India through the institutional **Antibiotic Steward programme**. These guidelines covering various clinical conditions that the medical professionals come across in the daily practice are followed in majority of the situations and are almost akin to the international standards. But there might be variations in the approaches that are suited to the real situations where the guidelines may vary as per the needs. However, the guidelines acceptable in majority of the medical institutions are presented here.

The readers are requested to get uptodate information from www.ncdc.moh.gov.in website.

1. Respiratory Tract Infections

Condition	Likely Causative Organisms	Empiric antibiotics (presumptive antibiotics)	Alternative antibiotics	Comments
Community acquired Pneumonia	***S.pneumoniae, H.influenzae, Legionella, Mycoplasma pneumoniae, Chlamydia pneumoniae, Moraxella catarrhalis***	**Mild to moderatecases** Amoxycillin- 500mg-1 g+clavulanic acid 125mg TDS oral . If IV indicated, ampicillin-sulbactam (1g+500mg)IV TDS **or** Ceftriaxone 2g IVOD **Severe cases:** Amoxycillin- clavulanate 1.25 gIV TDS **Or** Ceftriaxone 2gIV BID Duration 5-8 days	Piperacillin-Tazobactam 4.5gmIV 6 hourly or Imipenem 1g IV 6hourly **or** Cefoperazone-Sulbactam 3gm IV 12 hourly	If MRSA is a concern, add Linezolid 600mg IV/Oral BD If atypical pneumonia suspected, Doxycycline 100mg bd **or** Azithromycin 500 mg oral/IVOD
Hospital acquired pneumonia	S,pneumoniae, H.influenza, S.aureus, Gram-negative bacilli- P.aeruginosa, K.pneumoniae	Cefepime (2g IV 8th hourly), ceftazidime (2gIV8th hourly)	Piperacillin+Tazobactam 4.5gIV8th hourly Imipenem /Meropenem 1gIV 6th hourly	
Lung abscess, Empyema	***S.pneumoniae,E.coli, Klebsiella sp., Pseudomonas aeruginosa, S.aureus*, anaerobes**	Piperacillin- Tazobactam 4.5gmIV 6hourly or Cefoperazone-Sulbactam 3gm IV12 hourly	ADD Clindamycin 600-900mg IV 8hourly	3-4 weeks treatment required
Acute pharyngitis	Viral	None required		As most cases are viral no antimicrobial therapy required
	Group A ß-hemolytic Streptococci(GABHS), Group C, G Streptococcus,	*Oral Penicillin V 500mg BD* ***or*** *Amoxicillin 500 mgOral TDS for 10 days*	*In case of penicillin allergy. Azithromycin 500mg OD for 5days **or** Benzathine penicillin 12 lac units IM stat*	*Antibiotics are recommended to reduce transmission ratesand prevention of long term sequaelae such as rheumaticFever*
Ludwig's angina Vincent's angina	***Polymicrobial (Cover oral anaerobes)***	Clindamycin 600mg IV 8 hourly **or** Amoxicillin- Clavulanate 1.2gmIV	Piperacillin-Tazobactam 4.5gmIV 6 hourly	Duration based on improvement
Acute bacterial rhinosinusitis	*S. pneumoniae, H.influenzae, M. catarrhalis*	Amoxicillin- clavulanate 1gm oral BD for 7 days	Moxifloxacin 400mg OD for 5-7days	
Acute bronchitis	*Viral*	Antibiotics notrequired	-	-
Acute bacterial exacerbation of COPD And bronchiectasis	***S. pneumonia, H. influenza, M. catarrhalis***	Amoxicillin- clavulanate 1gm oral BD for 7 days	Azithromycin 500mg oral OD × 3 days	

2. Urinary Tract Infections

Asymptomatic bacteriuria NOT to be treated except pregnant women and immunocompromised patients. All cases ofdysuria may not be UTI. Refer to Obstetrics and gynaecology infections for treatment of asymptomatic bacteriuira inpregnant women.

Condition	Likely Causative Organisms	Empiric antibiotics (presumptive antibiotics)	Alternative antibiotics	Comments
Acute uncomplicated Cystitis	***E.coli, Staphylococcus saphrophyticus*(in sexually active youngwomen), *Klebsiella pneumoniae***	Nitrofurantoin 100mg BD for 7 days **or** Cotrimoxazole 960mg BD for 3-5days or Ciprofloxacin 500 mg BD for 3-5 days	Cefuroxime 250mg BD for 3-5 days	Get urine cultures done before antibiotic change, modify therapybased on sensitivities.
Acute uncomplicated *Pyelonephritis*	***E.coli, Staphylococcus saphrophyticus* (in sexually active young women), *Klebsiella pneumoniae, Proteus mirabilis***	Amikacin 1 g ODIM/IV or Gentamicin 7 mg/kg/day OD (Monitor renal function closely and rationalize accordingto culture report) Complete total duration of 14 days	Piperacillin-Tazobactam 4.5gIV 6 hourly or Cefoperazone+ Sulbactam 3g IV12 hourly or Ertapenem 1 g IV OD	Urine culture and susceptibilities need to be collected before starting antimicrobial treatment to guide treatment.
Complicated Pyelonephritis	***Escherichia coli, Klebsiella pneumonia, Proteus mirabilis, Pseudomonas aeruginosa, Enterococcus* sp.** Frequently multi-drug resistant organisms are present	Piperacillin- Tazobactam 4.5gmIV 6 hourly or Amikacin 1 g OD IV or Cefoperazone-Sulbactam 3gm IV12 hourly	Imipenem 1g IV 8 hourly or Meropenem 1gmIV 8 hourly	Get urine cultures before antibiotics & switch to a narrow spectrum agent based on sensitivities. Treat for 10-14 days. . Monitor renal function if aminoglycoside is used.
Acute prostatitis	**Enterobacteriaceae (*E.coli, Klebsiella sp.*)**	Doxycline 100 mg BD or Co-trimoxazole 960 mg BD.	In severe cases, Piperacillin-Tazobactam 4.5gm IV 6 hourly or Cefoperazone-sulbactam 3gm IV 12 hourly or Ertapenem 1 gm IV OD or Imipenem 1g IV 8 hourly or Meropenem 1gm IV 8 hourly	Get urine and prostatic Massage cultures before antibiotics & switch to narrow spectrum agent based on sensitivities and then treat total for 3-4 weeks. Use Ciprofloxacin (if sensitive)

3. Obstetrics and Gynaecological Infections

- Fluoroquinolones are contraindicated in first trimester
- Cotrimoxazole is contraindicated in 1st trimester.
- Doxycycline is not recommended in nursing mothers. If need to administer doxycycline discontinuation ofnursing may be contemplated.

Infections	Likely organism	Primary treatment (presumptive antibiotics)	Alternate treatment	Remarks
Asymptomatic Bacteriuria > 1,00,000 cfu (colony forming unit)/ ml bacteria of same species in 2 urine cultures obtained 2-7 days apart. Treat as per sensitivity result for 7days.	Escherichia coli, entrococcus species, Klebsiella, proteus, pseudomonas, enterobacter	Nitrofurantoin 100 mg Oral, BD for 7days or Amoxicillin 500mg Oral BD x 7-10 days .	Oral cephalosporins, TMP-SMX or TMP alone	Screen in 1st trimester. Can cause pylonephritisin up to 25% of all pregnant women. 30 % Chance of recurrence after empirical therapy
Group B streptococcal Disease, Prophylaxisand Treatment	**Group B Streptococci**	IV Penicillin G 5 million units. (Loading dose) then 2.5 -3 million unitsIV QID until delivery. or Ampicillin 2 gm IV (Loading dose) then 1 gm QID untildelivery	Cefazolin 2 gm IV (Loading Dose) andthen 1 gm TID Clindamycin 900 mg IV TID or vancomycin IV orteicoplanin for penicillin allergy	Prevalence very low so the prophylaxis may be required only on culture documented report Associated with high risk of pre-term labor, still birth, neonatalsepsis
Chorioamnionitis	Group B streptococcus, Gram negative bacilli, chlamydiae, ureaplasma and anaerobes, Usually polymicrobial		Clindamycin/ vancomycin/ teicoplanin and cefoperazone-sulbactum If patient is not insepsis then IV Ampicillin	Preterm Birth, 9-11% death rate in preterm infant's unfavourable neurologic outcome, lesser risk to terminfants.
Septic abortion	**Bacteroides, *Prevotella bivius*, Group B, Group A Streptococcus, Enterobactereaceae, *C. trachomatis, Clostridium perfringens*.**	Ampicillin 500 mg QID + Metronidazole 500mg IV TDS if patient has not taken any prior antibiotic (start antibiotic after sending cultures) If patient has been partially treated with antibiotics, send blood cultures and start	Ceftriaxone 2g IV OD	

Table *Contd...*

Infections	Likely organism	Primary treatment (presumptive antibiotics)	Alternate treatment	Remarks
		Piperacillin- Tazobactam or Cefoperazone-sulbactam till thesensitivity reportis available.		
Endomyometritis and Septic PelvicVein Phlebitis	**Bacteroides, Prevotella bivius,Group B, Group A Streptococcus, Enterobactereaceae, *C. trachomatis, Clostridium perfringens***		Same as above.	
Obstetric Sepsis during pregnancy	**Group A beta-haemolytic Streptococcus, *E.coli*, anaerobes**.	If patient is in shock and blood culture reports are pending, then start Piperacillin- Tazobactam or Cefoperazone-sulbactam till the sensitivity report is available and modify as per the report. If patient has only fever, with no features of severe sepsis start amoxicillin clavulanate oral 625TDS/IV 1.2 gm TDS Or Ceftriaxone 2gmIV OD+ Metronidazole 500mg IV TDS +/-gentamicin 7mg/kg/day OD if admission needed.MRSA cover may be required if suspected or colonized (Vancomycin/ Teicoplanin)		
Obstetric Sepsis following pregnancy	***S. pyogenes, E. coli, S. aureus S. pneumoniae,* Meticillin-resistant *S. aureus* (MRSA), *C. septicum* & *Morganella morganii*.**	Same as above	Sources of sepsis outside Genital tract Mastitis UTI Pneumonia Skin and soft tissue(IV site, surgical site, drain site etc.)	
Syphillis				Refer to STD program Guidelines
Tuberculosis in pregnancy	**Similar to NON PREGNANT population with tuberculosis**	Please refer RNTCP guideline WHO has advocated that, all the first line drugs are		Very small chance of transmission of infection to fetus.

Table *Contd...*

VIRAL INFECTIONS (NO ANTIBIOTICS TO BE GIVEN)				
Influenza In pregnancy (seasonal And H1N1) The best preventive strategy is administration of single dose of killed vaccine.	Oseltamivir 75 mg Oral BD for 5 days	Nebulization with Zanamvir respules (2)5 mg each, BD for 5 days	1. Tendency for severe including premature labor&delivery. 2. Treatment should begin within 48 hrs ofonset of symptoms. 3. Higher doses commonly used in non pregnant population (150mg) are not recommended in pregnancy due to safety concerns. 4. Chemoprophylaxis can be used in significant exposures. 5. Live (nasal Vaccine) is contraindicated in pregnancy.	Direct fetal infectionrare Preterm delivery andpregnancy loss.
Varicella	>20 wks of gestation, presenting within 24 hours of the onset of the rash, Aciclovir 800mg Oral 5 times a day IV acyclovir recommended for the treatment of severe complications,	VZIG should be offered to susceptible women < 10 days of the exposure. VZIG has no role in treatment once the rash appears. The dose of VZIG is 125 units / 10kg not exceeding625 units, IM.		Chickenpox during pregnancy does not justify termination without prior prenataldiagnosis as only. A minority of fetusesinfected develop fetal varicella syndrome.
	> 24 hrs from the onset of rash, antivirals are not found to be useful.			
PARASITIC INFECTIONS				
Acute Toxoplasmosis in pregnancy		If PCR (polymerase chain reaction) Positive - >18 weeks gestation and documented fetal infection by positive amniotic fluid PCR. Pyremethamine 50 mg Oral BD x 2 days then 50 mg OD + Sulphadiazine 75 mg/kg Oral x 1 dose then 50mg/kgbd + Folinic Acid (10-20 mg Oral daily) for minimum of 4 weeks or for duration of pregnancy.		
Malaria In pregnancy	As per national program			
Acute Toxoplasmosis in pregnancy		If PCR Positive - >18 weeks gestation and documented fetal infection by positive amniotic fluid PCR. Pyremethamine 50 mg Oral BD x 2 days then 50 mgOD + Sulphadiazine 75 mg/kg Oral x 1 dose then 50mg/kgbd + Folinic Acid (10-20 mg Oral daily) for minimum of 4 weeks or for duration of pregnancy.		

Table *Contd...*

PARASITIC INFECTIONS			
Malaria In pregnancy	As per national program		
GENITAL TRACT INFECTIONS			
Candidiasis	**Candida species**	Fluconazole oral 150 mg single doseFor milder cases- Intravaginal agents as creams or suppositories clotrimazole, miconazole, nystatin. Intravaginal azoles, single dose to 7-14 days.	Non-pregnant- If recurrent candidiasis, (4 or more episodes/year) 6 months suppressive treatment with fluconazole 150 mg oral once a week or clotrimazole vaginal suppositories 500 mg once a week.
Bacterial vaginosis	**Polymicrobial**	Metronidazole500mg Oral BD x 7 days Or metronidazole vaginal gel 1 HS x 5 days Or Tinidazole 2 g orally ODx 3 days Or 2% Clindamycin Vaginal cream 5 gm HS x 5 days	Treat the partner.
Trichimoniasis	**Trichomonas vaginalis**	Metronidazole 2 gm single dose or 500 mg Oral BD X7 days or Tinidazole 2 gm Oral single doseFor treatment failure – retreat with Metronidazole 500 mg Oral BD X 7 Days, if 2nd failure Metronidazole 2 gm Oral OD X 3-5 days	Treat sexual partner with metronidazole 2 gm single dose
Cervicitis/ Urethritis Mucopurulent gonoccocal	**Polymicrobial**	Ceftriaxone 250 mg IM Single dose + Azithromycin 1gm single dose OR Doxycycline 100mg BD x 7 day	
Pelvic Inflammatory Disease (Salpingitis & tubo-ovarian abscess)	***S. aureus*, Enterobacteriacae, gonococci, gardenella**	Outpatient treatment Ceftriaxone 250 mg IM/IV single dose plus +/- Metronidazole 500 mg BD x 14 days Plus Doxycycline 100 mg BD x 14 Days Inpatient Treatment Clindamycin +ceftriaxone till patient admitted then change to OPD treatment	Drainage of tubo-ovarian abscess wherever indicated Evaluate and treat sex partner
Mastitis without abscess	***S. aureus***	Amoxycillin clavulunate/Cephalexin 500 mg QID/ OR Ceftriaxone 2 gm OD OR MRSA- based on sensitivities AddClindamycin 300 QID or Vancomycin I gm IV 12 hourly /teicoplanin 12mg/kgIV 12 hourly x 3 doses followed by 6 once daily IV	
Mastitis with abscess		Drainage with antibiotic cover forMRSA Clindamycin 300 QID or Vancomycin 15mg/kg IV 12 hourly (maximum 1gm 12 hourly)/teicoplanin 12mg/kg IV 12 hourly x 3 doses followed by 6 mg once daily IV	

10

Standard and Approved Guidelines for Antibiotic use(Continued)

1) Gastrointestinal and Intra-Abdominal Infections

Condition	Likely Causative Org anisms	Empiric (presumptive) antibiotics/FirstLine	Alternativeantibiotics/ SecondLine	Comments
Acute Gastroenteritis *Foodpoisoning*	**Viral, Entero-toxigenic & Entero-pathogenic *E.coli*** ***S.aureus, B.cereus, C.botulinum***	None	None	Rehydration (oral/IV) essential
Cholera	***V.cholerae***	Doxycycline 300mg Oral stat Azithromycin Oral in children(20mg/kg) And pregnant women(1g)	Azithromycin1gm Oral or Ciprofloxacin500mgBD For 3 days	Rehydration(oral/IV) Is essential Antibiotics are adjunctive therapy.
Bacterial dysentery	***Shigella sp.*,Campylobacter,Non-typhoidal Salmonellosis, Salmonella dysentriae**	Ciprofloxacin 500 mg twice daily for 3 days Levoflozacin 500 mg twice daily for 3 days	Azithromycin1gODx3 days	For Campylobacter the drug of choice is azithromycin.
Travellers diarrhea	**Shigatoxin producing *E.coli and shegella,salmonella***	Antibiotic Treatment not recommended.		Antibiotic use associated with development of hemolytic uremic syndrome.
Amoebic dysentery	***E.histolytica***	Metronidazole 400mg Oral TDS for 7-10days	Tinidazole 2gm Oral OD for 3days	Add dicloxacin500 mg TDS for 10days
Giardiasis	***Giardialamblia***	Metronidazole 250-500mg oral TDS × 7-10d	Tinidazole 2gm oral × 1 dose	
Entericfever	***S. Typhi, S. Para typhi A***	Out patients: Cefixime20mg/kg/day for 14 days **or** Azithromycin 500 mg	Cotrimoxazole 960mg BD for 2 weeks (800+160)	Majority of strainsare susceptible to nalidixic aid.

Table *Contd...*

		BD for 7 days. Inpatients: Ceftriaxone 2g IVBD for 2 weeks +/- Azithromycin 500mg BD for 7 days		Ceftriaxone to be changed to oral cefixime when patientis are afebrile to Finish to duration of 14 days.
Biliarytract infections (cholangitis, cholecystitis)	**Enterobacteriaceae, *E.coli, Klebsiellasp.*)**	Ceftriaxone 2gm IV OD **or** Piperacillin-Tazobactam 4.5gm IV 8 hourly **Or** Cefoperazone-Sulbactam3gm IV12 hourly For 7-10 days	Imipenem 500mg IV6 hourly or Meropenem 1gm IV 8hourly For 7-10 days	Surgical or endoscopic intervention to be considered if thereis biliary obstruction. High prevalence of ESBL producing *E.coli, Klebsiellasp.* strain s. De-escalate therapy once antibiotic susceptibility isknown.
Hospital acquired diarrhea	***C.difficile***	Metronidazole 400mg oral TDS for10 days	Severe disease: start Vancomycin 250mg oral 6h empirically.	
Spontaneous bacterial Peritonitis	**Enterobacteriaceae (*E.coli, Klebsiella sp.)***	Cefotaxime1-2gm IV TDS **or** Piperacillin-Tazobactam 4.5gm IV 8 hourly **or** Cefoperazone-Sulbactam 3 gm IV 12 h	Imipenem500mg IV 6 hourly **or** Meropenem1gmIV 8hourly	Change to Ertapenem1 gm IV ODfor5-7 days Once the patient improves
Secondary peritonitis, Intra-abdominal abscess/GI perforation	**Enterobacteriaceae (*E.coli, Klebsiellasp.*), Bacteroides(coloni cperforation),Anaer obes**	Piperacillin-Tazobactam 4.5gm IV 8 hourly **Or** Cefoperazone-Sulbactam 3gm IV 12 hourly in severe infections In very sick patients, if required, addition of cover (fluconazoleiv 800 mg loading dose day 1, followed by 400mg 2nd day onwards) & s(vancomycin) / teicoplanin) may be contemplated	Imipenem1gIV8hourly **Or** Meropen em1gmIV8hourly **or** Doripenem500 mgTDS **or** Ertapenem1 gm IV OD	*Source control is important to reduce bacterial load.* If excellent source control – for 5- 7days; other wise 2-3weeks suggested.
Pancreatitis Mild-moderate		No antibiotics		

Table *Contd...*

Post necrotizing pancreatitis: infected pseudocyst; pancreatic abscess	***Entrobacteriaceae, Enterococci, S. aureus, S. epidermidis, anaerobes, Candidasp.***	Piperacillin-Tazobactam4.5gm IV 8 hourly empirically **or** Cefoperazone-Sulbactam3gm IV 8th hourly in severe infections	Imipenem-Cilastatin 500 mg IV 6 hourly **or** Meropenem1gm IV 8 hourly **or** Doripenem500mgIV 8h	Duration of treatment reduced, source control effected, and assess clinical improvement
		In severyly sick patients, if required, addition of cover (fluconazole iv 800 mg loading dose day1, followed by 400 mg2[nd] day onwards) & and for Enterococcus (vancomcin/ teicoplanin) may be contemplated For 7-10days		
Diverticulitis Mild-OPD treatment	***Gram- Negative Bacteria Anaerobes***	Amoxycillin-Clavulanate 625 mg TDS for 7days	Ciprofloxacin + Metronidazole for 7 days	
Diverticulitismo derate	***Gram-Negative Bacteria Anaerobes***	Ceftriaxone 2gm IV OD + metronidazole 500 mg IV TDS or Piperacillin-Tazobactam 4.5 gm IV 8 hourly empirically or Cefoperazone-Sulbactam 3gm IV 8 hourly		BL-BLI agents have very good Anaerobic cover, so No need to add metronidazole.
Diverticulitis Severe	***Gram-Negative Bacteria Anaerobes***	Meropenem1gmIV 8hrlyorImipenem Cilastatin500mgIV6 hourly		Duration based on improvement
Liver Abscess	***Polymicrobial***	Amoxycillin-clavulanate/ 3rd generation cephalosporin + Metronidazole 500mg I.V. TID /800mg oral TID for 2 weeks	Piperacillin-Tazobactam IV	Ultrasound guided Drainage indicated In largea bscesses, Signs of mminent Rupture and no Response to Medical treatment.

2) Central Nervous System Infections

Condition	Likely Causative Organisms	Empiric antibiotics (presumptive antibiotics)	Alternative antibiotics	Comments
Acute bacterial Meningitis	***S. pneumoniae, H. influenzae, Neis seriameningititidis***	Ceftriaxone 2g IV 12 hourly/ Cefotaxime 2 g IV 4-6 hourly 10-14 days treatment	Chloramphenicol if patient is allergic to penicillin	Antibiotics should be started as soon as the possibility of bacterial meningitis becomes evident, ideally within 30 minutes. Do not wait for CTs can or LP results. No need to add vancomycin as primary agent, as ceftriaxone resistant *Pneumococcus* is not common in India. *Listeria* is also rare in India and ampicillin is also not indicated Adjust therapy once pathogen and susceptibilities are known.
Meningitis- Post— neurosurgery or Penetrating headtrauma	***Staphylococcus epidermidis, Staphylococcusaureus, Propionibacterium acnes, Pseudomonasaeruginosa, Acinetobacter baumanii***	Meropenem 2gm IV 8 hourly ANDVancomycin 15mg/kg IV 8 hourly For14 days.		May need intraventricular therapy in severecases
Meningitis with basilar skull fractures	***S.pneumoniae, H.influenzae***	Ceftriaxone 2gm IV 12 hourly For14 days		Dexamethasone 0.15 mg/ kg IV 6 hourly for 2- 4days (1st dose with or before first antibiotic dose)
Brain abscess, Subdural enpyema	**Streptococci, Bacteroides, Enterobacteriaceae, *S. aureus***	Ceftriaxone 2 gm IV 12 hourly **or** Cefotaxime 2 gm IV 4-6 hourly **AND** Metronidazole 1gm IV 1-2 hourly Duration of treatment to be decided by clinical & radiological response, minimum two months required.	Meropenem 2gm IV8 hourly	Exclude TB, Nocardia, Aspergillus, Mucor If abscess <2.5cm & patient neurologically stable, await response to antibiotics. Otherwise, consider aspiration/surgical drainage and modifyantibiotics as per sensitivity of aspirated/drained secretions.

3) Cardiovascular Infections

Condition	Likely causative Organism	Empiric antibiotics (presumptive antibiotics)	Alternative antibiotics	Comments
Infective Endocarditis: *Native valve (awaiting cultures) Indolent*	**Viridans Streptococci, other Streptococci, Enterococci**	Penicillin G20 MUIV divided doses, 4 hourly **or** Ampicillin 2g miv 4 h AND Gentamicin 1 mg/kg 8 hr Duration:4- 6weeks	Vancomycin15mg /kg IV 12 hourly (maximum 1g 12 hourly), teicoplanin 12 mg/kg IV 12hourly x 3 doses followed by 6-12 mg/kg once daily IV depending upon severity +Gentamicin1m g/kg IM or IV8 hourly Duration:4- 6weeks **or** Daptomyc in 6mg/kg IV once a day Duration:4- 6weeks	*Ifpatientisstable, ideally wait blood cultures.* Antibiotic choice as per sensitivity results. Guidance from Infectious disease specialist or clinical microbiologistis recommended
Infective Endocarditis: Native valve (awaiting cultures) In Severe Sepsis	***S. aureus*** **(MSSA or MRSA) Risk for gram-negative bacilli**	Vancomycin 25- 30mg/ kg loading followed by15- 20mg/kg IV 12 hourly (maximu m 1gm 12 hourly)/ teicoplan in 12mg/kg IV 12 hourly x 3doses followedby6- 12mg once daily IV depending upon severity AND Meropenem 1gm IV 8h Duration:4- 6weeks	Daptomycin 6 mg/kg IV once a day AND Meropenem 1gm IV 8th hourly Duration:4- 6weeks	Modify antibiotics based on culture results and complete 4-6 weeks of antibiotics
Infective Endocarditis: Prosthetic Valve awaiting Cultures		Vancomycin15 mg/kg IV 12 hourly (maximum 1gm 12 hourly)/ teicoplan in 12mg/kg IV 12 hourly x 3doses followed by 6- 12mg once daily IV depending upon severity + Gentamicin 1mg/kgq12hIV	Daptomycin can be used in place of Vancomycin/ Tei coplanin for patients un responsive to **or** intolerant of Vancomycin/Teicoplanin **or** with Vancomycin/ Glycopeptide- resistant isolates	Antibiotic choice as persensitivity. Guidance from Infectious disease specialist or microbiologist is recommended.

4) Skin & Soft Tissue Infections

Condition	Likely Causative Organisms	Empiricantibiotics (presumptive anti biotics)	Alternativeantibiotics	Comments
Cellulitis	***Streptococcus pyogenes*** **(common),** ***S.aureus***	Amoxicillin-Clavulanate 1.2gm IV TDS/625mg oral TDS or Ceftriaxone 2gm IV OD	Clindamycin 600-900mg IV TDS	Treat for 5-7days.
Furunculosis	***S.aureus***	Amoxicillin- Clavulanate1. 2gm IV/Oral 625 TDS or Ceftriaxone 2gm IV OD Duration–5-7days	Clindamycin 600-900mg IV TDS	Get pus cultures before starting antibiotics
Necrotizing fasciitis	***Streptococcus pyoge nes, S. aureus,*** **anaerobes, enterobacteriaceae,**	Piperacillin-Tazobactam 4.5gm IV 6 hourly or Cefoperazone-Sulbactam 3gm IV 12 hourly AND Clindamycin 600-900mg IV 8 hourly Duration depends on the progress	Imipenem 1g IV 8 hourly **or** Meropenem 1gm IV 8 hourly AND Clindamycin 600-900mg IV TDS/linezolid 600 mg IV BD/daptomycin 6mg/kg/day	Early surgical intervention crucial

11

Evidence based Medicine – An Insight

Overview and Introduction

At any given time, value based clinical practice is essential for the best therapeutic outcomes ensuring the precision, efficacy and safety during the course of the treatment. This can be substantiated by ensuring and adopting evidence-based medicine (EBM) which in turn brought about by application of the best available research in clinical cases. This ensures an integration of evidence with experience with expertise of the physician meeting the patient's requirements.

Definition of EMB

EMB is the conscious, explicit and judicious use of current best evidence in making decisions about the care of individual patients. It can be further explained as an integration of individual clinical expertise with the best available external clinical evidence from systematic research.

The second definition comes from **McMaster university website**: **EBM is an approach to health care that promotes the collection, interpretation and integration of valid, important and applicable patient – reported, clinician – observed and research – derived evidence**. The best available evidence, moderated by patient circumstances and preferences, is applied to improve the quality of clinical judgements.

Main steps for applying EBM to clinical practice

1. Defining a clinically relevant question - It is an issue which the health care provider (physician, pharmacist, clinical expert) addresses with the patient. Here the attending health care provider should be able to understand the patient's problem, the clinical presentation, history of the clinical condition (both present and past) including family history, the current treatment if any he is receiving and other important data related to the clinical condition which includes the laboratory and diagnostic tests he had undergone if available.
2. Searching for the best scientific evidence.
3. Critically appraising the evidence.
4. Applying the evidence
5. Evaluating the performance of EBM – Scientific evidence includes study outcomes and opinions. Not all the data has the same strengths. Recommendations from an expert are not as robust as the results of a set of well – conducted study. Thus, in evidence-based medicine, the levels of evidence or data should be graded according to their relative strengths. **Stronger evidence should be given more weight while making clinical decisions.**

Stratification of evidence: The evidence can be stratified according to the following levels.

1. **Level IA:** Evidence obtained from a Meta – analysis of multiple, well conducted, and well – designed randomized trials. Randomized trials provide some of the strongest clinical evidence, and if these are repeated and the results combined in a Meta – analysis, then the overall results are assumed to be even stronger.

2. **Level IB:** Evidence obtained from a single well conducted and well-designed randomized control trail. The randomized controlled study, when well designed, and well – conducted, is a gold standard for clinical evidence.
3. **Level IIA:** Evidence obtained from a single well-designed and executed non-randomized controlled study. When randomization does not occur, there may be more bias introduced into the study.
4. **Level IIB:** Evidence from at least one well – designed case – control or cohort study. In this, not all clinical questions can be effectively or ethically studied and assessed as with a randomized controlled study.
5. **Level III:** Evidence from at least from one non – experimental study. Typically level III evidence would include case series as well as not well – designed case control or cohort studies.
6. **Level IV:** Evidence from a single descriptive or qualitative study
7. **Level V:** Expert opinions from respected authorities on the subject based on their clinical experience.

Diagnostic test: Apart from assessing the clinical condition a patient based on the level of evidence as envisaged above, diagnostic tests are used to determine the cause of illness in symptomatic persons and can be helpful in patient management by evaluating the severity of disease, determining prognosis, detecting disease recurrence or selecting appropriate medication or other therapies.

Levels of evidence can also be represented as follows (Representative Hierarchy)

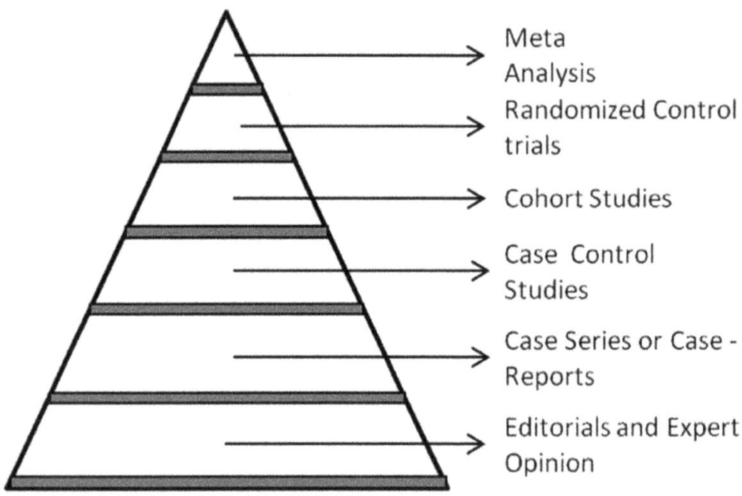

Application of EBM in clinical practice

All the clinical studies or scientific evidence can be classified into one of the above categories.

The clinician must then use their professional, clinical experience to extrapolate the scientific evidence as it applies to the specific patient under observation. Most clinical studies have specific inclusion and exclusion criteria, as well the specific population studies (demographic studies like age, gender, physical and mental status). More often than not, the patient being treated by the clinician will have one or more differences from the population in the study. The medical provider must then use their clinical judgment to determine how the variations between the patient and the study populations are important or not and how they affect applying the study results to the specific patient. The best choice for the attending physician would be to adhere to the guide lines specified in the levels of evidence in the descending order (Levels 1 to 5) the strongest evidence being at the level 1 though it is not always possible to stick on to that. Evidence at the level 2 is also mostly acceptable.

Evidence medicine now routinely defines the standard of care for many clinical conditions which is followed universally. The existing guidelines should be improved and applied based on the latest randomized controlled trials and consolidated into newer practicing guidelines.

This sums up that when faced with two treatment options, patients should receive the treatment that was more effective, safe, and reproducible based on randomized clinical trials. Treatments shown to be inferior, on average, in randomized clinical trials are assumed by many to be inferior to all patients.

Evaluating evidence about Treatment

One of the most common problems facing physicians is the need to assess the validity of new treatments being developed as well as validity of traditional treatments that have been used for years. For example, how long after discharge from the hospital should treatment with antimicrobial agents continue for the patient who had been hospitalized for pneumonia? What is the value of plasmapheresis in thrombotic thrombocytopenic purpurea?

Patient's role in EBM

Searching for the best evidence and applying it have the ultimate goal of providing better patient care. The process should also involve informing the patient of the available options and offering options based on good evidence. Effective communication, geared toward the patient's level of health literacy, is crucial to ensure that the patient makes an informed decision. Alternatively the treatment choices could also be discussed with the patient's family members. Using a certain therapy or implementing a diagnostic test may be inconvenient, or the patient may develop a certain side effect that he or she is not willing to accept.

Judgment and Merits of EBM

It is generally accepted that informal physicians (those aware of the evidence for therapeutic outreach) who combine their own clinical experience with up – to – date scientific evidence may offer better outcomes than physicians who unanimously choose treatments shown to be effective, on average, in clinical trials. Quality metrics also plays an important role in the application of evidence based medicine. For instance, reimbursable quality metrics that target 100% adherence to specific measures may be clinically appropriate for all patients in certain instances - e.g., childhood vaccinations – but may not be suitable for all patients in other instances – e.g., use of β - blockers in patients with prior MI, which experienced clinicians, may opt not to prescribe universally because of presence associated comorbidities or other contraindications The need to skillfully apply evidence – based medicine occurs because many clinical scenarios do not present clear choices. For example, current guidelines for ST – elevation MI (STEMI) state patients presenting STEMI should undergo PCI rather than thrombolysis if PCI can happen within 90 minutes at a center that offers PCI or within 120 minutes if the patient needs to be transferred. An emergency physician working in a hospital without a capable PCI facility who sees a paticnt with STEMI must decide:

1. Follow guidelines and transfer the patient to a nearby PCI center or 2. Deviate from guidelines and give thrombolysis immediately? The second choice would be better even though there is a deviation from the guidelines because of a possible risk to the patient while transferring to a PCI centre before an effective intervention is contemplated. **Ultimately, the successful application of evidence – based medicine is an art that requires first and foremost, an awareness of the evidence, and also an ability to determine how well the evidence applies to any given patient.**

Brief Account of representative Hierarchy

Meta-Analysis

It is a valid, objective, and scientific method of analyzing and combining results of different studies (clinical trials), in order to obtain more reliable results. A meta analysis is conducted mainly on randomized control trials which have a high level of evidence. A meta analysis is a statistical analysis that combines the results of multiple scientific studies addressing the same question with each individual study reporting measurements that are expected to have some degree of error. It is often an important component of systematic reviews of the trials made from different sources. Literature search is first step, and is very important for meta analysis, as incomplete literature may bring about incorrect results. Meta analysis is done by identifying a common statistical measure that is shared among studies, and calculating a weighted average of that common measure. The statistics of meta analysis would be conducted with software such as Stata or Review manager.

Randomized control trial: It is a prospective experimental design that randomly assigns participants to an experimental or control group. It is a comparative, quantitative, and controlled study/experiment performed with random allocation of interventions in series of individual groups (study groups Vs control groups) that also rules out bias. It is the most rigorous and robust research method of determining whether a cause-effect relation exists between an intervention and the outcome among the groups. All the potential compounding factors are divided equally among the groups that later be compared (structural equivalence). These factors include age, weight, gender, and other associated factors which may affect the patient's response. High quality evidence can be generated by performing a randomized control trial while evaluating the effectiveness and safety of an intervention, which will yield to systematic review and meta analysis providing a solid base for practicing 194g evidence generated by such studies.

To give an example of randomized control trial one can consider a situation wherein a new drug is being tested and its' efficacy to be known by comparing its response to that likely to be produced by a placebo. For example if 100 patients are being randomized 50 will get the drug and 50 will receive a placebo and the study outcomes compared at the end of the study period.

Double blind clinical trial

In controlled trials double blind usually refers to keeping the study participants, those involved with their management including the investigators, and those collecting and practicing clinical data unaware of the assigned treatment, so that they should not be influenced by that knowledge. This is to ensure exclusion of selection bias. If randomization included which is the usual case it becomes **randomized double blind clinical trial.**

Cohort Studies

Cohort studies are types of observational studies also known as longitudinal studies in which a cohort or a group of individuals sharing some characteristic (age, occupation, exposure to drug or vaccine, pregnancy) are followed up over a time, collecting data and the outcomes measured at one or more occasions after their exposure to a factor of interest. In the studies a possible relationship between the cause and the effect can be assessed and a possible conclusion made based on the study results. Cohort studies may be prospective or retrospective. In the **prospective cohort studies** data is collected over time to compare the occurrence of outcome of interest in those who were exposed to the risk factor and those who are not. For example a study could be made to correlate the occurrence of cancer between smokers and non smokers at different age groups, different occupations, and different social statuses. Similarly the risk of occurrence of heart disease between smokers and non smokers could also be studied and so also the risk of heart disease based on BMI. In **retrospective cohort studies** also known as historic studies, retrospective collection and compilation of data is made out to compare the incidence of a disease, a clinical condition, or a health related issue between those who were earlier exposed to a risk factor and those who were not to determine the factors' influence in the outcomes. The same examples as mentioned in the prospective studies could also be made out in the retrospective studies. Both the types are longitudinal in nature and extend over a period of few years. Prospective studies are more rewarding, more reliable and most likely conclusive.

Case control studies

These studies are observational studies and comprise an experimental design that compares a group of participants possessing a condition of interest to a very similar group lacking the condition. Here, the participants possessing the attitude of study such as disease, are called "case" and those without are called the control. The case control studies help to find the likely risk factors for an associated clinical condition. They are quick to perform, economical, and easy to design and implementation. They are retrospective studies because researchers create case and control groups after outcomes for the subjects (disease Vs no disease) are known. They are mostly useful for the evaluation of outbreaks and rare clinical conditions. They are ideal for the preliminary investigation phase, where scientists screen potential risk factors. As such they point the way for more thorough, time-consuming and expensive studies which are likely to clinch much more evidence for better research results. They are equally beneficial when current state of science knows little about the connection between the risk factors and the medical condition. However, case studies cannot establish causality and provide lower quality evidence than other experimental designs such as randomized controlled studies. They also cannot estimate incidence or prevalence rates for a disease. One example in this category is to study the incidence of Kaposi sarcoma in individuals who have been exposed to HIV infection and those who were not exposed to the infection. At another incidence one can find out the risk factors involved in cases of acute gastroenteritis due to consumption of contaminated drinking water or the roadside eatables

Case reports and case series

Case reports and case series are descriptive studies that recount a patient scenario complete with pertinent medical information such as laboratory values, medications given, and clinical diagnosis made. A case report includes a detailed discussion of unique medical scenario of a single case or event in light of the current available literature and provides an evaluation of the findings without comparison. **Case series** describe "a group of patients with similar diagnosis or undergoing a similar procedure followed over time". Although case reports and case series are at the lowest end of hierarchy of evidence, they provide valuable information to practicing physicians and policy makers because they typically describe previously unrecognized diseases or unusual variants of a known disease process. They help in alerting the health community to the presence of a new disease. Classical examples that include in this category are the recent episodes of CORONA VIRUS-19 infection starting with the identification of the clinical symptoms, progression of the disease, pathogenesis, diagnosis, laboratory testing and many types of treatment options administered, and identification of treatment failures that resulted in millions of deaths and recoverable and unrecoverable complications associated with the disease and the treatment given. The case studies and case reports also helped to identify many variants of the virus that resulted in the discovery of Vaccines for the prophylactic use against the virus. Earlier, similar studies pertaining to reporting the incidence of opportunistic infections in HIV infected homosexual people came to light and alerted the health officials to the presence of HIV infection in the community.

Editorials and expert opinions

Every scientific journal has an editorial board that helps in publishing scientific articles, research reviews and expert opinions that are aimed at research guidance and development. These publications are authoritative, scholarly, credible, and highly informative that help researchers or the practicing physicians gain knowledge about the advances made in a particular field and serve as guide to follow them or better them for their own research studies. Every speciality in the medical field has its own group of journals to help guide research and to make advancements and also help furthering the knowledge in the specified fields.

Some of the journals for Pharmacology and Pharmacy courses

The following are **some** of the journals that help guide the PG students in their pursuit to gain the recent and up to date information in the fields of pharmacology and pharmacy. The students are advised to follow the journals as per their interest and as per the suggestions of the faculty at their respective institutes.

- Indian journal of pharmacology: Indian journal of pharmaceutical sciences
- Journal of pharmacology and pharmacotherapeutics: Indian journal of pharmacy and pharmacology : Indian journal of hospital pharmacy

- International journal of pharmacy and pharmaceutical sciences: Clinical pharmacology and therapeutics: British journal of Pharmacology: British Medical journal: Journal of American Medical association: Asian journal of pharmacy and pharmacology

Medscape: Medline: Medicus: are also helpful

Cochrane: Cochrane is one of the most trusted source of information for all medical professionals, researchers, research data analysts, practicing professionals, and medical post graduate students undertaking thesis work for PG and post doctoral studies.

Cochrane produces systematic reviews of primary research in human health care and policy. Each Cochrane review addresses a clearly formulated question; for example- Can antibiotics help in alleviating the symptoms of sore throat?

It provides all the relevant information through **search box.** It provides featured reviews, podcasts, systematic reviews. **Cochrane library** is a rich source of information through its website which contains a data base for the needed information on any topic concerning medical and health related topics.

"Cochrane summarizes the findings so people making important decisions –you, your doctor, the people who write medical guidelines- can use unbiased information to make difficult choices without having to first need every study out there"

Sifting the evidence, The Guardian, 14th September 2016

Conclusion

Clinical practice guidelines are systematically developed statements that aim to help physicians and patients reach the best health care decisions. Appropriately prepared guidelines incorporate validity, reliability, reproducibility, clinical applicability and flexibility, clarity, development through a multidisciplinary process, scheduled reviews and documentation. Thus, evidence based clinical practice guidelines represent statements developed to improve the quality of care, patient access, treatment outcomes, and appropriateness of care, efficiency and effectiveness and achieve cost containment by improving cost benefit ratio. EBM is a universal approach for any clinical condition and the ultimate choice rests with the physician who uses his expertise before undertaking any clinical treatment or intervention.

12

Adverse Drug Reactions and Pharmacovigilance

Overview

Adverse drug reactions (ADRs) and drug allergies – as a result of ADRs – make a significant health concern, complicating 5 to 15% therapeutic outcomes. They may result in diminished quality of life, increased physician visits, health care costs, hospitalizations, and even death. **WHO** had identified the following descriptions to understand ADRs.

- An **adverse drug reaction (ADR)** is an unwanted or harmful reaction experienced following the administration of a drug or combination of drugs under normal conditions of use and is suspected to be related to the drug. An ADR usually requires the drug to be discontinued or the dose reduced.
- An **adverse event** in harm that occurs while a patient is taking a drug, irrespective of whether the drug is suspected to be the cause or not.
- A **side – effect** is any effect caused by a drug other than the intended therapeutic effect, whether beneficial, neutral or harmful. The term side – effect is often used interchangeably with 'ADR' although the former implies an effect that is less harmful, predictable, and may not even require discontinuation of therapy (ankle oedema with vasodilators, cough with ACE inhibitors)
- **Serous ADRs** are those which result in life – threatening outcomes and mortality, require inpatient hospitalization or extension of hospital stay, causes persistent or significant physical, mental disability/incapacity and likelihood for congenital/teratogenic effects.
- **Drug toxicity** describes adverse effects of a drug that occur because the dose or plasma concentration has risen above therapeutic range, either unintentionally or intentionally (drug abuse) – Examples include the use of barbiturates and general anesthetics causing CNS and respiratory depression; lithium toxicity due to prolonged use, Digoxin causing cardiac irregularities in excessive doses
- **Drug abuse** is the misuse of recreational or therapeutic drugs that may lead to **addiction** or **dependence**, serious physiological injury – hepatotoxicity in chronic alcoholism; psychological harm – abnormal behavior patterns, hallucinations with the use of ketamine and with other psychotomimetic drugs like amphetamine derivatives.

Classification of ADRs

Type A: These ADRs are expected undesirable effects which are predicted and dose – dependent. They are augmentation of known pharmacologic effects of the drug, the incidence of which is high, but mortality is less. Reduction in dose or change over to other drug medication can reverse the ADR. Examples include orthostatic hypotension to antihypertensive drugs (Vasodilators, ganglion blockers, α – receptor blockers); hypoglycaemia due to antidiabetic drugs; dryness of the mouth and retention of urine due to anticholinergic drugs.

There may be secondary effects to drugs other than the pharmacological effects. Examples include the development of super or suprainfection (fungal infections) due to the use of broad spectrum antibiotics causing candidiasis of oropharynx and external genetelia, pseudomembronous colitis; haemorrhage due to anticoagulants; bradycardia due to β – blockers; ototoxicity and nephrotoxicity due to aminoglycosides; hepatotoxicity due to pyrazinamide, INH and rifampicin; rhabdomyolysis due to simvastatin; hypoplacia of teeth due to tetracyclines; syncope and headache due to nitrates.

Type B: ADRs with bizarre effects

Adverse reactions occur in some people, unpredictably. They are independent of the dose and are due to unusual attributes of the patient reacting to the drug. They often have high morbidity and mortality rate and are usually uncommon. Examples include anaphylactic reaction due to penicillin, acute malignant hyperthermia due to halothane and other volatile general anesthetics or succinylcholine, and myopathy or rhabdomyolysis due to statins. These reactions are also called **idiosyncratic reactions; immunological reactions.**

Type C: ADRs due to long term drug use

These ADRs occur due to chronic usage of drugs. Examples include iotrogenic cushing syndrome with glucucorticoids; orofacial dyskinasia, signs and symptoms of Parkinsonism (drug induced parlinsonism) due to phenothiazines, butyrophenones, reserpine and all dopamine antagonists; retinopathy due to ethambutol, systemic lupus erythematosus with hydralazine, gastritis and gastric ulcer due to long term use of NSAIDs, and Candidiasis due to the use of broad-spectrum antibiotics.

Type D: ADRs with delayed effects

Adverse reactions of this type occur due to prolonged exposure to the drug either in the patients or their children years after treatment. Examples include craniofacial malformations in infants whose mothers had taken isotretinoin during pregnancy, and clear cell or adenocarcinoma of the vagina in the female children whose mothers had taken estrogens during pregnancy, or teratogenicity with thalidomide.

Type E: ADRs with end – of use effects

Adverse reactions occur due to abrupt ending of a drug use (**withdrawal response**). Example include sympathomimetic effects after sudden withdrawal of clonidine, β – blockers; adrenocortical insufficiency after sudden stoppage of glucocorticoids and withdrawal seizures occurring after sudden withdrawal of phenytoin, carbamazepine, alcohol and opioids.

Factors associated with ADRs

Drug related factors: Majority of ADRs occur as a result of the extension of the desired pharmacological effects of a drug, often due to the substantial variability in the pharmacokinetics and pharmacodynamics seen among patients. Pharmacological, immunological and genetic factors are involved in the pathogenesis of ADRs. Factors that predispose to pharmacological ADRs include dose, drug formulation, pharmacokinetic or pharmacodynamic abnormalities, and the drug interactions. The metabolic conversion of drugs to metabolites is one of the important factors for ADRs. For example, **Acetaminophen (paracetamol)** is converted to a highly reactive intermediate metabolite, ***N – acetyl – P – benzoquinonimine (NAPQI)*** which gets accumulated when the drug is given in large doses at shorter intervals and results in hepatotoxicity.

Patient related factors

Age: All drugs can produce ADRs, nut not all patients develop the same level and type of ADRs. Age is a very important factor which affects the occurrence of ADRs. Elderly patients with multiple medical problems who are taking multiple drugs, those who have an earlier history of ADRs, and those with a reduced capacity to eliminate drugs are at high risk for ADRs. Similarly, pediatric patients are also vulnerable for ADRs because drugs are less likely to be studied extensively in these extremes of age, and drug absorption and metabolism are more variable and less predictable in both of these age groups.

Gender: The biological differences of males and female affect the action of many drugs. The anatomical and physiological differences are body weight, body composition, GI tract factors, liver metabolism, and renal function. Women in comparison to men have lower body weight and organ size, more body fat, different gastric motility, and lower glomerular filtration rate. These differences can affect the way the body deals with drugs by altering pharmacokinetics and pharacodynamics of drugs including drug absorption, distribution metabolism, and elimination. For example, the severity and frequency of ADRs due to antiretroviral drugs is more in females than in men. Similarly women are more prone than men to develop torsades-de pointes ventricular tachycardia during the administration of drugs that prolong cardiac repolarisation (sotalol, amiodarone, dronedarone) . Pharmacodynamic differences between men and women are particularly seen with cardiac and psychotropic drugs. Female gender is a risk factor for hepatotoxicity.

Maternity status: Pregnancy has an impact on drug treatment as not only the pregnant women but also the fetus will be exposed to ADRs of the drug. There are certain physiologic changes that occur during pregnancy which might affect drug pharmacokinetics and pharmacodynamics that might result in ADRs. The effect of drugs on each trimester is different depending on the degree of fetal development. Drug teratogeniciy is most likely to occur when drugs are taken during the first trimester of pregnancy, when fetal organ are formed. For drugs taken during the second and third trimesters, ADRs are usually manifested in the neonate (birth to 1 month) or infant (1 month to 1 year) as growth retardation, respiratory problems, infection or bleeding. Teratogenic drugs like isotretinoin, phenytoin, antihistamines like doxylamine and tetracyclines are contraindicated during pregnancy.

Similarly, consuming alcohol during pregnancy can lead to fetal alcohol syndrome. Smoking during pregnancy can result in lower birth weights in neonates. Thalidomide once used for sedation during pregnancy results in phocomelia or seal limbs in the fetus. Other drugs which have potential teratogenic effects include ACE inhibitors, cyclophosphamide and methotrexate.

Pre-existing illness: Pre-existing hepatic or renal disease can exacerbate or precipitate ADRs. This is usually due to the longer stay of the drugs in the body. Reduced metabolism or excretion due to the pre-existing disease condition makes the patients more susceptible to augmented ADRs even to the standard doses, for example potassium sparing diuretics like amiloride or spiranolactone are likely to cause hyperkalemia in patients with impaired renal function. In patients with hepatic dysfunction, warfarin action is greatly increased due to slow metabolization of the drug. Acetaminophen can precipitate hepatotoxicity of a toxic metabolite, N – acetyl – P – benzoquinonimine. Nephrotoxicity is more likely to occur with the use of aminoglycosides in patients with pre-existing renal disorder.

Dose dependent ADRs: These types of reactions are dose – related and occur usually when higher doses are given or inadvertently taken. For example, ACE inhibitors can cause fall of blood pressure due to higher doses. Anti-diabetic drugs can cause hypoglycaemia in higher doses. Barbiturates can cause CNS and respiratory depression in a dose dependent way.

Genetic factors: The presence of genetic abnormalities can adversely affect the drug action and bring about different adverse reactions. The examples include- Glucose – 6- Phosphate dehydrogenase deficiency (G_6PD) can result in haemolytic anaemia in certain races with the use of drugs such as primaquine, sulphonamides and sulfones. G_6PD is an enzyme found in the cytoplasm of all cells in the body. It is an in-house keeping enzyme that plays a vital role in preventing cellular damage from reactive oxygen molecules. Erythrocytes in particular are vulnerable for oxidative stress and damage due to their role in oxygen transport. Inherited deficiencies ofG_6PD can result in acute haemolytic anemia during the times of increased free radical accumulation leading to oxidative stress and antimalarial drugs can precipitate the oxidative stress in the absence of G_6PD. Other example where genetic factors play an important role in the cause of ADR is the presence of a typical (pseudocholinesterase/butyrylcholinesterase) in some people who are prone to develop respiratory distress and apnea when administered with depolarizing muscle relaxants like succinylcholine and mivacurium. Pseudocholinesterase or butyrylcholinesterase is responsible for hydrolysis of succinylcholine or mivacurium. Atypical pseudocholinesterase or the lack of it can increase the levels of the two drugs in the blood and increase their pharmacological action and produce respiratory distress or apnea. Other example of genetic factors influencing the drug effects include slow and fast acetylation of INH, while slow acetylation results in hepatotoxicity(due to accumulation of INH) and fast acetylation leads to peripheral neuropathy (due to pyridoxine deficiency).

Preventing ADRs: while some ADRs are unpredictable such as anaphylaxis in a patient after one previous uneventful exposure to penicillin, many are preventable with adequate foresight and monitoring. Two important aspects can be considered while taking steps to prevent ADRs

A. An earlier known susceptibility of the patient to a particular medication, thereby modifying the prescription modalities to avoid any possible ADR to the prescribed drug.
B. Susceptibility factors such as age, gender, pregnancy states and ethnicity can help predict the risk of an ADR occurring.

ADR Reporting program: In a robust health care system it is always imperative and essential to have a well-defined and well documented system to report ADRs which is carried out by healthcare professionals such as pharmacists, physicians, and monitoring authorities. ADR programs encourage surveillance, facilitate documentation, promote reporting, provide mechanisms for monitoring the safety of the drug use, and stimulate the education of healthcare professionals.

Goals of an ADR program: The primary goal of an ADR program should be to raise awareness of the risks associated with ADRs, identifying ADRs that have occurred, and reduce their risk of associated harm. A continuous or ongoing ADR program can provide benefits to the organization, patients, pharmacists and other healthcare professionals with the following end of the effort outcomes.

1. Improve the patient care and decrease length of the hospital stay by ensuring safer use of drugs and appropriate follow up.
2. Educating healthcare professionals and patients about drug effects and increasing their awareness regarding ADRs
3. Providing an indirect measure of the quality of drug therapy through identification of potential ADRs and anticipatory surveillance for high – risk drugs or high – risk patients.
4. Complementing organizational risk management activities and efforts to minimize liability in the event of occurrence of ADRs during drug therapy.
5. Assessing the safety of drug therapies
6. To identify medication errors responsible for ADRs.
7. Characterizing ADR incidence in prescribed groups or organizations, populations, gender wise, patient mix, drugs used, modalities utilized to assess risk and patient harm.

Pharmacovigilance: Pharmacovigilance can be considered as synonym for ADR reporting mainly for reporting of the safety of a drug in use. Pharmacovigilance is the science and activities relating to the detection, assessment, understanding and prevention of ADRs or medicine – related problems. Before a medicine is authorized for use, evidence of its safety and efficacy is limited to the results from clinical trials, where patients are selected carefully and followed up very closely under controlled conditions. This means that at the time of a medicine's authorization, it has been tested in a relatively small number of selected patients for a limited length of time. After authorization and approval by competent drug controlling authorities the medicine may be used in a large number of patients over extend periods either alone or in combination with other medicines. Any drug can produce a short term ADRs as long as it is used for limited periods. The drug can also produce ADRs when used for extended periods for months and years in chronic illnesses and aged people. It is therefore essential that safety of all medicines should be monitored throughout their use. Medication errors such as overdose, misuse, and abuse of a drug as well as drug exposure during pregnancy and breast feeding are also of interest, and should be monitored even without an adverse event, because they are likely to result in an adverse reaction. Hence, it is very essential to collect data of drug safety with regard to its possible role in the event of ADR. Information received from patients and health care providers via pharmacovigilance programs and agreements, as well as other sources such as the medical literature, plays a critical role in providing the data necessary for the pharmacovigilance to be operational and to be effective. The **post marketing surveillance** can be defined as reporting of ADRs identified and recorded after the approval and marketing of a drug after the drug enters the market for its regular use. It is the responsibility of the manufacturer of the drug (pharmaceutical companies) to provide an authentic, recorded and readily accessible data of ADR for periodical scrutiny of the safety of the drug by the drug approval and licensing authorities. It is a continuous process to increase awareness for safe drug use by the consumers.

ADR reporting in India

Understanding the compelling need for a stable ADR reporting system in India, ministry of health and Family welfare, Government of India launched a robust techno – science-based system in the form of **Pharmacovigilance program of India (PvPI)** in July 2010, initially housed at AIIMS, New Delhi as the national coordination center (NCC). Further, in order to safeguard the health of Indian population and take PvPI to greater heights and implementing this program in a more effective way, the Ministry of Health and Family welfare, Government of India recasted and widened this program that resulted in the creation of **adverse reaction monitoring canters (AMC)** and functioning under India Pharmacopoeia Commission (IPC) located at Ghaziabad, UP initially. Currently there are 395 AMCs encouraging proper reporting of ADRs through ADR – reporting forms.

The mission, vision and objectives of PvPI are as under:

Mission – To safeguard the health of Indian population by ensuring that the benefits of use of medicine outweigh the risks associated with its use.

Vision – To improve patient safety and welfare of Indian population by monitoring safety of medicines, thereby reducing the risk associated with their use.

Objectives

- To create a nation – wide system for patient – safety by ensuring drug safety.
- Indentify and analyze new signals (ADRs) from the reported cases (for study of possible or likelihood of ADRs if a similar drug being introduced into the market)
- Analyze the benefit – risk ratio of marketed medications.
- Generate evidence – based information on safety of medicines.
- Communicate safety information on use of medicines to various stakeholders for preventing/minimizing the risk.
- Collaborate with other national centers for exchange of information and data management.
- Provide training and consultancy support to other pharmacovigilance canters across the globe.
- Promote rational use of medicines.
- Emerge as a National center of Excellence for pharmacovigilance activities.

Course of steps in ADR reporting

Pharmacovigilance program of India (PvPI) has been initiating an intensive and concerted effort to gather scientific information on Adverse Drug – reaction monitoring from hospitals to evaluate the benefits and risks of the medicines. The gathered Adverse event/Adverse experience data are collected, collated, and analyzed for ADRs at NCC – PvPI, with Indian Pharmacopoeia Commission (IPC) serving a major source of evidence – based scientific support which in turn provided to the National regulatory authority, the central Drugs standards Control organization (CDSCO) for regulatory interventions.

Recognizing the strengths and progressive journey of PvPI in the area of Pharmacovigilance, it is a matter of great honor and pride for the nation that NCC – PvPI has been recognized as the "WHO" collaboration canter for pharmacovigilance in public health programs and Regulatory Services . PvPI is also working in collaboration with other national health programs being run in the country such as National Tuberculosis Elimination Program (NTEP), National AIDS control organization (NACO) and National vector Borne Disease control program (NVBDCP), universal immunization program (UIP) etc;

Several tools and methods have been introduced by PvPI including suspected ADR reporting form (for Health care Professionals), Medicines side effects reporting form (for consumers) in different Indian languages, Mobile APP (ADR PvPI), PvPI helpline and others. NCC – PvPI organizes regular training programs including skill development programs on pharmacovigilance to enhance knowledge, skills and practice of stakeholders and to promote quality and safety of medicines manufactured and marketed in India.

ADR reporting centers

ADRs can be reported at the following canters in the duly filled forms by any of the stakeholders in healthcare system.

Peripheral pharmacovigilance (PV) center: It is a primary ADR information gathering canter. It includes small medical centers, private hospitals, dispensaries, nursing homes and pharmacies. ADRs are recognized and synchronized by Regional pharmacovigilance canter (RPCs) or zonal pharmacovigilance canters (ZPCs). Every state, union territory and few leading medical colleges in India have this peripheral canter.

Regional PV center (RPV): It is regarded as a secondary PV canter. It is located in a medical college having relatively large facilities. They are indentified and coordinated by Zonal canters. There are five such regional centers in India

Zonal PV centers: It is regarded as Tertiary PV canter and generally located in metro city's medical college having attachment of sufficient facility. It is identified by CDSCO and acts as first ADR data collection canter. Zonal canter for North and East Zone is AIIMS, New Delhi. Central **Drug standard control organization (CDSCO)** has zonal and sub – zonal offices located at Ahmedabad, Hyderabad, Ghaziabad, Jammu, Kolkata, Mumbai, Navi Mumbai, Chennai, Kochi and Bangalore.

Processing of ADR: All ADR reports from various sources are collected at the AMCs. PV staff at AMC study, validate and prioritize the report and perform provisional causality assessment. The assessed ADR forms are then directed toward the authorized coordinating canter for further proceedings.

The AMC's staff maintains a record of all the activities of the canters under their jurisdiction and carries out ADR monitoring of drugs as per the standard watch list. The coordinating canters then conduct a final causality evaluation and feed the reports into PV database. These canters also prepare an aggregate report of ADRs collected at said time interval and send it to WHO - UMC. The finding of PV analysis is then implemented and integrated into general population health program.

Events to be reported in ADRs: The events that are reported as ADRs include life – threatening event or death, hospitalization of the patients, congenital anomaly, medically significant event (if the event is considered by the physician), lack of efficacy by a medical device or drug product, all suspected drug interactions, and all known and unknown, serious, non – serious, frequent or rare reaction caused due to use of vaccine or drug.

Persons concerned in reporting of ADRs: All persons involved in health care like medical specialists, pharmacists, dentists, midwives, nursing staff, all patients, patient's relatives, witness or any common person after medical confirmation can report ADRs after filling the concerned ADR reporting form. It is a voluntary process as well as specialized health care system (ADR reporting form included below). The hierarchy of ADR reporting is as follows.

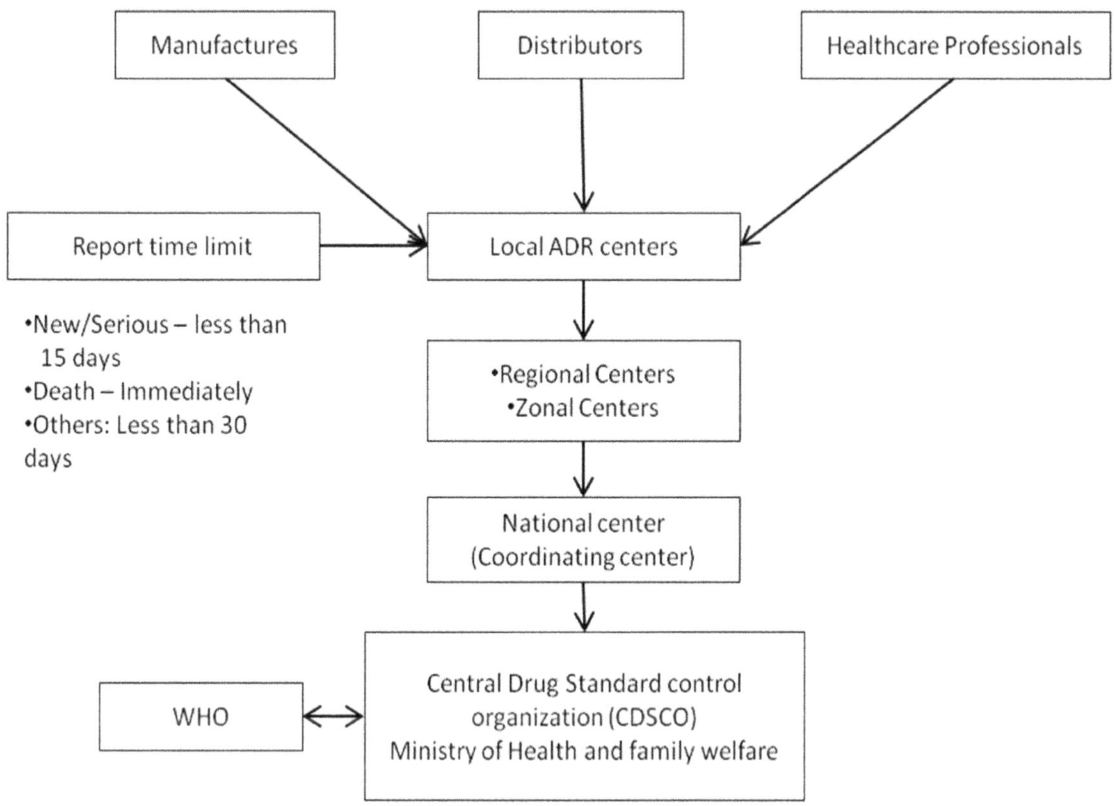

Some important ADRs associated with the drug use requiring close observation

- Coronary steal phenomena – Isoflurane, Dipyridamole
- Carbamezepine – Cleft lip, cleft palate
- Valproic acid – Neural tube defect
- Thalidomide – Phocomelia
- Toxic ambylopia – Ethambutol
- Fatal myocarditis – clozapine
- Idiosyncretic hepatic necrosis in infants – sodium valproate
- Clear cell cancer – Diethylstilbestrol
- Daytime blindness – trimethadione
- Pseudoporphyria – piroxican
- Drug induced myasthenia gravis – d – penicillamine
- Drug related eosinophelia and systemic symptoms – Allupurinol
- Osteogenic sarcoma – Teriparatide

- Peripheral oedema – Amlodipine, pioglitazone
- Bleeding – Anticoagulants
- Skin reactions – sacubitril/ valsartan, Tramadol, glimipride, gatifloxacin
- Teratogenic effects- Retinoids use in pregnancy
- Hypotension/Hypertension – Prednisolone, ACE inhibitors, diuretics, α – blockers, nitrates and other vasodilators.
- Respiratory and cardiac depression- Haloginated general anaesthetics
- Tachycardia, dizziness – Prazocin, Thyroxin,
- Gastritis – Risodronate, Alendronate, NSAIDs, Warfarin, aspirin
- Myopathy – Atorvastatin, Rosuvastatin, Simvastatin
- Cardiac irregularities – Digoxin
- Thrombcytopenia – Antimalignancy drugs
- Anaphylaxis- Penicillin
- Livido reticularis – Amantadine
- Fanconi syndrome – Tetracyclines
- Peripheral neuropathy resembling motor - neuron disease-Dapsone
- Acute hepatic necrosis in pregnancy – Tetracyclines
- Gray baby syndrome – chloramphenicol
- Fetal aplasia cutis – carbimazole or methimazole in pregnancy
- Hemorrhagic cystitis – Ifosamide
- Purple toe syndrome – warfarin
- Dry cough – ACE inhibitors, imipramine
- Blurred vision, dryness of mouth - Amitryptiline

National Coordination Centre for Pharmacovigilance Programme of India
Ministry of Health & Family Welfare, Government of India
Sector-23, Raj Nagar, Ghaziabad-201002
Tel.: 0120-2783400, 2783401, 2783392, Fax: 0120-2783311
www.ipc.nic.in

ADVICE ABOUT REPORTING

A. What to report?

- Report serious adverse drug reactions. A reaction is serious when the patient outcome is:
  - Death
  - Life-threatening
  - Hospitalization (initial or prolonged)
  - Disability (significant, persistent or permanent)
  - Congenital anomaly
  - Required intervention to prevent permanent impairment or damage
- Report non-serious, known or unknown, frequent or rare adverse drug reactions due to Medicines, Vaccines and Herbal products etc.

  Note- Adverse Event Following Immunization can also be reported in Serious AEFI case Notification Form available on http://www.ipc.gov.in)

B. Who can report?

- All healthcare professionals (Clinicians, Dentists, Pharmacists and Nurses etc) can report adverse drug reactions

C. Where to report?

- Duly filled inSuspected Adverse Drug Reaction Reporting Form can be sent to the nearest Adverse Drug Reaction Monitoring Centre (AMC) or directly to the National Coordination Centre (NCC) for PvPI.
- Call on Helpline (Toll Free) 1800 180 3024 to report ADRs or directly mail this filled form to pvpi.ipc@gov.in
- A list of nationwide AMCs is available at:
  http://www.ipc.gov.in, http://www.ipc.gov.in/PvPI/pv_home.html

D. What happens to the submitted information?

- Information provided in this form is handled in strict confidence. The causality assessment is carried out at AMCs by using WHO-UMC scale. The analyzed forms are forwarded to the NCC through ADR database. Finally the data is analyzed and forwarded to the Global Pharmacovigilance Database managed by WHO Uppsala Monitoring Centre in Sweden.
- The reports are periodically reviewed by the NCC-PvPI. The information generated on the basis of these reports helps in continuous assessment of the benefit-risk ratio of medicines.
- The Signal Review Panel of PvPI to review the data and suggest any interventions that may be required.

E. Mandatory fields for suspected ADR reporting form

- Patient initials, age at onset of reaction, reaction term(s), date of onset of reaction, suspected medication(s) and reporter information.

For ADRs Reporting

- E-mail:pvpi.ipc@gov.in
- *PvPI Helpline (Toll Free):1800 180 3024(9:00 AM to 5:30 PM, Monday-Friday)*
- *ADR Mobile App: "ADR PvPI"*

1

Mineralocorticoid Receptor Antagonists and their Clinical uses

Overview

Aldosterone is the main mineralocorticoid steroid hormone produced by zona glomerulosa of the adrenal cortex in the adrenal gland. It is mainly responsible for conservation of sodium in the kidney and elsewhere in salivary glands, sweat glands, and colon. It plays an important role in the homeostatic control of blood pressure, plasma sodium (Na^+) and potassium (K^+) levels. It acts through mineralocorticoid receptors in the distal tubules and collecting ducts of the nephron. It influences the reabsorption of Na^+ and excretion of K^+ in the kidney, thereby indirectly influencing water retention or loss, blood pressure and blood volume. When deregulated, aldosterone is pathogenic and contributes to the development and progression of cardiovascular and kidney disease. Aldosterone has exactly the opposite function/effects of atrial natriuetic peptide (ANP), BNP (brain natriuretic peptide), and C-type natriuretic peptide CNP) hormones all secreted in the heart. Aldosterone is part of renin – angiotensin – aldosterone mechanism which plays an important role in the overall mechanism for the control of blood pressure and body fluid balance.

Aldosterone acts through mineralocorticoid receptor (MR) which is an intracellular steroidreceptor.

Aldosterone mechanisms in cardiovascular and renal diseases

Mineralocorticoid receptor (MR) over production causes kidney and CV damage through inflammation and fibrosis. The following steps explain the role of aldosterone in the genesis of renal and cardiovascular (CV) disease conditions (CKD, nephropathy, cardiac hypertrophy, and hypertension). In cardiorenal diseases the MR pathway becomes over activated through multiple mechanisms, with an increase of gene expression of NADPH oxidase, proinflammatory cytokines and pro – fibrotic mediators leading to inflammation and fibrosis. This will result in the following

Renal damage -	Glomerular damage,Proteinuria Tubular injury, Reduced renal blood flow,Kidney injury (overall kidney injury)
Vascular damage	Vascular remodelling, Endothelial dysfunction, Increased vascular stiffness
Myocardial damage	Myocardial hypertrophy, Ventricular remodeling, Reduced coronary blood flow,Ischemia/ infarction, Myocardial injury

By blocking MR over activation, MR antagonists have been found to be very effective in treating heart failure, refractory hypertension, and diverse nephropathies, namely diabetic nephropathy.

They inhibit the action of aldosterone at the mineralocorticoid receptor, preventing receptor activation which in turn prevents inflammation, cardiac remodeling, and an improved proteinuria.

Renin - Angiotensn - Aldosterone machanism and systmic effeat prouduced

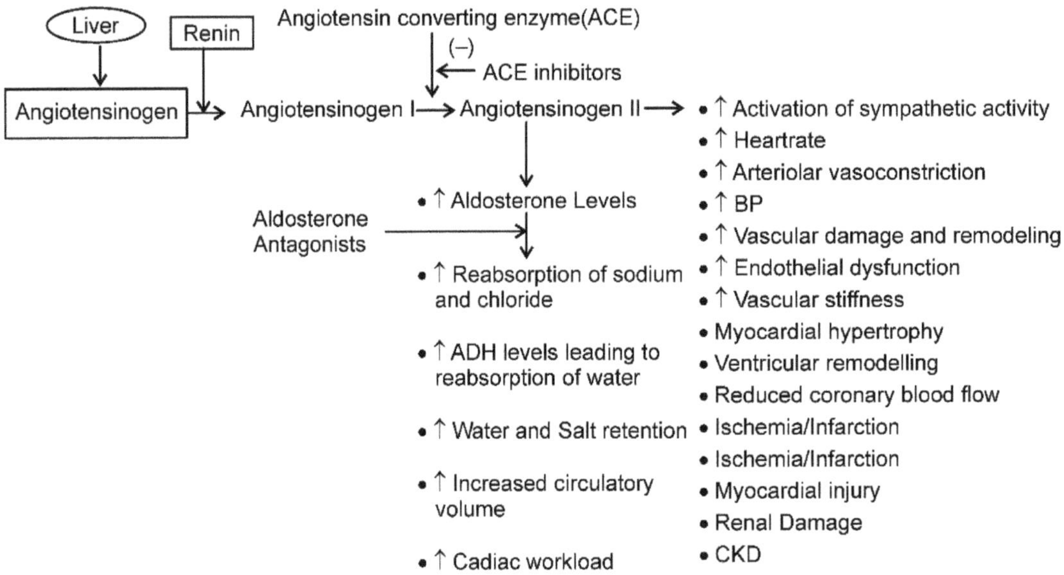

Classes of MR Mineralocorticoid antagonists (MRAs) and differences in properties

Broadly MRAs can be classified as

1) Steroidal and 2) Non - steroidal

S.No.	Properties	Steroidal	Non - Steroidal
1	Structural properties	Flat – Spironolactone Eplerenone Canrenone	Bulky – Finerenone Esoxerenone Apararenone
2	Potency to MR	Spiranolactone – High Eplerenone – Low	High
3	Selectivity to MR	Spiranolactone – High Eplerenone – Low	High
4	Anti-inflammatory and antifibrotic effects	Low	Moderate to High
5	Chances of Hyperkalaemia	High	Low
6	Better renovascular and CV outcomes	Moderate to High	High
7	Sex hormone – relatedside effects (gynacomastia)	Seen	Few
8	Diuretic action	Minimal	Minimal
9	Distribution in tissues	Predominantly inKidney	Equally distributed inthe kidney and heart

Role of MRAs in congestive heart failure

Treatment with MRAs have been demonstrated to improve clinical outcomes in patients of heart failure with reduced ejection fraction (HF_rEF) with mild to severe symptoms, and also in patients with left ventricular dysfunction after myocardial infarction (MI). Addition of eplerenone (25 – 50 mg/day) to standard therapy with ACE inhibitor or AT1 receptor antagonists, β – blockers, digoxin, and diuretics resulted in reduced morbidity and mortality leading to reduced hospitalizations of patients with LV dysfunction (EF < 40%) after a recent episode of MI. Eplerenone improves LV dysfunction and EF more effectively when given in combination therapy.

Mechanisms of action of MRAs in heart failure

MRAs act through different mechanisms to antagonize the effects of aldosterone and thus can cause a decrease of myocyte growth, decreased superoxide synthesis, and reduced oxidative stress, a decrease of endothelial dysfunction, decrease of collagen activation, decrease of platelet aggregation and better clinical outcomes, and reduced hospitalizations for HF. The beneficial effects of fenerenone are more than eplerenone, and the chances of hyperkalemia are also less.

Chronic kidney disease (CKD)

MRAs are the essential element in the treatment CKD due to their anti – inflammatory and antifibrotic effects. CKD is defined as "abnormalities in kidney structure or function which are present for more than 3 months. CKD is defined as a progressive kidney disorder which is present with GFR, ≤ 60ml/mL/min/ 1.73m^2 for more than 3 months, urinary albumin-creatinine ratio more than30 mg/g. CKD is classified by the cause, glomerular filtration rate (GFR) category, and albuminuria category. Proteinuria is a noted risk factor for the progression of CKD. Renin-angiotensin system (RAS) blockers are efficient and commonly used as reno protective and antialbuminuric drugs. However, they are not singularly enough to reduce proteinuria and slow down the progression of renal failure. The advantage of MRAs therapy is that an appreciable reduction in proteinuria, which results in a delay of the progression of renal failure and may contribute to a slower rate of decline in GFR.

Conclusion

Higher levels of proteinuria are a significant risk factor in progression of kidney disease in diabetic and non – diabetic patients. Several studies demonstrated that MRA therapy causes a significant reduction in proteinuria, which results in a delay of progression in renal failure. In addition, the combination of MRA with ACEI/ARB results in a significant reduction of urine albumin andcreatinine levels (albumin/creatinine ratio) compared to the values seen only with ACEI/ARB treatment.

The results of the studies have also shown that treatment may be a beneficial to reduce cardiovascular mortality in CKD patients as this is a leading cause in the end-stage renal disease. Spironolactone has been shown to be effective in reducing left ventricular hypertrophy (LVH) and can be safely used provided hyperkalemia is well controlled. Currently, the drug with the greatest promise in reducing cardiovascular risk in patients with CKD particularly associated with diabetes mellitus is finerenone.

2

Effective Management of H. Pylori Infection and the Role of Potassium – Competitive Acid Blockers

Overview

With the high rate of incidence of acid gastric disorders like peptic ulcer disease, gastroesophageal reflux disease (GERD), non – steroid anti-inflammatory drug – induced GI damage, ulcers in Zolinger Ellison syndrome, and the possible role of H. Pylori in these conditions, it has become necessary to find the best possible and effective drugs including the ones which can eradicate H. Pylori and result in successful clinical outcomes. It has been customary to use antacids (aluminum hydroxide, magnesium trisilicate, magnesium hydroxide), H2 receptor blockers (famotidine, nizatidine), prostaglandins (misoprostol), mucosal protective agents (sucralfate, colloidal bismuth compounds), and anticholinergic agents (mepenzolate) for treating acid peptic disorders. However, the use of Proton pump inhibitors (rabeprozole, esomeprazole and others)) has completely changed the line of treatment of acid peptic disorders because of their effectiveness over the earlier drug choices.

However, there are certain drawbacks or limitations for the use of proton pump inhibitors over a period that include the following

1) Short half – life (0.5 to 1.5 hours)
2) Destruction in an acid environment requiring acid protection
3) Inhibition of only activated proton pumps
4) Requiring 4 – 5 cycles of administration before achieving full effect
5) Clinical variability to CYP2C19 polymorphisms (independent of enzyme activity)
6) Chronic and repeated use may cause vitamin and mineral deficiencies, including Vitamin B12, Vitamin C, calcium, iron and magnesium.

A new class of drugs known as potassium competitive acid blockers like vonoprazon havechanged the course of treatment guidelines of acid peptic disorders like peptic and duodenal ulcers, GERD, NSAID induced gastritis, and gastric distress, and ulcers in Zolinger Ellision syndrome the effectiveness of which has increased in the antibiotic-based combination therapy for the eradication of H. Pylori infection.

Vonoprazan

Vonoprazon inhibits acid secretion by acting on the proton pump (H^+/K^+ ATPase) at a different site by competitively blocking the availability of K^+ in the proton pump thereby inactivating the pump altogether and thereby decreasing the acid secretion more effectively than the conventional PPIs.

Pharmacokinetics

It is absorbed with or without food with a C_{max} in the range of 1.5 to 2.0 hours. It has a half – life of 7.7 hours. Its high Pka(>9) promotes accumulation in canalicular space of partietal cells, where it competitively inhibits active and resting proton pumps. Intragastric pH above 4 is maintained both during day and night times.

Benefits of Vonoprazan

1) Rapid and sustained acid inhibition effects day long.
2) No need to get converted to active moiety unlike conventional PPIs
3) Stable in acid medium and does not need enteric coating
4) Can be taken with or without food
5) Rapid absorption, quick onset of action and rapid reach of peak plasma levels
6) Maximum acid inhibitory action from day one.
7) Metabolism through CYP3A4 and little drug interactions
8) No evidence of QT/QTC prolongation or arrhythmogenic effects with maximal and supramaximal doses.
9) Better tolerated in triple therapy with antibiotics for eradication of H. Pylori than thecombination of PPIs and antibiotics
10) Significantly better in the healing rate of erosive esophagitis (98.7%) as compared to lansoprazole 30mg (87.5%) at 8 weeks
11) H. Pylori eradication of 87.9% as compared to 71.6% (Esomeprozole), 62.9%(Rabiprazole), 57.3% (lansoprazole).

This is particularly advantageous for eradication of H. Pylori due in part to lack of antibiotic resistanceand to a substantial increase of antibiotic effectives

Dosage of Vonoprazan

1) Gastric ulcer 20mg once a day for 8 weeks.
2) Duodenal ulcer 20mg once a day for 6 weeks.
3) GERD and erosive gastritis 20mg single dose/day for 4 to 8 weeks.
4) Prevention of recurrence of Peptic ulcer or duodenal ulcer during NSAIDs treatment, 10mg single dose/day.
5) Adjuvant to H. Pylori eradication 20mg twice a day along with clarithromycin 500mg twice a day, Amoxacillin 500mg twice day for a duration of 7 – 10 days only.

   It is available in Indian markets under brand name 'VONZAI' and being used as substitute to conventional PPIs

Adverse effects

Except for minor GI adverse effects like diarrhea, or constipation, no major adverse effects were noticed including hepato or neurotoxicity during the study period and later in clinical use.

3

Parkinsonism and the Newer Drugs of Choice

Overview of Parkinson's Disease

Parkinsonism or Parkinson's disease (PD) is a chronic neurodegenerative disorder, the classic features of which were originally described by British physician Parkinson in the year 1917. The biochemical defect in PD has been described as imbalance between dopamine (DA) and Acetylcholine (Ach). In normal state, there is a balance between the excitatory effects of Ach and inhibitory effects of dopamine within the extrapyramidal motor system. But as the nigrostriatal degeneration progresses, a state of dopamine depletion and cholinergic excess takes place. Additionally, imbalances of other neurotransmitters (GABA, Glutamate, NAD, 5-HT) occur and neuronal degeneration within other subcortical structures such as locus ceruleus and hypothalamus also follow that characterize the disease. The profound reduction in striatal dopamine disrupts the complex motor circuit of extrapyramidal motor system that is composed of basal ganglia (striatum and globus pallidus) and substantia migra. The end result of striatal dopamine depletion is the expression of aberrant motor movements.

Cardinal motor and clinical features

Cardinal motor features of PD include bradykinasia, muscular rigidity (limbs and trunk), resting tremors which decrease during voluntary movements (occurring in hands, arms, legs, jaw and face) and postural instability leading to disturbances of gait with a tendency to fall. As the disease progresses, there is difficulty in walking, and completing simple tasks and increased salivation and constipation. There may be associated symptoms of depression or emotional changes. Untreated, the patient may die of aspiration pneumonia or pulmonary embolism.

Drug–induced Parkinsonism

Symptoms of Parkinsonism appear with the use of dopamine antagonists like phenothiazines, butyrophenones, metoclopramide, and reserpine. Symptoms can also be caused by selective serotonin reuptake inhibitors (SSRTs), amiodarone, valproic acid, and long – term use of diltiazem.

Differences between degenerative Parkinonism and Drug-induced Parkinsonism

- Drug-induced parkinsonism often affects both sides of the body equally, whereasdegenerative Parkinsonism is always asymmetric, affecting one side of the body more than the other
- Degenerative Parkinsonism is typically accompanied by various non-motor symptoms, some of which, such as depression, sleep disorders, loss of smell, and constipation appear earlier in the disease course than the motor symptoms of the clinical condition
- Drug-induced Parkinsonism typically encompasses only the motor symptoms like tremor including resting tremor. The other feature of drug-induced parkinsonism is increased salivation

Receptor mechanisms in Parkinson's disease

Dopamine receptors

There are two main subgroups of dopamine receptor: D1 – like and D2 – like.The former contains D1 and D5 receptor subtypes and the latter contains D2, D3 and D4 subtypes.

D1 receptor subgroup is coupled to stimulatory G proteins (Gs) and facilitates the formation of second messengers c-AMP and IP3, D2 receptor subgroup is coupled to inhibitory G proteins (GI) and decrease the formation of c-AMP and IP3. D1 receptors are the most abundant and widespread in areas receiving dopaminergic innervation (the striatum, limbic system, thalamus, and hypothalamus). **D2 receptors are also widespread in these areas as well as the pituitary gland and involved mostly in the pathogenesis of PD**. D3 and D4 are present in the limbic system. All the dopamine receptor – D1, D2, D3 and D4 are involved in PD, though D2 type playing a little more prominent role.

Adenosine

Adenosine is a molecule present in all body fluids and tissues and acts through A1, A2A, A2B, and A3. A2A receptors are found in the dopaminergic pathways and uniquely interact with dopamine to induce motor symptoms of the disease.

Classes of drugs of drugs used in Parkinsonism

1) Drugs which increase dopamine levels – levodopa, peripheral decarboxylase inhibitors –carbidopa
2) Dopamine receptor agonists – Bromocriptine, pergolide, ropinirole, and pramipexole
3) Endogenous dopamine releasers – Amantadine
4) COMT inhibitors – Tolcapone, Entacapone. Opicapone
5) MAO-B inhibitors – Selegiline, rasagiline, safinamide
6) Cholinergic antagonists – Benzatropine, biperidine, orphenandrine, procyclindine, trihexyphenidyl, Adenosine A (A2A) receptor antagonists- Istradephylline
7) Adenosine receptor blocker (A2A)-Istradphylline

While the mechanisms of actions, clinical indications, adverse effects of all the classes of drugs – 1,2,3,4, part of 5 (selegeline, rasalgiline) are known earlier, this topic mainly is devoted to safinamide (MAO-B inhibitor) and Istradefylline and other newer developments in the treatment of Parkinsonism.

Safinamide

Safinamide, is a MAO-B inhibitor and used as add – on treatment for patients with Parkinson's disease who are currently taking levodopa/ carbidopa and experiencing 'off' episodes frequently.

Monoamine-B(MAO-B) is expressed predominantly in the brain and is responsible for the metabolic degradation of catecholamines (NAD, Dopamine). Selegiline is a selective irreversible inhibitor of MAO-B. Safinamide is a reversible MAO-B inhibitor and increases the dopamine levels in the brain with blockade of voltage-dependent Na+ and Ca+ channels It also causes a reduced reuptake of dopamine with additional antiglutaminergic effects. It improves motor symptoms in PD with an antidyskinetic effect through its effect on glutamate release. It is given as a adjuvant therapy along with a levodopa and carbidopa combination to minimize the 'wearing – off' phenomena. The usual combination therapy includes carbidopa 25mg/Levodopa 100mg, 1 tablet 3 times a day + 50mg of safinamide 1 tablet/day. Safinamide is available under brand name 'Xafinast'

Progress of the disease

Motor fluctuations in PD reflect the short plasma half – life of 150minutes for levodopa alone, 90 minutes when given with carbidopa with reduced ability of the striatum to store and buffer striatal dopamine, and the variable absorption of oral levodopa reflecting delayed gastric emptying.

In the early stages of PD, levodopa is effective because after being converted to dopamine in thebody, striated dopaminergic transmissions are restored, thereby eliminating symptoms of PD.

However, as PD progress, more dopamine terminals are lost, and the striatum is unable to store dopamine in terminal vesicles and buffer synaptic terminals to control the symptoms. Due to continued changes in levodopa plasma concentration levels and progressive neuronal death in the nigrostriatal system, up to 50% of patients with PD develop mild motor fluctuations and dyskinasia within 2 years of the initiation of therapy. ***Over time, patients with PD on levodopa will experience adecrease in response to treatment with shorter response time, referred to as wearing – OFF phenomena.***

For the control of 'OFF' effects during the therapy with levodopa there are on demand ***rescue therapies*** available that include subcutaneous or sublingual apomorphine and inhaled formulation of levodopa (Powder form). The other alternative is the use of **Safinamide** in combination with **opicapone** (peripheral COMT inhibitor). The combination of safinamide (100mg) and opicapone (50 mg) given once daily complement each other by a reduction of necessity of oral levodopa intakes and cover "**OFF**" times.

Istradefylline

It is an adenosine A2 (A2A) receptor blocker and given as add – on treatment to levodopa/carbidopa in adults with Parkinson's disease experiencing '**off**' episodes and given orally in doses of 20 to 40mg once daily as an adjuvant. It reduces the over activity of the striatal pathway, restoring the balance of basal ganglia.

4

Migraine Treatment – Newer Treatment Options

Overview and Clinical Presentation

Migraine is a complex disorder characterized by recurrent episodes of headache most often unilateral and in some cases associated with visual or sensory symptoms – collectively known as **aura** that arise most often before the cranial pain starts. It is most commonly seen in women. The features of aura may precede or accompany the headache phase or may occur in isolation. It usually develops over 5 – 20 minutes and lasts for nearly one hour. Aura consists of visual feature mostly but may also be associated with motor or sensory features. The visual features consist of a band of absent vision with a shimmering or glittering zigzag border.

Migraine consists of triad of paroxysmal headache, nausea/ or vomiting and the feature of aura as mentioned earlier. Typically, a classical migraine attack starts with nonspecific prodromal symptoms of malaise and irritability followed by severe, throbbing, hemicranial headache with photophobia and vomiting.The headache is thought to be caused by vasodilation of extracranial vessels with subsequent activation of nociceptive transmission in the brain stem trigeminal nucleus. There is **release of calcitonin gene – related peptide (CGRP)** which is responsible for vasodilatation. There is also participation of other peptides like substance P and neurokinin A. Extravasation of plasma and plasma proteins into perivascular space causes perivascular edema resulting in mechanical stretch of pain nerve ending in the dura. The onset of headache is sometimes associated with a marked increase in amplitude of temporal artery pulsations.

Management

Migraine treatment involves **acute (abortive)** and **Preventive therapy (Prophylactic therapy).** Acute treatment aims to reverse or at least stop the progression of headache that has started already. Preventive treatment, which is given even in the absence of a headache, aims to reduce the frequency and severity of migraine attack.

Abortive therapy

Numerous abortive medications are available. Simple analgesics alone or in combination with other compounds have provided relief to mild to moderately serve headaches. Acute treatment is most effective when given within 15 minutes of pain onset and when pain is mild. Analgesics used for abortive purposes include acetaminophen, NSAIDs and narcotic analgesics like oxycodone, and metoclopramide/domperidone can be given IV to control nausea and vomiting.

Dihydroergotamine (DHE)

Dihydroergotamine (DHE) is now available as nasal spray with 1.5mg/ spray for the acute attack of migraine, apart from its earlier injectable (IV route) preparation given in 1 mg doses. DHE 1 mg IV+ metoclopramide 10 mg is a usual combination in an acute attack of migraine which is effective to relieve the acute symptoms and also preventing the likely association of nausea and vomiting in the episode. Sumatryptan 6 mg given subcutaneously is highly effective in controlling the acute symptoms of migraine.

1. **Nonselective β-blockers and tricyclic antidepressants and other drugs used for migraine prophylaxis**

   Nonselective β-blockers like propranolol, timolol, and tricyclic antidepressant drugs like amytriptiline have been found to be effective for prophylaxis in patients who experience frequent episodes of migraine. Antiepileptic drugs like valproic acid, gabapentine, and topiramate are also effective prophylactic agents. Similarly, calcium channel blockers like verapamil and flunarazine have been found to efficacious for migraine prophylaxis.
2. **Methysergide, a 5-HT antagonist:** is also useful in doses of 4-10 mg /day as prophylactic agent for migraine. The following strategy can be used to manage an acute attack depending upon the severity of the headache.

Moderate Headache - NSAIDs, opioids, acetaminophen, aspirin, ergotamine with caffeine, isometheptene, naratriptan, rizatriptan, sumatriptan, zolmitriptan, almotryptan, frovatriptan, eliptrypton.

Severe Headache - Naratrytan, Rizatryptan, Sumatryptan, frovatryptan, dihydroergotamine (DHE), Dopamine antagonists.

Triptans - (Sumatryptan, Zolmitriptan, Naratriptan, Rizatriptan, Eletriptan, Almotriptan, Frovatryptan) activate 5 – HTIB and 5 – HTD receptors on the presynaptic trigeminal nerve endings to inhibit the release of vasodilating peptides like calcitonin gene – related (CGRP) which is responsible for vasodilation, the characteristic feature of migraine and which is responsible for throbbing headache. They cause vasoconstriction. Triptans reduce the nociceptive transmission in the brain stem trigeminal nucleus and diminish central sensitization. They reduce nausea and vomiting by deactivation of central tryptaminergic system.

Newer additions for migraine treatment

Ditans

Lasmiditan is a 5–HTF1 receptor agonist. Ditans do not elicit vasoconstrictive effect, whereas triptans cause vasoconstriction via agonist action at 5 – HT1B/1D receptors. It is given in a dose range of 50mg – 200mg/orally once daily depending upon the frequency and severity of the migraine episodes. It can be given in patients with CV diseases unlike triptans which are likely to produce prinzmetal angina and other CV symptoms like ventricular arrhythmias. Pain freedom period post – dose is 4 to 6 hours.

Gepants

Gepants (**Rimegepant, ubrogepant, atogepant**) are calcitonin gene – related peptide (CGRP) receptor antagonists. They block the vasodilation that CGRP causes which is associated with migraine pain and are used to abort an acute attack of migraine. Ubrogepant comes as an oral dissolvable tablet and gets dissolved instantly and then swallowed. The dose is 75mg once daily. All the three drugs allow a pain freedom of 2 hours.

Zavegepant is a third generation gepant given intranasally

It is a high affinity, selective and structurally unique, small molecule CGRP receptor antagonist. It inhibits neurogenic inflammation caused by trigeminal nerve release of CGRP. It also inhibits the pathological dilation of intracranial arteries. It is given transnasally in a dose of 10 mg/spray in one nostril at a time. The dose can be repeated once/day.

Monoclonal antibodies

These are fully grown humanized immunoglobulin G1(IgG1) monoclonal antibodies that block CGRP receptor and prevent the inflammatory responses seen in migraine and indicated as prophylactic agents for prevention of migraine attacks

Eptinezumab is a monoclonal antibody that target CGRP α and β and given as IV infusion in a dose 100mg once in three months.

Erenumab

It is available as single dose prefilled sureclick autoinjector in 70mg/mL and 140mg/ mL doses. It is indicated for preventive treatment of migraines and given subcutaneously in the prescribed doses once monthly. The other drugs that belong to this category include **fremanezumab**, and **galcanezumab,**

Monoclonal antibodies have high efficacy for prophylactic use in migraine. They also have longer periods of pain free states when compared to the rest of the drugs used for prophylaxisof migraine.

5

Hyperkalemia – Role of Potassium Binders

Overview

Hyperkalemia is a potentially life – threatening metabolic problem caused by inability of the kidneys to excrete potassium, impairment mechanisms that move potassium from the circulation into the cells, or a combination of these factors. The triggering cause of acute episodes of hyperkalemia include overdose of drugs affecting K+ homeostasis and also due to dehydration. In patients with diabetic nephropathy, hyperkalemia may be caused by the syndrome of **hyporeninemic hypoaldosteronism**.

The presence of typical ECG findings is suggestive of hyperkalemia of acute origin and can be confirmed by the elevated levels of serum potassium levels greater than 5.5 or 6.5 mEq/L or nearing 7.0 mEq/L.

Disorders causing Hyperkalemia

1. Disorders leading to hyperkalemia caused by impaired renal excretion of potassium – acquired hyporeninemic hypoaldosteronism; Addison's disease, congenital adrenal hyperplasia, mineralocorticoid deficiency, primary hypoaldosteronism or hyporeninemia, pseudohypoaldosteronism, renal insufficiency or failure, systemic lupus erythematosus and type - 4 renal tubular acidosis.
2. Disorders leading to hyperkalemia caused by shift of potassium into extracellular space – Diabetic ketoacidosis, damage to tissue from rhabdomyolysis caused by statins, burns or trauma; familial hyperkalemic periodic paralysis; hyperosmolar states (uncontrolled diabetes, glucose infusions); insulin deficiency or resistance, and tumor lysis syndrome.
3. Agents/drugs that may cause hyperkalemia – Amiloride, triamterene and other potassium sparing diuretics, amino acids, ACE inhibitors or AT1 receptor antagonists, azole antifungals, β – blockers, cyclosporine, digoxin at toxic levels, fluoride toxicity, glucose infusions or insulin deficiency, heparins, NSAIDs, potassium supplements, succinylcholine, tacrolimus, trimethoprim and pentamidine.

Diagnosis

The initial diagnostic approach begins with clinical history, review of medications, and physical examination followed by laboratory investigations as early as possible.

The presenting symptoms include muscle cramps, muscular weakness or flaccid paralysis and characteristic ECG findings such as tall peaked 'T' wave, loss (flattening) of 'P' wave, prolongation of PR interval, widened QRS complex. These ECG changes progress to a state of ventricular arrhythmias if remedial measures are not taken immediately. The immediate laboratory tests included serum electrolytes, creatinine, and blood urea nitrogen. A spot urine test for potassium, creatinine and osmoles should be obtained to calculate the **fractional excretion of potassium gradient** (trans-tubular potassium gradient) which is an assessment of renal potassium handling with a normal value of six to nine, rising at times to 11 after an increase of potassium intake. Values lower than five in the face of hyperkalemia suggest an inappropriate renal response to high potassium, a very low value suggests hypoaldosteronism.

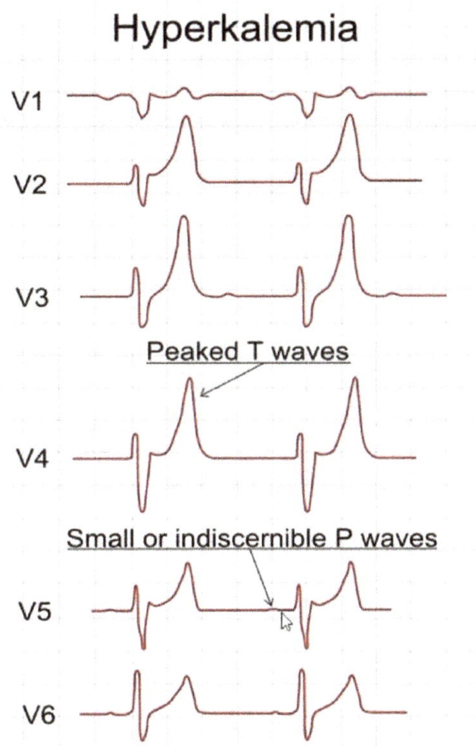

Management of hyperkalemia

Urgent treatment of hyperkalemia includes stabilizing the myocardium to protect against arrhythmias and shifting potassium from the vascular space into the cells. After the serum potassium level is reduced to safe levels, treatment focuses on lowering total body potassium. The following lines of therapy are more appropriate to manage a case of hyperkalemia.

Medication	Recommended doses for hyperkalemia	Route of administration	Onset of action
Calcium	10 mL.Calcium chloride or calcium gluconate	IV	Immediate 1 – 3 min
Insulin (Short – acting)	10 units	IV	1 – 3 min
Albuterol	10 – 20mg	Inhalation	30 min
Frusemide	40 – 80mg	IV	15min
Sodium polystyrene sulfonate	15 – 60g	Oral	>2hr
(Available sorbitol – free)	30 – 50g	Rectal	>7hr
Patiromer	8.4 – 25.2g	Oral	7hr
Sodium Zirconium cyclosilicate	10g 3times a day initial dose for two days, 10g once a day later	Oral	>7hr

1. **IV calcium** is indicated when the serum potassium is >6.5m Eq/L regardless whether ECG changes are present. The immediate goal of acute management in hyperkalemia is the stabilization of the cardiac membrane potential. **Calcium antagonizes the effects of hyperkalemia** through effects on the threshold potential and the speed of impulse propagation at the cellular level. It should be noted that calcium has no effects on the serum potassium levels and does not lower them. It does not facilitate or promote the intracellular shift or elimination of potassium. **It is given mainly for the purpose of preventing any possible development of ventricular arrhythmia**.
2. **Insulin**: Insulin accelerates the intracellular movement of potassium into muscle cells by binding to its receptor on skeletal muscle. Once this occurs, the abundance and activity of ATPase increases on the cell membrane and there is rapid shift of potassium from extracellular compartment into intracellular compartments thereby leading to a decrease of serum K+ levels quite effectively.
3. **B2 agonists** – Albuterol (salbutamol) inhalation can be considered in non-acute situations to lower potassium. Albuterol stimulates Na^+K^+ ATPase, which results in intracellular shift of potassium. Use of albuterol has been shown to decrease serum potassium levels by 0.3 to 0.6 mEq/L within 30 minutes and the decrease lasts for 2 hours. Doses from 10 to 20mg utilized in hyperkalemia are much higher than those used to treat acute bronchospasm. Due to the higher doses used and the potential β1 receptor stimulation may cause tachycardia.
4. **Diuretics:** Following the use of methods to shift potassium into the cells, strategies should then be undertaken to eliminate excess potassium. In patients with adequate kidney function, loop diuretics (frusemide and bumetanide) in combination with thiazides can be used for the excretion of potassium. Onset of action is 15 to 30 minutes.
5. **Sodium polystyrene sulfonate (SPS):** It is insoluble polymer cation - exchange resin which can be given either orally or per rectum. It causes an exchange of sodium with potassium in the GI tract. But it is associated with some bowel necrosis because of the presence of sorbitol in it.
6. **Potassium binders**: **Patiromer and Zirconium cyclosilicate (SZC)** are the new class of drugs that are being used to treat hyperkalemia on a long term basis soon after the emergency treatment with calcium, insulin, β2 agonists and diuretics is successful thereby preventing the development of complications for an acute state of hyperkalemia. Patiromer is a nonspecific binder of potassium in the colon that exchanges calcium for potassium whereas SZC selectively binds potassium in exchange for sodium and hydrogen ions in the small and large intestine

Comparison of Novel potassium binders – [Patiromer and Zirconium cyclosilicate]

	Patiromer	SZC
Mode of action	Nonspecific cation binding in exchange for $Ca^{+}2$	Selective K+ binding in exchange for Na^+ and H^+
Time to Normokalemia	Achieves normokalemia as early as 1 week depending on severity of hyperkalemia	84% of patients normokalemic within 24 hours
Onset of effect	K^+ levels reduced significantly 7 hours after 1st dose	Median time to normalization 2.2 hours
Drug – drug interactions	Other oral drugs administration at least 3 hours before or after patiromer	Other oral drugs administered at least 2 hours before or after SZC
Location of K^+ binding	Distal colon predominantly	Likely to be upper and lower GI tract

Table *Contd...*

	Patiromer	SZC
Safety and tolerability	Well tolerated but may cause hypomagnesemia and GI adverse effects like mild to moderate constipation	Well tolerated but may cause edema and mild to moderate GI adverse effects
Effective in maintaining normokalemia in the presence of drug actions through RAAS inhibition	RAAS inhibitors can be continued	RAAS inhibitors can be continued
Dose and route of administration	8.4g orally once a day, adjusted in weekly intervals based on K^+ levels (Maximum of 25.2g/day)	10g 3 times a day given orally for 2 days followed by 10g once a day as maintenance dose adjusted as per K^+ levels

Conclusion

Hyperkalemia is an emergency clinical condition when the serum K^+ levels cross 6.5 mEq/L. The first line of treatment is aimed at prevention of cardiac irregularities – ventricular arrhythmia by giving calcium IV. This is followed by the use of insulin plus glucose given IV (glucose to prevent a possible hypoglycomia), β2 agonists and frusemide to facilitate a decrease of K^+ by effecting shift of potassium into the intracellular compartments in the skeletal muscle. Then the use of potassium binding agents patiromer and zirconium cyclosilicate facilitates a sustained loss of potassium, lowering the serum potassium levels for a considerable period of time and to prevent recurrent acute episodes of hyperkalemia.

6

The Role of Dual GIP/GLP-I Receptor Agonism in the Management of Diabetes and Overweight

Overview

In the existing scenario of alarming increase of incidence of diabetes mellitus globally there is a need for efficient and safe therapy to improve such metabolic diseases as obesity and type-2 diabetes.

Type – 2 diabetes(T2D) is a complex disease and a common pathway appears for most people with T2D and obesity. Obesity is a triggering factor for diabetes associated with insulin resistance. In individuals who are obese, non-esterified fatty acids, glycerol, hormones, and pro-inflammatory cytokines that could participate in development of insulin resistance are released by adipose tissue. Besides, endoplasmic reticulum stress, adipose tissue hypoxia, oxidative stress, lipodystrophy, and genetic background have a role in insulin resistance. It is generally accepted that people with T2D who are obese and insulin-resistant have a more central distribution of fat excess (visceral fat). The body fat instead of confining to subcutaneous tissue is distributed to skeletal muscle and liver (insulin target tissues). Visceral fat accumulation not only promotes low-grade inflammation at the systemic level but also favors ectopic fat accumulation mainly in the liver and skeletal muscle.These mechanisms lead to development of reduction of insulin action in these tissues which lead to insulin resistance. There is an overall decreasing β-cell functionality and also a core need to promote insulin secretion by different mechanisms as a part of therapeutic approach to treat T2D.

An effective treatment of obesity and diabetes simultaneously is the most preferred choice to reduce CV and stoke risk in those who are obese with associated T2DM.

The development of dual GIP-GLP1R co-agonists that bind to either one or other receptor (sequence-mixed dual agonists) has emerged as an innovative therapeutic strategy for both obesity and type-2 diabetes.

Incretin hormones

Incretins are hormones that work to increase insulin secretion. There are two main incretin hormones in humans. GLP-I (glucagon-like Peptide-I) and GIP (glucose dependent insulotropic peptide, also known as gastric inhibitory peptide. Both the hormones are secreted by the endocrine cells, GLP-1 through L-type cells, GIP through K-type cells that are located in the epithelium of the small intestine (duodenum and upper jejunum GIP). GLP-1 and GIP act through their specific receptors (GLP-1R and GIP-R). Glucose in the small intestine stimulates incretin release. Incretins are carried through the circulation to the target tissue, the pancreatic β-cells. Incretin stimulation of β-cells causes them to secrete more insulin in response to meals (post pandreal increase of insulin). Hence it is observed that reduced incretin effect is responsible for the glucose intolerance seen in diabetes.

Based on the clinical experiences and several clinical trials it was found that GLP-I agonists like exenatide, dulaglutide, liraglutide, lexisenaside, albiglutide and semaglutide were shown as potent insulotropic agents and found a place prominently in the treatment of type 2 diabetes. But the role of GIP in its effectiveness for the clinical use in type 2 is not fully understood till recently. However, its role came out with clarity in the study of pancreatic hormonal status post bariatric surgery, (a procedure performed to help patients who are severely overweight lose excess fat in order to lower the risk of severe, life threatening health conditions such as heart disease, stroke, high blood pressure, non-alcoholic fatty liver disease, sleep apnea, and T2DM) wherein there is an increase in various gut hormones such as GLP-I, GIP and peptide YY (PYY) all of which cause stimulation of insulin secretion. In addition, it was also observed that they have effects to reduce body weight by various mechanisms. These findings led to the development of dual –peptide agonists which target not only GLP-I receptor but also that of GIP receptors. However, it was also observed that while GLP-I is a very powerful incretin hormone that stimulates insulin secretion in both healthy and patients with TD2, GIP elicits a significant stimulation of insulin secretion in healthy subjects, but the effect is less in patients of TD2.

It is also observed that GLP-I lowers glucagon secretion while GIP increases the same through stimulation of pancreatic α cells.

The following chart gives the physiological effects brought about by both GLP-I and GIP (pleiotropic actions of GLP-I and GIP in T2D)

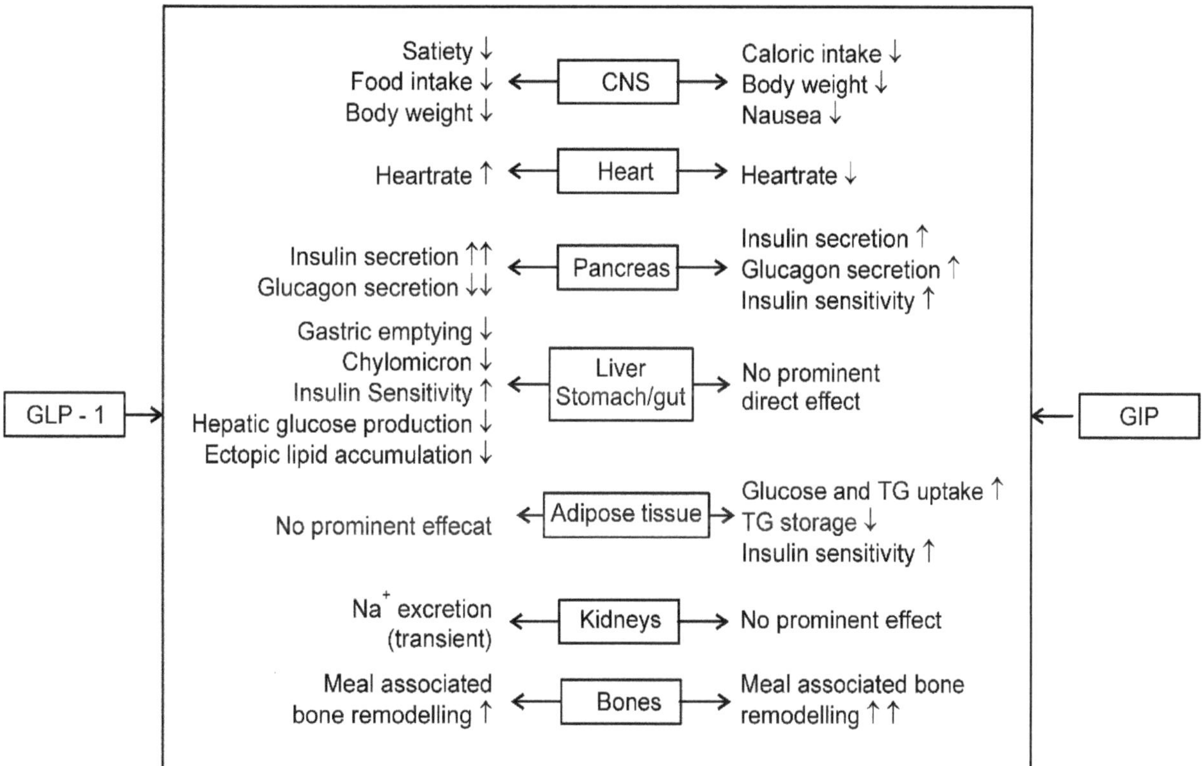

Pleiotropic acton of GLP Iand GIP in T_2D

Observations of incretin hormonal effects post bariatric surgery		
1. Pancreas →	↑ Sensitivity of β cells	**Overall effects**
2. Stomach→	↑ PPY (Pancreatic Peptide Y)	Increased formation of GLP- I,
3. Intestines→	↓ Ghrelin	GIP, glucagon and peptide YY
4. Adipose tissue→	↑ GLP	lowered
5. Brain→	↓ GIP	**Provides a more sustained**
	↓ Leptin resolution, leptin resistance	**glycemic control and body**
	↓ NPY (Neuro pepticle Y)	**weight reduction**

These findings suggest the beneficial effects of bariatric surgery (Roux-en-Y Gastric Bypass (RNY)) as the most ideal procedure in the control of T2D associated with excess body weight.

With continued efforts in the development of newer antidiabetic agents, unimolecular GLP- IR/GIP-R dual agonists (twin cretins) can provide added efficacy especially among obese individuals with T2D. The simultaneous activation of GLP-IR and GIP- R might have greater, multiplicative effect on glucose lowering abilities than either agent alone. GIP is responsible for a substantial portion of postpandreal insulin secretion in T2D and mild hyperglycemia in early disease. These hormones seem to work in tandem, GLP-I inhibits of glucagon secretion when plasma glucose concentration is high, while GIP acts at lower glucose levels. Thus, GIP functions as both ally and a rival in T2D, depending upon the glucose status, the stage in the natural history of the disease, and the GLP-I presence in the system. Because GLP-I and GIP may act synergistically on pancreatic β-cells, simultaneous activation of both the pathways may have additional benefits on β-cell functionality. Additionally, GIP also causes a weight reduction apart from the one produced by GLP-I.

Tirzepatide

Tirzepatide known as **'twincretin'** is a first-in-class and the only GLP-I and GIP receptor agonist that can significantly reduce glycemic levels and improve insulin sensitivity, as well as reducing body weight by more than 20% and improving lipid metabolism.

Therapeutic benefits of Tirzepatide

1. **Insulin secretion and insulin sensitivity:** Tirzepatide has shown significant improvement in insulin secretion and insulin sensitivity compared to semaglutide. It induces insulin in response to meal (primarily by hyperosmolality of glucose in the duodenum) to facilitate the metabolism of carbohydrates, fats and proteins. It works to stimulate first and second phase insulin secretion and reduces glucagon levels, both in a glucose dependent manner. Tirzepatide is also shown to delay gastric emptying, lower fasting and postpandreal glucose concentration, decrease food intake and reduce body weight in patient with type 2 diabetes.
2. **Hb A1c levels:** Tirzepatide (5mg, 10mg and 15mg) demonstrated significantly lowered HbA1c and body weight in comparison to insulin glargine, insulin degludec and as add on therapy with metformin or metformin+ SGLT-2inhibitor according to surpass-1, surpass-2, surpass-3, surpass-4 trials at the end of 52 weeks of treatment (up to 25% lowering from the base level at 15mg weekly doses).

Indications

Tirzepatide is indicated as an adjuvant to diet and exercise to treat T2 diabetic patients who are overweight and not adequately responding to the first line antidiabetic drugs like metformin, sulfonylurea, GLP-I agonists, SGLT-2 inhibitors or DPP-4 inhibitors.

Route of administration and dosage

It is highly bound to albumin in the plasma, which prolongs its half-life (5 days). Hence given once weekly as subcutaneous injection.

As initiation therapy it is started at a lower dose of 2.5mg/SC once weekly and given for 4 weeks. Then the dose is increased to 5mg/SC week and further increased to a maximum dose of 15mg per week.

Adverse effects

Hypoglycemia, nausea, vomiting, clyspepsia, abdominal pain and occasional hypersensitivity reactions

Availability

It is available as 2.5mg/0.5ml, 5mg/0.5ml, 7.5mg/0.5ml and 10mg/0.5ml for subcutaneous administration.

7

Oxerin Peptides – Antagonists – their Clinical Applications

Overview

Orexins (orexin A and orexin B) comprise two neuropeptides produced by orexin neurons in the lateral hypothalamus and released by extensive projections of these neurons throughout the central neurons system. Oxerins bind and activate their associated G – protein coupled orexin type-I receptors (OX1Rs) and orexin–2 receptors (OX2Rs) and act on numerous physiological processes, such as sleep-wake regulation, feeding, reward, emotion, and motivation. Orexinl(OX1Rs) markedly increase wakefulness by their direct action on the locus coeruleus and Cingular Cortex, while OX2Rs are selectively expressed in tuberomammilary nucleus, hypothalamic paraventricular nucleus and nucleus accumbens. Narcolepsy usually results from loss of orexin neurons and their corresponding peptide levels and action through respective receptors. Narcolepsy not only produces day time sleepiness, but also dysregulation of REM sleep during sleep cycle. Orexins also thought to play some role in the normal control of appetite. Orexin neurons may also contribute to the behavioral and autonomic responses consequent to stress. It has been found that orexins also play a role in the pathophysiology of psychiatric disorders, depression, sleep disorders, anxiety and drug addiction. By blocking both the receptors by antagonists it is possible to find suitable, alternative and even effective agents for majority of the conditions.

Orexin receptor antagonists include selective OXIR antagonists (SORA1s), selectiveOX2Rs antagonists (SORA2s) and dual OXI/2R antagonists (DORAs), based on their receptor selectivity are used in the treatment of these disorders based on both preclinical and clinical evidence. SORA2s and DORAs have more pronounced efficacy in the treatment of sleep disorders, whereas SORA1s may be promising for the treatment of anxiety and drug addiction. Many reviews have indicated that orexin system is involved in the regulation of reward, motivated behaviors, and stress related psychiatric disorders.

Orexin antagonists

Suvorexant was the first dual OX1/2R antagonist approved for clinical use to treat insomnia. Another dual antagonist (DORA) Remborexant has been shown to be effective for similar use (insomnia). **Seltorexant** and **Lemborexant** are the other OX1/OX2R antagonists that are developed in the recent past and have shown promising clinical effects in the management of sleep disorders, psychiatric disorders associated with insomnia, and as adjutants in the treatment of cocaine addiction along with deaddiction treatments.

Clinical uses of orexin receptor antagonists

Sleep disorders, especially primary insomnia

The discovery of selective orexin neuron loss in narcolepsy sparked great research interest in the sleep field and raised the possibility of an alternative approach of treating the symptoms of insomnia with orexin receptor antagonists. OX1Rs and OX2Rs play distinct roles in gating NERM and REM sleep. OX2Rs are the pivotal receptors that regulate wakefulness and NREM sleep, whereas REM sleep is controlled by both the receptor subtypes.

DORAs block the activity of both OX1Rs and OX2Rs and result in a rapid transition to sleep. Suvorexant inhibits the wakefulness blocking orexin neurons of the arousal system. It promotes sleep primarily by increasing REM sleep duration and reducing the latency to REM sleep. It also improves sleep maintenance. Dependence and abuse liability are also less unlike barbiturates, benzodiazepines, and so also are the respiratory depression or change in the balance or gait. **Suvorexant** has an onset of action of 1hr after administrator with a half-life of 12.2hr. It is given orally in doses of 10mg/day 1hr before going to bed and also can be increased to 20mg. It has very minimal adverse effects profile. Dose related somnolence and CNS depression have been reported with the use of suvorexant.

Lemborexant is another dual OX1R/OX2R antagonist indicated for insomnia characterized by difficulties with sleep onset and/or sleep maintenance. It has an onset of action in 15-20 minutes, peak plasma levels reached in1-3 hr after administration and has an elimination half- life of 17hr (5mg) 19hr (10mg). It is given orally in a 5mg dose immediately before going to bed, with at least 7hr remaining before planned time of awakening.

8

Renal Denervation

Overview

Hypertension is a significant cause of morbidity and mortality worldwide and plays an important role in the etiopathogenesis of many clinical conditions like ischemic heart disease, cardiac failure, renal failure and stroke. However, many individuals fail to achieve proper blood pressure control despite lifestyle modifications and maximal medical therapy. Renal sympathetic overactivity has been proposed as a significant driver issuch cases. *One potential treatment is renal denervation (RND),* a minimally invasive catheter – based technology that uses *radiofrequency energy* to obliterate the renal nerves adjacent to the afferent and efferent renal arteries. It involves the use of a catheter to position electrodes (typically 4 spaced approximately 6mm apart in a spiral sequence) that generate heat using medium – frequency alternating current. The heat generated causes obliteration of the sympathetic renal nerves. More recently, several studies suggest that *catheter – based ultrasound ablation* is a better option for RND as an alternative to radiofrequency ablation due to deeper penetration of ultrasoundenergy and more competitive renal nerve ablation. Another approach other than the two consists ofintroduction of a small catheter with 3 tiny concentrically placed micro needles embedded in it. When the catheter is properly positioned the micro needles are extended, penetrating the renal artery wall into the perivascular space, and a small amount of liquid neurotoxin (typically a total of 0.6mL of absolute ethanol) is injected through the 3 needles simultaneously which results in renal denervatrion

Present status of Renal denervation

- A clinical consensus statement on the use of renal denervation (RDN) for the treatment of hypertension (HTN) was recently put forth by the European society of cardiology council (ESC) on hypertension and European Association of cardiovascular interventions.
- The European statement concludes that RND may be used in adult patients with uncontrolled resistant hypertension. Specific parameters for eligible patients include office/ hospital BP≥160/≥90 mm confirmed by 24-hour ambulatory systolic BP(SBP)≥150 mmHg or daytime SBP ≥ 140 mm Hg, treatment with ≥3 antihypertensive drugs, and eGFR ≥ 40 mL/min/1.73m^2.
- It is mainly indicated in uncontrolled and persistent hypertension not responding to physical activity, dietary modifications and the use of specific antihypertensive drugs for considerable periods and those likely to develop complications if blood pressure is not controlled within the reasonable levels.
- The European statement also concludes that RDN may be possible treatment option for patients who are unable to tolerate long – term treatment with antihypertensive drugs and for patients who express a preference to undergo RDN is a shared decision – making process.
- **RDN has been shown to effectively lower BP for at least 3 years**. A global study had shown RND demonstrated decreases in both office/hospital and 24 – hour ambulatory SBP sustained over 3 years, and a 26% relative risk reduction in major cardiovascular events.
- Safety of catheter – based RDN procedures bas been demonstrated through multiple meta – analyses.
- RDN is only valid for patients suffering from primary hypertension

The RDN status in India

- The first RDN procedure was successfully performed at CIMS hospital, Ahmedabad using the simplicity TM renal denervation system of Medtronic's Inc. It was further used successfully at Apollo hospital, Indore and Metromed International cardiac center, Calicut, Kerala. The observations include
    1. The treatment is minimally invasive; does not require open surgery and it takes 40 – 60 minutes and performed under local anesthesia.
    2. Patients aged between 18 and ≥80 years are eligible to undergo if their systolic blood pressure of 160 mm Hg – 170 mm Hg and are on the regular use of minimum 2 drugs for the treatment of hypertension for the past 3-4 years without much specific reduction of BP towards normal levels.

9

New Drug Approvals and Treatment Guidelines Approved in the Recent Past

1. **Olanzapine Samidorphan**

   Olanzapine is a second – generation antipsychotic with established efficiency in several psychiatric diseases. It acts through 5-H-T2A, D2,H1, and M1 receptors. It is commonly prescribed to treat **schizophrenia** both for acute attack and for maintenance therapy and usually given in doses of 10-30mg/day. The target symptoms for which the antipsychotic drugs seem to be especially effective include agitation, combativeness, hostility, hallucinations, delusions, insomnia, anorexia, poor self – care, negativism, and social withdrawal. Olanzapine is also useful to treat schizo effective disrobers which area a combination of schizophrenia and affective disorders.

   But the main adverse effects of olanzapine include weight gain and metabolic effects (insulin resistance leading to onset of diabetes mellitus. **Samidorphan** is a novel opioid antagonist that bindsto μ, K and δ – opioid receptors and is hypothesized to reduce cravings for high calorie foods thus attenuating antipsychotic – induced weight gain. The combination of olanzapine and samidorphan is approved by the FDA in June 2021 and has since being given for schizophrenia and bipolar disorder.

   The recommended dose for both the drugs – olanzapine and samidorphan is 10mg each/day which can be increased to 15mg (olanzapine) and 10mg (samidorphan) over a period. The same dose is applicable to treat bipolar disorder also.

2. **Drospirenone /ethinylestradiol**

   Drospirenone 3mg/(progestin) and ethinylestradiol(estrogen) 20 micrograms or 30 micrograms is a new unique oral contraceptive formulation that combines in a novel dosing regimen- the lowest dosage of ethinyl estradiol commonly used today with drospirenone.

   Ethinyl estradiol reduces gonadotropin releasing hormone (GnRH) from hypothalamus, reduces gonadotropin (FSH and LH) release from pituitary, thereby preventing ovulation and corpus luteum formation. The combination of the two drugs also brings about a change in the cervical mucus which becomes viscid and scanty thus inhibiting sperm penetration and motility, changes in the endometrium, and secretion in the uterine tubes, all of which prevent fertilization and a possible implantation.

   Drospirenone is the progestin used in the combination and it is a spironolactone analog with anti – mineralocorticoid and antiandrogenic activity.

   The combination drug is available as a 28 tablet pack, 21 of which contain the medication and the rest contain an inert substance. One tablet is taken – each day for 28 days and continued for 28 days. The cycle starts on the 5th day of the menstrual and continued for 28 days. Withdrawal bleeding occurs at the end of the 21 – day active medication.

   The combination preparation is also useful to treatment premenstrual syndrome/disorder andacne.

3. **American diabetic association (ADA)** suggests new blood pressure and lipid targets for people with Diabetes
    1. A document of ADA for the standard of care in diabetes for the year 2023 suggests the following guidelines to keep morbidity and mortality of diabetic people under control.
    2. The blood pressure should be controlled and adjusted to the level of 130/80 mmHg.
    3. LDL cholesterol levels below 70 mg/dL
    4. Weight loss as one of the primary preventive measures
    5. Use of **finerenone** for the use of people with chronic kidney disease (CKD) andassociated/Primary condition of diabetes mellitus.
    6. Regular monitoring of HbA1c of >6% with suitable drug dosage adjustments.
    7. Guidance and screening of peripheral artery disease
    8. The new targets of lipid levels for people with diabetes between the ages of 40-75years who are at increased CV risk factors, Including those with one or more atherosclerotic risk factors, high – intensity statin therapy is recommended to reduce LDL cholesterol by 50% or more of baseline and to a target of less than 70mg/dL. To achieve this, adding **ezetimibe** or a **PCSK of inhibitor like Evolocumab, alorocumab, Evinacumab** along with the maximally tolerated statin dose is highly recommended.
    9. Another recommendation calls for the addition of SGLT inhibitor **(dapagliflozin**, **empagliflozin, canagliflozin, sotagliflozin**) for kidney protection in people with estimated GFR $\geq$ 20mL/min/1.73^{2}cm and urinary albumin $\geq$ 200mg/g, albumin/creatine ratio of 30mg/g for more than 3 months.

4. **Dasiglucon**

    Dasiglucon is a glucagon receptor agonist which increases blood glucose concentration by activating hepatic glucagon receptors, thereby stimulating glycogen breakdown and release of glucose from the liver. It is used as a **anti-hypoglycemic agent** indicated for the treatment of severe hypoglycemia in patients with diabetes in whom the blood glucose levels fall significantly due to overdose of antidiabetic drugs

    Dasiglucon is given in a dose of 0.6mg subcutaneously (through autoinjector and prefilled syringe)

5. **Drugs for heart failure with reduced ejection fraction (EF)**

    (a) Omecamtiv Mecabryl (selective myocin activator) has been shown to improve cardiac function in patients with heart failure with a reduced ejection fraction. It augments cardiac contractility by effectively binding to cardiac myocin, thus increasing the number of force generators(myocin heads) that can bind to the actin filament and initiate a power stroke at the start of the systole. Short term IV administration of the drug improved cardiac performance in early clinical trials.

    It increased the left ventricular systolic ejection time, and stroke Volume, decreased left ventricular systolic and diastolic volumes with a suggested beneficial reversal of cardiac remodeling and reduced Plasma natriuritic peptide levels and heart rate.

    (b) Vericiguat, a novel soluble guanylate cyclase(sGC) stimulator, is approved for the treatment of heart failure with reduced ejection fraction. Decreased nitric oxide(NO) availability, sGC desensitization to NO, sGC deficiency, and reduced cGMP signaling are potential contributing factors for HF-disease progression. Vericiguat works via stimulation of sGC in the critical NO-sGC-cGMP Pathway.

    It is indicated for the treatment of the adult with symptomatic chronic HF and EF less than 45% following a hospitalization for HF or need for outpatient IV diuretics.

    A starting dose of 2.5mg is administered orally once daily with food. The dose is the doubled approximately every two weeks to reach the target maintenance dose of 10mg once daily with food.

6. **Istradefylline:** It is indicated as adjuvant therapy to Levodopa and Carbidopa in Parkinsons disease to treat "off" episodes, caused when the existing medicines are ineffective and lead to an increase in PD symptoms. It is a selective D2 receptor agonist which is supposed to reduce the overactivity of the straital pathway, restoring the balance of besal ganglia. It is available as 20 and 40mg tablets. Adenosine is an endogenous A2 receptor agonist and Istradefylline blocks A2 receptor and simultaneously also acts as a D2 receptor agonist and thus inhibits the actions of adenosine and promoting the movement(locomotion).
7. **Daclatasvir:** It is indicated for the treatment of Hepatitis-C infection and used along with sofosbuvir. It is available in 30, 60 mg tablets given once daily
8. **Abiraterone:** It is an androgen antagonist used along with prednisolone or methylprednisolone to treat castration-resistant metastatic prostate cancer and given in 25 mg tablets twice daily
9. **Pitavastatin:** It is a statin and acts by inhibiting HMG-COA reductase enzyme thereby preventing the production LDL cholesterol and triglyserides with a moderate increase in HDL cholesterol and used in dyslipidemias. It is given orally in 2 mg/ day
10. **Carbotegravir:** It is an integrase strand Transfer inhibitor used in combination with Rilpivirine for the treatment of HIV infection. It is given orally in doses of 30 mg/day
11. **Paliperidone:** It is a second generation antipsychotic (atypical antipsychotic). It is used in Schizophrenia, Schzoeffective disorders, It is very effective in treating positive symptoms (hallucinations, delusions) and negative symptoms (social withdrawal, ambivalence) of Schizophrenia. It is also indicated in major depressive disorders, delusional disorder, severe agitation, Tourette disorder, acute mania, and personality disorder.
12. **Tenegliptin:** It is an antidiabetic drug and acts by inhibiting dipeptidylpeptidase enzyme (DPP-4 inhibitor) which is responsible for the breakdown of GLP-1 thereby increasing its availability and used in T2D
13. **Umeclidinium:** It is a long acting muscarinic antagonist approved for the maintenance treatment of COPD. It is also approved as a combination drug along with **Vilanterol** and fluticasone for the same indication. It is found to be effective for bronchitis and emphysema. It is a power for inhalation each actuation containing 62.5 mcg inhaled once daily.

    Vilaterol is long acting β2 adrenergic agonist used in combination with other bronchodilators for the management of COPD, including chronic bronchitis and emphysema. It is a highly selective β2 agonist with a faster onset of action than salmeterol

    Mechanism of action: It increase intracellular adenylcyclase which catalyzes the conversion of ATP to cyclic AMP which causes relaxation of bronchial smooth muscle, and inhibition of release of hypersensitivity mediators from mast cells in the lungs. It is available as 22 mcg metered dose powder for inhalation as aeroso, usually in combination of fluticasone and or Umiclidinium.
14. **Risperodone injectable** (extended release) –bi-weekly long acting formulation used as atypical antipsychotic for the treatment of Schizophernia.
15. **Lenacapavir:** It is a long acting HIV-1 capsid inhibitor for use in combination with other anti- retroviral HIV drugs for the treatment of HIV-1 infection in heavily treatment experienced people with multidrug resistant HIV-1 infection.
16. **Bexagliflozin**: It is a sodium-glucose cotransporter-2 (SGLT-2) inhibitor indicated as adjutant to diet and exercise to improve glycemic control in adults withT2D.
17. **Elacestrant:** It is an estrogen receptor antagonist indicated for the treatment of ER-positive, HER-2 negative, and ESR-1 mutated breast cancer in women with disease progression following at least one line of endocrine therapy. It is given orally in single daily doses of 345 mg.

18. **Daprodustat:** It is an oral hypoxia-inducible factor propylhydroxylase inhibitor (HIP-PH-1) indicated for the treatment of anemia in those patients with chronic renal disease(CKD) who are on dialysis treatment for ≥ 4 months. It stabilizes hypoxia inducing factor required for the synthesis of endogenous erythropoietin from kidneys. It increases serum tranferrin and total iron binding capacity. It also decreases serum tranferrtin levels, transferritin saturation, and hepcidin. It is given orally in daily doses of 4 mg which can titrated upwards to 8-12 mg/day as per the needs.

19. **SARS- Covid-2 and Covid- 19 medications:** In the acute phase of Covid infection there is an acute surge of cytokines that include IL-8, Gamma interferon (greatly produced by T lymphocytes) which in turn stimulates macrophages, and these make many cytokines that include IL-1B, IL-6, TNFα, granulocyte-macrophage colony stimulating factor (GM-CSF) all of which play important role in the genesis of inflammatory reaction in Covid-19.

    25-40% Covid positive patients are asymptomatic. The others have mild, a bad-flu-like illness that may keep Covid-19 positive patients in bed for periods of 2-3 weeks. Out of these 20% need hospitalizations for respiratory symptoms.

    Fever, dry cough, congestion, nausea, vomiting, headache, loss of taste and smell, muscle and body aches, and diarrhea are seen early on primarily. Hypoxia develops later that necessitates O2 administration. C-reactive protein levels rise and also lactic dehydrogenase.

    Tocilizumab is the usual monoclonal antibody which controls cytokine surge along with dexamethasone. Anakirna (IL1 recdeptor antagonist) and Emapalumab are also effective in controlling the cytokine surge. Many antiviral drugs were found to be effective if used early on the symptoms of Cocod-19. They include **Nirmatrelvir** (Paxlovid developed by Pfizer) is a protease inhibitor given orally in a dose of 300 mg in combination with **ritonavir**100 mg for 5 days.

20. **Molnupiravir:** It is new antiviral drug for cases of patients who do not require hospitalizations andsuffering from mild to moderate infection with Covid-19. The treatment with molnupiravir has tobe initiated within first few days of diagnosis of symptoms and the drug does not work towards the more severe end of the spectrum, and even in moderate cases if started late. It is given oral in doses of 800 mg twice daily for 15 days

21. **Remdesivir:** It is a nucleotide prodrug of an adenosine analog. It is effective in Covid-19 patients who have mild to moderate symptoms and likely to progress to severe stage and need hospitalization due to different causes. It is usually given in hospitalized patients who require monitoring of vital functions, who require ventilator support and to arrest further progression which is likely to lead to respiratory failure and mortality. It is available as power to be reconstituted for administration by IV route. The loading dose is 200 mg given as single injection followed by 100 mg/day for a total of 7-10 days.

22. **Cefideracol:** It is a new antibiotic active against multidrug-resistant Gram negative bacteria. It is a cephalosporin with different molecular structure- catechol substituted siderophone side chain. It is active against Psedomonas aeuginosa, Klebsiella pneumoniae, Proteous mirabilis, acinobacter, proteus, enterobacter, aerobic Gram-negative bacteria including carbapenem-colistin resistant bacteria and has no action against Gram-positive bacteria.

    It binds to penicillin- binding protein-3 and disrupts cell wall synthesis. It is highly stable against hydrolysis by various β-lactamases, including severe serine β-lactamases and metallo-β-lactamases.

    It is indicated in highly complicated cases of Urinary tract infections, hospital acquired bacterial pneumonia, and ventilator-assisted/associated bacterial pneumonia all cause by Gram-negative bacteria. It is given IV in 2 g doses 8th hourly.

23. **Lefamulin:** There had been an imperative need for the development of new antibiotics due to alarming increase of rates of bacterial resistance due to antibiotic misuse in the recent past. Lefamulin is one such antibiotic developed recently which was found to be effective in community acquired pneumonia. It is a

pleuromutilin (obtained from pleuromutilin fungus clitophilus scyphoides) inhibits bacterial protein synthesis binding to unique sites of peptidyl transferase center of 50 S bacterial ribosomal sub unit

It is a broad spectrum antibiotic effective against G-positive and Gram-negative organisms that include *Streptococcus pneumoniae, Hemophylus influenza, Morexella catarrhalis, Legionella pneumophila, Mycoplasma pneumoniae, and Chlamydophila pneumoniae*

It is mainly in community acquired pneumonia and given as 600 mg oral tablet once daily or as 150 mg/15mL infusion given in doses of 2g 12th hourly for 5-7 days.

24. **Ocrelizumab:** It is a humanized monoclonal antibody that targets CD20-positive B cells (Immune cells) that play a key role in the progression of multiple sclerosis. It is indicated in relapsing or primary progressive forms of multiple sclerosis. The first dose of 300 mg is given IV infusion over 2.5 hours, followed by an additional 300 mg given as IV infusion 13 days later. Subsequent doses of 300 mg given every 6 months as IV infusion.

25. **Interferon beta-1a:** It is a monoclonal antibody used to treat relapse forms (relapse-remitting forms) of multiple sclerosis in doses of 30mcg IM once in a week

26. **Aprocitenton:** It is an endothelium receptor antagonist that inhibits the binding of endothelins (ET) to $\mathbf{ET_A}$ **and** $\mathbf{ET_B}$ receptors and inhibit the activity of endothelin $\mathbf{ET_1}$, thereby relaxing vasoconstriction and causing vasodilatation which causes fall of blood pressure. ET_1 is potent vasoconstrictor and also acts as a driver for the aldostrone production which is implicated in the cause of systemic hypertension. Aprocitenton is given in doses of 12.5 mg in combination with other antihypertensive drugs to treat chronic or malignant hypertension not amenable to the combination therapy with other drugs.

27. **Insulin Icodec:** Insulin icodec is novel, long acting insulin analog designed to cover basal insulin requirements with once- weekly subcutaneous administration. A number of in vivo assays measuring receptor binding, intracellular signaling as well as cellular metabolic and mitogenic responses were used to characterize the biological properties insulin isodec. In order to study the pharmacological properties of insulin-isodec in individuals with Type-2 diabetes, a randomized double-blind, double-dummy, active-controlled, multi dose, dose-escalation trial was conducted.

    The long half-life of isodec (196 hours) was achieved by introducing modifications to the insulin molecule aiming to obtain a safe, albumin-bound circulating depot of insulin (icodec), providing protracted action and clearance (a slow insulin receptor mediated clearance). Addition of a C_{20} fatty diacid- containing side chain imparts strong, reversible albumin-binding, while three amino acids substitutions (A_{14} E, B_{16} H and B_{25} H) provide molecular stability. In vitro cell-based studies showed that insulin icodec activates the same dose-dependent IR—mediated signaling and metabolic responses as native human insulin. The long half-life facilitates the administration of Insulin-icodec once in weekly in doses of 70U given subcutaneously.

28. **Lobeglitazone** (a thiazolidinedione derivative) 0.5mg + **Glimepiride** (sulfonylurea derivative) 1mg Given to effectively control Type-2 diabetes mellitus

29. **Lenacapavir** is a long-acting anti HIV-1 drug indicated in treatment experienced adults with multidrug – resistant infection and provides hope of accelerating efforts to end AIDS as per UNAIDS (United Nations programme on HIV/AIDS). It is released recently in to the market. It is administered as follows.

    Day 1 : 927 mg given Subcutaneously (SC) + 600 mg PO

    Day 2 : 600 mg PO

    Maintainance - Every six months (26 Weeks from last injection) +/- 2 Weeks: 927 mg SC

30. **Plazomicin** is a new aminoglycoside derived from sisomicin and has the same mechanism of action as other aminoglycosides inhibiting 30 S ribosomal submit, It is indicated for the treatment of complicated uninary tract injections including pyelonephritis caused E. coli, klebsiella pneumoniae, proteins mirabilis, Enterobacter cloacae. It is given IV is a dose of 500 mg / 10 ml infused over for 30 minutes for 4-7 Days.

10

Oral Anticoagulant Reversal

Bleeding is a common side effect of anticoagulant use. However, the majority of bleeding events are not life threatening and can be managed effectively by appropriate interventions needed on hand. It is always imperative for the doctors to locate the site of bleeding, evaluate laboratory studies (including blood counts and coagulation studies), close monitoring the vital signs and initiate the appropriate therapy at the earliest. Local measures such as compression can be useful in case of skin-bleeds and epistaxis. Similarly blood transfusion can be given to maintain blood volume and prevent development of shock. Ultimately, the decision to reverse the anticoagulant events should be taken as early as possible to prevent hemorrhagic complications.

Indications for anticoagulant use

Oral anticoagulants both Vitamin k antagonists (VKTS) like warfarin, acenocoumarol, dicoumarol, anisindione) and direct acting oral anticoagulants(DOACs) like epixaban, edoxaban, betrixaban are indicated in many clinical conditions like atrial fibrillation, venous thromboembolism, prosthetic cardiac valve placement, intracardiac thrombi, and mechanical support devices such as left ventricular assist devices.

Complications of oral anticoagulants

The patients put on oral anticoagulants are at increased risk of morbidity and mortality. The common complications that arise due to oral anticoagulant use include intracranial hemorrhage including spontaneous intracranial hemorrhages, epistaxis and bleeding from gums(oral cavity). Critical sites of hemorrhage include intracranial and pericardial areas, hemorrhage in the airway, haemothorax, retroperitoneal areas and intra-abdominal locations.

Interventions needed After confirming the diagnosis using endoscopy for GI bleeding, CT scan and MRI for intracranial bleeding and a history of the usage of aspirin and NSAIDs.

The following interventions required.

1. Assessment and control of acute major bleed and stabilizing the patient.
2. Identifying the concomitant usage of medicines and comorbidities.
3. To assess the need for dosage adjustment of the anticoagulant in use after the control of the bleed.
4. To maintain the vital functions with the supportive therapy and to find out the options for treating or reversing the anticoagulant hemorrhages.

Management of Vitamin K Antagonist – related bleeding

In the setting of a life-threatening bleed related to vitamin K antagonists use, rapid reversal of the VKA drug effects and replenishing clotting factors is a priority. To achieve that goal, a 10 mg dose of vitamin K is given IV along with 4 – factor prothrombin complex concentrate (4F-**Pcc**) or fresh frozen plasma (FFC) to achieve an INR of 1.5, depending on the site of the bleed.

Management of Direct oral anticoagulant – related bleeding (DOACs)

DOACs are now widely used in the treatment of venous thromboembolism(VTE) and various thromboembolic disorders. Unlike VKAs, standard coagulation test such as activated partial thromboplastin time(aPTT) and prothrombin time(PT/ INR) are unreliable markers of anticoagulant effect in DOAC-treated patients.

Till recently there were no specific antidotes or reversal agents for DOAC related acute bleeding except for supportive treatment and infusion of clotting factors. Dabigatran (a direct thrombin inhibitor) reversal can be achieved by the administration of 25-50 units/kg/IV dose of activated **prothrombin complex concentrate (PCC)**. Dabigatran reversal can also be achieved by the administration of **indarucizumab**, a humanized monoclonal antibody fragment(Fab) given in dose of 5G IV, provided as 2 separate vials each containing 2.5g/50ml.The need for the administration of Idarucizumeb occurs for emergency surgery or urgent procedures or in the event of life-threatening or uncontrolled bleeding.

For the reversal of **Factor X a inhibitors (epixaban**) a combination **of Andexamet alfa (a modified recombinant human factor Xa decoy protein)** that binds and sequesters apixaban or rivaroxaban) and **4 – factor PCC** can be used. Adenexamet alfa is given in a dose of 400mg/IV followed by infusion of 4mg/min for up to 2 hours and the dose of 4-factor PCC is 25-50 units/kg/given IV. Anticoagulant therapy can be resumed as soon as medically appropriate conditions are restored. Adenexanet alfa therapy can cause thromboembolic events, including ischemic events and cardiac events that are likely to occur during andenexanet alfa therapy and within 30 days of treatment.

11

Benign Prostatic Hyperplasia and Prostatic Malignancy-Newer Treatment Choices

Overview and Pathophysiology

Benign prostatic hyperplasia (BPH) is a common disorder in which the prostrate is abnormally enlarged and that usually occurs in men aged 60 years and above. The enlargement is characterized by nodular hyperplasia and cellular hypertrophy in the transitional zone, beginning in periurethral gland. As the prostrate continues to grow, the tissue begins to compress urethra which leads to lower urinary tract symptoms. This ultimately results in the inability to completely empty the bladder that results in urinary retention which further causes urinary incontinence. BPH is often complicated by hematuria, bladder or kidneys infection, bladder calculi, hydronephrosis and renal insufficiency. BPH is associated with proliferation of prostatic cells, decrease of prostatic cell apoptosis and an elevation of angiogenesis in the prostatic gland thus increasing prostatic mass of the gland.

The altered levels and balance of androgens such as testosterone, and estrogens, gonadotropins are most likely the primary causative factor of BPH. Changes in autocrine and paracrine growth factors such as insulin-like growth factor, epidermal growth factor, nerve growth factor, fibroblast factor, IGF binding proteins, and transforming growth factor-beta also seem to contribute to the disorder. Simultaneously, the potent androgen dihydrotestosterone (DHT) accumulates in the prostrate due to conversion of testosterone to DHT by type II 5-alfareductase. DHT and androgen receptors connect to each other in cell nuclei and end up resulting in BPH. **5α-reductase type 3 is an important biomarker of malignancy in the prostrate.** As age advances, serum levels of testosterone decline but the estrogens are converted to testosterone which in turn converted to DTH. Age related geriatric changes take place which include muscle weakness due to decreased muscle mass, loss of libido and the risk of hyperplasia of prostrate

Clinical features of BPH

A patient having BPH may present with symptoms such as urinary frequency, trouble starting urination, a weak or interrupted urine outflow, dribbling at the end of urination, nocturia, urinary retention and incontinence, painafter ejaculation or during urination, urinary tract or renal infections and hematuria.

Diagnosis of BPH: The diagnosis of BPH is based on diagnostic tests which comprise urine analysis, a prostate-specific antigen test **(PSA test)**, urinary outflow test, postvoid residual volume test, urodynamic tests, cystoscopy, digital prostatic examination, transurethral ultrasound and biopsy.

Medical management of BPH: The classes of drugs that could be used in benign prostatic hyperplasia include:

1. α_1-selective adrenergic receptor blockers	Prazosin, Alfuzosin, Tamsulosin, Terazosin, Silodosin
2. Phosphodiesterase inhibitors	Tadalafil, Sildenafil Avanafil, Vardenafil,
3. 5 – α – reductase inhibitors	Finasteride and Dutasteride
4. Combination therapies	Finasteride and Tadalafil

1. **α_1 – selective adrenergic inhibitors** – These group of drugs block α_1 receptors located in the smooth muscle of trigone and sphincter in the base of the bladder and prostate (prostatic urethra and prostatic capsule) and prevent contraction of the smooth muscle and help in decreasing the outflow resistance that occurs in prostatic hyperplasia. Thus, they relieve lower urinary tract symptoms (LUTS) and decrease the progression of BPH. Further, they eliminate hematuria secondary to BPH, improve bladder emptying, reverse acute urinary retention, and reduce urinary urgency or hesitancy and other symptoms associated with BPH. **The most preferred drugs in this category include terazosin, doxazosin, tamsulosin, alfuzosin and silodosin.**
2. **Phosphodiesterase inhibitors** – Tadalafil is a Phosphodiesterase-5 (PDE_5) inhibitor that inhibits the breakdown of cGMP and cause an increase in its levels at the effector sites. Thus, there is relaxation of the smooth muscle of the trigone and sphincter in the base of the bladder and prostate (prostatic urethra and prostatic capsule). This is followed by relief from LUTS.
3. **5 – α – reductase inhibitors** – In the hyperplasia of the prostate, the potent androgen dihydrotestosterone (DHT) binds intracellular androgen receptors in the prostate leading to an increase in transcription of proteins that are responsible for increased cellular proliferation. As the gland enlarges, it compresses the prostatic urethra, producing the symptoms of lower urinary tract (LUTS). **Finasteride, dutasteride** act by preventing the conversion of testosterone to DHT thereby blocking the action of DHT and prevent prostatic cellular proliferation and enlargement followed by relief of lower urinary tract described earlier.
4. **Combination therapies** – Alpha blockers+5-alpha–reductase inhibitors can cause improvement of the lower urinary tract symptoms associated with BPH. This is particularly useful in patients with moderate to severe LUTS with an increased risk of progression. Similarly a combination of 5- alpha-reductase inhibitor + PDE_5 inhibitors is also other option. In patients with overactive bladder and prostatic hyperplasia a combination of three drugs that includes **muscarinic receptor antagonist (tolterodine, trospium, solifenac)** or a **β_3 agonist (Vibegron, mirabegron)** is a better choice.

   Prostatic cancer: Prostatic cancer is frequently a very slow growing disease, often causing no symptoms until it is in advanced stage. At that point, symptoms may include difficulty in starting urination, week and interrupted flow of urine, and frequent urination, especially at nights (nocturia) the symptoms of which might be similar to the ones caused by BPH (LUTS). Manifestations of metastatic and advanced prostate cancer may include weight loss, loss of appetite, anemia, bone pain, neurological deficits from spinal cord compression, lower extremity pain and edema due to obstruction of venous and lymphatic tributaries by nodal metastasis. **Androgens bind to androgen receptor (AR) protein** in prostate cancer cells. Once activated, AR stimulates the expression of specific genes that cause cancer cells to multiply. In early phase of androgen-dependant prostate cancer high androgen levels are required for cancer growth cells. As such, treatments that decrease androgen activity can inhibit cancer cell growth.

   Diagnosis is based on digital rectal examination and prostate specific antigen (PSA) levels which are increased from a normal level of o-4mcg/L to an abnormal level of 4 mcg/L. However, PSA levels may not be an accurate diagnostic criterion. The other diagnostic tests include transrectal ultrasound, biopsy, MRI, CT, and bone scan to diagnose metastatic cancer.

Pharmacological management

1. Androgen receptor antagonists such as flutamide, nilutamide, bicalutamide and apalutamide
2. Antiandrogens like cyproterone, cyproterone acetate are the androgen antagonists used in the treatment of prostatic cancer which exhibit a negative feedback on hypothalamo-pituitary axis and inhibit LH, resulting in diminished production of testosterone.
3. Bicalutamide and nilutamide are more effective in the treatment of metastatic prostate carcinoma in combination with **GnRH analogs (leuprolide, goserelin, gonadorelin, nafarelin, histrelin and triptorelin).**
4. Docetaxel and paclitaxel are the anticancer taxane derivatives that can be used to treat advanced and late stage prostatic cancer or metastasized cancer and that does not respond to hormone treatment.

12

Bronchial Asthma-Role of Leukotrein Antagonists and Other Drugs

Bronchial asthma

It is a chronic inflammatory respiratory condition characterized by hallmark symptoms of intermittent dyspnea, cough, and wheezing. The development of asthma, often in childhood involves a complex interplay of genetic, environmental factors with a history of atopy. The hallmark symptoms can be exacerbated by triggers ranging from allergens to viral infections. The most significant risk factors for adult onset include tobacco smoke, occupational exposure, acute rhinitis, or a history of atopy. The other factors that can contribute to asthma and airway hyperreactivity include the following

- Exposure to environment allergens, such as house dust mites, animal allergens, cockroach allergens, and fungi
- Physical activity or exercise
- Exposure to fossil fuel exhausts, smoke from any origin,
- Exposure to cold and humid weather.
- Conditions such as hyperventilation, GERD, and chronic sinusitis
- Hypersensitivity to aspirin and NSAIDs
- Use of β-blockers, including ophthalmic preparations
- Expose to irritants such as household sprays (perfumes), paint fumes
- Industrial exhausts
- Emotional factors

Pathophysiology

Asthma is a syndrome characterized by diverse inflammatory mechanisms present in the airway cells. These mechanisms lead to airway inflammation, intermittent airflow obstruction, and bronchial hyperresponsiveness. The activation of mast cells by cytokines and other mediators plays pivotal role in the development clinical features of bronchial asthma. Following expose to triggering allergens, there is release of IgE antibodies due to an over expression of T-helper2 lymphocytes (Th2 lymphocytes). Cytokines produced by Th2 lymphocytes include IL-4, IL-5, and IL-13, which promote IgE and eosinophilic responses in atopy. Once produced, these specific IgE antibodies on mast cell surfaces are activated following attachment to allergens and release mediators like histamine, PGD2, cystenyl leukotreins C4(LTC4), D4(LTD4), and E4 (LTE4), by degranulation (mast cell degranualation). Leukotreins cause the smooth muscle cells of the bronchi to contract. This is followed by infiltration of eosinophils, basophils, monocytes, denditric cells, neutrophils, which all contribute to later phase of asthma. The narrowing of airway lumen throughout the tracheobronchial tree is caused by the contraction of airway smooth muscle, thickening of the airway wall due to edema, mucus plugging in the airway passages, and airway remodeling which collectively contribute to the clinical presentation of a case of bronchial asthma.

Leukotrein antagonists

Leukotrein antagonists play an important role in the treatment of bronchial asthma both as prophylactic and therapeutic agents.

They include leukotrein synthesis inhibitor Zileuton and leukotrein receptor antagonists like montelukast, zafirlukast, and pranlukast.

Montelukast, zafirlukast and pranlukast are cysteinyl leukotriene receptor antagonists indicated to prevent and treat chronic bronchial asthma. Leukotrienes are eicosanoid inflammatory mediators derived from β-arachidonic acid. Neither montelukast nor zafirlukast has a role as rescue medication during an acute asthmatic attack. Pranlukast is another cysteinyl -LT1 receptor antagonist that is also used to treat bronchial asthma. All the three antagonists inhibit the receptor mediated effects of cysteinyl leukotreins LTC_4, LTD_4, LTE_4. Zileuton is a potent and selective inhibitor of 5- lipooxygenase activity

Mechanism of Action

The main indication for leukotriene receptor antagonists is in treating chronic asthma. Leukotrienes are synthesized from arachidonic acid by the action of 5-lipoxygenase in many inflammatory cells in the airways. Arachidonic acid is released from cell membrane phospholipids mainly by phospholipase A2. The cyclooxygenase pathway produces thromboxane and prostaglandins from arachidonic acid. Corticosteroids inhibit phospholipase A2 and subsequent synthesis of eicosanoid inflammatory mediators, including both prostaglandins and leukotrienes. Non-steroidal anti-inflammatory drugs such as aspirin inhibit cyclooxygenases and further formation of prostaglandins. ***Zileuton inhibits 5-Lipoxygenase***

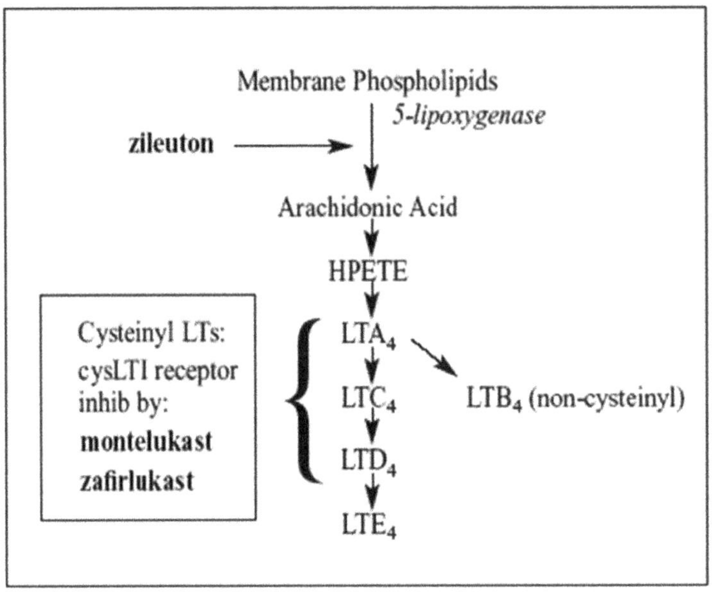

There are two groups of leukotrienes: One with and the other without amino acid moieties._ Leukotriene B4 carries hydroxyl moiety only and binds to BLT receptors (Leukotriene B4 receptor). The signaling pathway via G protein-coupled BLT receptor activation produces a potent chemotaxis response. Cysteinyl leukotrienes (LTC4, LTD4, and LTE4) have amino acid moiety and bind to cysteinyl leukotriene receptors (CysLT1 and CysLT2). Bronchoconstriction, vascular permeability, eosinophil recruitment, and chronic inflammation are mediated through the G protein-coupled activation of cysteinyl leukotriene receptors. Montelukast and zafirlukast are antagonists to cysteinyl leukotriene CysLT1 receptors but not CysLT2 receptors). Pranlukast selectively binds to LTD4 and inhibits it. Research has shown that eosinophils are the main source of cysteinyl leukotrienes, and cysteinyl leukotrienes are very important in eosinophil recruitment. Earlier studies have shown that ***cysteinyl leukotrienes also play an important role in airway remodeling in chronic asthma.*** Asthma is the most common chronic lung disease characterized by reversible bronchoconstriction, inflammation, and airway remodeling that results in hyperresponsiveness.

Sympathomimetic agents such as beta-adrenergic receptor agonists are the therapeutic choice for treating acute bronchoconstriction. They activate beta two adrenergic receptors and relax airway smooth muscle cells. **Short-acting beta2-selective** agonists include albuterol, levalbuterol, terbutaline, metaproterenol, and pirbuterol. They sustain bronchodilation for 3-4 hours.

Long-acting beta2-selective agonists with 12-hour durations of action include salmeterol and formoterol. **Ultra-long-acting** beta-agonists include indacaterol, olodaterol, vilanterol, and bambuterol and patients need to take either of them only once a day. Because beta-agonists do not inhibit inflammatory responses, they do not have a role as monotherapy for controlling persistent asthma. They are frequently a second agent added to inhaled corticosteroids. Based on the inflammatory mechanism of asthma, several pharmacological agents with different modes of action have undergone development to treat this endotype of asthma (asthma types which have distinct pathophysiologic mechanisms at a cellular and molecular level). Exposure to allergen stimulates IgE synthesis driven by CD4+ T helper type 2 cells. The IgE antibodies bind to their receptors on the tissue mast cells and blood basophils. On re-exposure to an allergen, the allergen cross-links the IgE antibodies on the immune cell surface (mast cell and basophil cell surface). It triggers the release of preformed mediators of anaphylaxis and the synthesis of inflammatory mediators. **Cromolyn or nedocromil** may prevent mast cell degranulation. However, these drugs are not commonly used in asthma treatment these days because they are less effective than inhaled corticosteroids. Histamine, tryptase (an enzyme found mainly in mast cells) and arachidonic acid metabolites such as leukotrienes C4 and D4, and prostaglandin D2 are released and cause acute smooth muscle contraction and increased vascular permeability. Three to six hours later, more sustained bronchoconstriction occurs in the late asthmatic response. There are suggestions that the cytokines produced by type 2 immune response mediate late asthmatic response. Advances in understanding the molecular heterogeneity of asthma have revealed the importance of type 2 immune response mediated by T helper type 2 cells in the pathology of eosinophilic asthma. **Omalizumab** is a monoclonal antibody that can reduce the amount of circulating IgE, IL-4, IL-5, and IL-13 that mediate type 2 immune responses. Anti-IL-5 antibody **mepolizumab** minimizes the number and activity of eosinophils in the airway mucosa**. Dupilumab** is an anti-IL-4, IL-13 receptor antibody (monoclonal antibody)

Indications

Montelukast ,zafirlukast, pranlukast are cysteinyl leukotriene receptor antagonists. Leukotrienes are eicosanoid inflammatory mediators derived from arachidonic acid. Montelukast's indications include the prophylaxis and chronic treatment of asthma, the prevention of exercise-induced bronchospasm, and the relief of symptoms of allergic rhinitis. Montelukast monotherapy is not recommended for first-line therapy for allergic rhinitis. Instead, monotherapy with an intranasal glucocorticoid is a strong recommendation in the initial treatment of patients with moderate/severe seasonal allergic rhinitis who are 12 years of age or older and have had no prior treatment. The role of montelukast in an effective treatment for eczema remains inconclusive. Parents of asthmatic children prefer montelukast because the once-a-day oral dosage is more convenient than inhaler use. It also avoids the clinical concerns regarding the side effects of long-term use of corticosteroids, such as growth retardation and metabolic abnormalities.

Zafirlukast indications include the prophylaxis and chronic treatment of asthma in children five years and older and adults. It is used off-label for allergic rhinitis and the prophylaxis of exercise-induced bronchospasm.

The first-line therapy for the prophylaxis of exercise-induced bronchospasm is inhaled short-acting beta-agonist such as albuterol (solbutamol and levosolbutamol). Daily use of inhaled corticosteroid or leukotriene receptor antagonists, such as montelukast, zafirlukast or pranlukast is recommended in patients with exercise-induced bronchospasm who earlier inhaled preventative short-acting beta-agonist but continue to have symptoms or who develop tolerance to continued usage of short-acting beta-agonist. **Both montelukast and zafirlukast have no role as rescue medication during an acute asthmatic attack. Instead, inhaled beta-agonist induces immediate bronchodilation**

Administration

Montelukast administration is via the oral route, without regard to food or meals. It should be taken as a single dose in the evening in patients with asthma. For the treatment of allergic rhinitis, administration can be either morning or evening. It should be taken at least two hours before exercise to prevent exercise-induced asthma. **Patients should not take another dose within 24 hours**. The usual oral dose of Montelukast is 10 mg once daily, and that of zofirlukast is 20 mg twice daily. Pranlukast is given in single daily doses of 112.5 or 225 mg.

Zafirleukast's bioavailabilty. gets reduced by 40% when taken orally and hence should be taken 2 hours after or 1 hour before meals.

Adverse Effects

Montelukast is relatively well-tolerated and generally safe. The most commonly observed side effects in patients aged 15 years and over were headaches, influenza infection, abdominal pain, cough, and dyspepsia. In children, diarrhea, nausea, laryngitis, pharyngitis, sinusitis, otitis, and viral infection may occur. Neuropsychiatric disorders, including depression, aggression, suicidal ideation, insomnia, anxiety, and nightmares, may occur. Allergic granulomatous angiitis (Churg-Strauss syndrome) may also correlate with the use of montelukast, although there is not yet an established causal relationship. There are some reports of serious adverse events due to angioedema, hypersensitivity, fatigue, confusional state, abnormal dreams, epilepsy, aggression, immune system disorder, hemorrhage, excoriation, eosinophil count increase, pain in extremity, and abdominal pain. In an animal study, it did not produce teratogenic effects at doses much higher than the maximum daily dose in humans. **Zafirlukast is generally well tolerated, and associated adverse events are minimal.** Headache, upper respiratory tract infection, and gastrointestinal disturbances such as nausea, vomiting, dyspepsia, abdominal pain, diarrhea, and malaise are common adverse effects. Rarely the elevation of liver enzymes, acute hepatitis, and hyperbilirubinemia has been linked to zafirlukast.

In spite of many adverse effects mentioned above both Monteleukast and Zafirleukast are well tolerated in all age groups and have definitive role in different allergic conditions including bronchial asthma.

Contraindications

Both montelukast and zafirlukast are contraindicated in patients with hypersensitivity to the drug or any component of their formulation.

Contraindications to zafirlukast also include patients with acute episodes of asthma or hepatic impairment.

Monitoring

Depression, aggression, and other behavioral changes have correlations with the leukotriene receptor antagonists. Careful monitoring is necessary for patients treated with leukotriene receptor antagonists.

Zafirlukast may cause severe but rare acute liver damage. It is a major substrate of the cytochrome P450 CYP2C9 enzyme. Patients receiving concomitant therapy with drugs such as alpelisib, dabrafenib, enzalutamide, erythromycin, loxapine, lumacaftor, rifapentine, terfenadine, and warfarin require monitoring for potential drug interactions.

Toxicity

Both montelukast and zafirlukast have a wide margin of safety. Patients who had taken an overdose had no adverse symptoms, a rash, and GI upset and had an uneventful course of recovery.

When overdosed, unabsorbed drug is removed using active charcoal and by instituting supportive therapy, if needed.

13

Emergence of New Antidiabetic Drugs and their Extended Clinical uses

Overview

Diabetes is a metabolic disease characterized by elevated levels of blood glucose, which leads overtime to serious damage to the heart, blood vessels, eyes, kidneys, and nerves (**microvascular and macrovascular complications**). Type2 diabetes is the most common in occurrence usually seen in adults, manifests when the body insulin levels fall short of meeting the metabolic requirements and associated with other comorbidities such as atherogenic CV risk factors, hypertension, and obesity. In the past three decades the prevalence of type2 diabetes has risen dramatically in countries of all income levels. Type1 diabetes, once known as juvenile diabetes or insulin dependent diabetes, is a chronic condition in which the pancreas produces little or no insulin by itself. For people living with diabetes, access to affordable treatment, including insulin, is critical to their survival. There is a globally agreed consensus to target a reduction in the incidence from the present level to half and to reduce by equal proportion obesity by 2025. Globally 422 million adults were living with diabetes in 2014, compared to 108 million in 1980. The global prevalence (age standardized) of diabetes has nearly doubled since 1980, rising from 4.7% to 8.5% in the adult population. In 2015, an estimated 1.6 million deaths were directly caused by diabetes mellitus. As per Indian council of Medical research India Diabetes study, the prevalence of diabetes is 10.1 crores (2023 status)

Diabetes is associated with accelerated atherosclerosis leading to increased risk and incidence of myocardial infarction (MI), stoke and peripheral artery disease. Diabetes is also the leading cause of adult blindness(retinopathy), end-stage renal disease or chronic kidney disease (CKD) and non-traumatic amputations. Compared to death rates for cardiovascular disease, stroke and cancer, which have remained stable or even declined since the mid1980s, death rates for diabetes have increased by 20-30%.

If glycaemic controls are achieved satisfactorily by therapeutic and non-therapeutic approaches, it is possible to slowdown the progression of atherosclerosis, stabilize rupture-Prone plaques and prevent arterial thromboembolism and can prevent cardiac deaths due to MI. Similarly, the incidence of retinopathy and nephropathy can be minimized. Further, the lower the HbA1c, the lower is the risk of cardiovascular (CV) events. The risk factors for pre-diabetics and type2 diabetics include a family history(Parent or sibling) of prediabetes or type2 diabetes, obesity, hypertension, hypercholesterolemia, physical inactivity, smoking, gestational diabetes which is generally reversible after the delivery.

For the control of diabetes and its progression to complications with increased morbidity and mortality there are as many a types of treatment choices that include insulin preparations including the newer additions, sulfonylureas, thiazolidinediones, biguanides, GLP-1 receptor agonists, DPP-4 inhibitors, SGLT-2 inhibitors. Apart from achieving good glycemic control, GLP-1 receptor agonists, SGLT-2 inhibitors and DPP-4 inhibitors have shown significant CV benefits that have markedly increased their use in congestive heart failure, CKD and diabetes associated with obesity. An attempt is made here to explain the role played by some of the non-insulin anti-diabetic drugs with reference to glycemic control, CV and renal benefits.

Glucagon-like petide- 1 receptor agonists(GLP-1 agonists)

Antidiabetic actions

GLP-1 receptor agonists (Exenatide, exenatide LAR, dulaglutide, liraglutide, albiglutide, lixisenatide, taspoglutide, semaglutide) have anti-diabetic action, by an increase of or augmentation of glucose dependent insulin secretion, increase of pancreatic β-cell function, β-cell mass, reduced β-cell apoptosis, decrease of glucagon secretion, decreased glucose production in the liver by reducing hepatic gluconeogenesis, and increased uptake by skeletal muscle and adipose tissue. GLP-1 receptor agonists are considered as incretins which are released in the small intestine and carried to the pancreatic beta cells the stimulation of which causes the releases of insulin.

Weight effects

GLP-1 receptor agonists cause a weight loss due to decreased appetite and neuroprotection through central mechanisms and it is known they cause a net weight loss of 5.5 kg over a period of 20 weeks of treatment.

Cardiovascular effects

On a molecular level insulin resistance causes substantial changes in the energy metabolism in cardiomyocytes, leading to the loss of substrate flexibility and increased fatty acid oxidation which is accompanied by lipid accumulation, impaired mitochondrial membrane potential and reduced ATP production. These processes not only affect cellular energy levels, but are also accompanied with cardiac fibrosis, myocardial stiffness, inflammation, apoptosis, ultimately leading to structural organization and a decrease in heart function. Over a period of years these deregulatory changes manifests clinically as arrhythmias and heart failure with preserved ejection fraction (HFpEF) and latter leading to increased failure with reduced ejection fraction(HFrEF).

The cardioprotection of GLP-1 agonist is in line with Metformin, SGLT-2 inhibitors, DPP4 inhibitors and shown as reduced fibrosis, increased glucose uptake, increased autophagy, reduced lipid accumulation, reduced myocardial stiffness, reduced inflammation, reduced apoptosis in the cardiomyosites, improved cardiac output, reduced incidence of arrhythmias, and reduced infarct size. In addition, GLP-1 agonists reverse atherosclerosis and cause modest decrease in systolic blood pressure, decreased body weight and all put together provide better outcomes in diabetic patients with associated congestive heart failure. A stronger CV benefit was induced by Liraglutide, Semaglutide, Albiglutide and Dulaglutide which are highly homologous with endogenous human GLP-1(ineretin), compared to the structurally distinct Exenatide and Lixisenaside. **CV benefits may be restricted to patients with established CVD**. This had been proved in many cardiovascular outcome trials(CVOTs)- Liraglutide effect and action in diabetes evolution results(LEADER), SUSTAIN-6 trial to evaluate cardiovascular and other long term outcomes with Semaglutide in subjects with type-2 DM,

EXSCEL (exenatide study of cardiovascular event lowering) trial, with once-weekly extended release preparation showing CV benefits had shown no difference in 3-point MACE (major adverse cardiac events) like cardiac deaths, MI, stroke in comparison to other GLP-1agonists.,

Some currently available GLP-1 analogs and their doses given in the following table.

Name of the Drug	Dose	Route of administration
Exenatide	5mcg/twice/daily, 2 mg ER/SR once weekly	Subcutaneous
Dulaglutide	0.75 mg once weekly	Subcutaneous
Liraglutide	0.6 mg/day, titrated on weekly basis to a maximum of 1.8 mg/day	Subcutaneous

Table *Contd...*

Name of the Drug	Dose	Route of administration
Lixisenatide	20 mcg/day	Subcutaneous
Taspoglutide	20 mg once weekly	Subcutaneous
Semaglutide	3,7 or 14mg once daily (oral) 0.25 mg/weekly for 4 weeks, 0.5mg/ week For further 4 weeks and maintained there after	Subcutaneous
Efpeglenatide	4 – 6 mg weekly	Subcutaneous

SGLT 2 inhibitors

Antidiabetic action

SGLT2 inhibitors (sodium-glucose co-transporter 2 inhibitors) like Dapagliflozin, Canagliflozin, Empagliflozin, Remogliflozin, Sergiliflozin, Ertugliflozin) act by inhibiting a carrier protein, sodium-glucose co-transporter 2(**SGLT-2)** responsible for glucose reuptake in the proximal renal tubule thus facilitating its elimination in the urine. This is followed by a decrease of blood glucose levels. They also have an additional action of increased insulin sensitivity, uptake of glucose in muscle cells, decreased gluconeogenesis, and improved first-phase insulin release from the beta cells.

CV effects

SGLT 2 inhibition leads to **cardioprotection** by different mechanisms. SGLT2 inhibitors elicit a decrease arterial stiffness, systolic blood pressure, cardiac preload/afterload, cardiac wall stiffness stress and an improved cardiac efficiency. They demonstrated their efficacy in reducing the incidence of heart failure with both preserved (HFpEF), and reduced (HFrEF) ejection fraction, decreased hospitalizations for HF and causing a decrease of major adverse cardiovascular events(MACE) like MI, stroke, end stage kidney disease is high risk patients with or without diabetes.

Renal effects

Chronic kidney disease(CKD) or chronic renal failure is a term that includes all degrees of decreased renal function which is one of the leading causes of morbidity and mortality is patients of diabetes. The most common observation in CKD is a decreased glomerular filtration rate(GFR) of less than 60 mL/ min/ 1.73m^2), increased albuminuria (albumin elimination> 30 mg/24hr or albumin: creatinine ratio >30 mg/g for more than 3 months, electrolyte and other abnormalities due to tubular disorders, histologic abnormalities and structural abnormalities.

SGLT2 inhibitors cause an immediate functional reduction of GFR, reduce blood pressure and preserve kidney and heart function in the long term, despite a lesser anti-hyperglycemic effect. GFR reduction reduces the tubular transport work and metabolic demand, thereby improving renal cortical oxygenation. This is due to improved renal mitochondrial function in response to SGLT2 inhibition. They also reduce the risk and severity of acute kidney injury in Type2 diabetics. Dapagliflozin Empagliflozin, Canagliflozin reduce the hyperfiltration seen in diabetic patients at the onset of the therapy and **slow the decline in eGFR in the long-term**. This early decline in eGFR is reversible followed by better preservation of GFR, decreased albuminuria and decreased creatinine levels. Initial GFR reduction is not a serious concern as it gets adjusted within 4 to 12 weeks with improvement of overall renal function in due course. Diabetic patients with established heart failure and with chronic kidney disease, are strongly recommended with the use of SGLT2 inhibitors.

Some currently available SGLT-2 inhibitor and their doses.

Name of the drug	Dose (Oral)
Dapagliflozin	5mg once daily
Canagliflozin	100mg once daily
Empagliflozin	10mg once daily
Sotagliflozin	400mg in two divided doses
Ertugliflozin	5mg once daily

Sotagliflozin is a dual inhibitor of both SGLT 1 and 2. SGLT 1 inhibition improves glucose homeostasis by reducing dietary glucose absorption in the intestine and by increasing the release of incretins (GLP-1 agonists)

SGLT2 expressed in proximal renal tubular is responsible for the majority of the reabsorption of filtered glucose from the tubular lumen; SGLT2 inhibitors reduce glucose reabsorption and lower the renal threshold for glucose thereby increasing glucose excretion.

DPP-4 inhibitors (Saxagliptin, Sitagliptin, Linagliptin, Vidaglyptin, Teneligliptin)

Anti diabetic actions

Dipeptidylpeptidase – 4 enzyme is responsible for degradation of various biologically active peptides including endogenous GLP-1 and GIP(glucose-dependent insulinotropic peptide). By inhibiting DPP-4, these drugs lower the blood glucose levels. They do not cause weight loss or weight gain.

Cardiovascular effects

DPP-4 inhibitors are not found to offer any significant CV benefit and they do not increase or decrease the CV events compared to a placebo. A large population cohort study evaluated major adverse CV events(MACE) which was a composite of MI and hospitalizations for stroke, heart failure and hypoglycaemia. These patients were on a combination treatment for diabetes with sulfonylurea and DPP-4 inhibitor and were found to have a moderate reduced risk of stroke, but not MI or hospitalization for stroke.

Renal effects

DPP-4 inhibitors have been found to provide some renoprotective effects, and given that nephropathy is a common complication of diabetes, these agents could be beneficial in patients suffering from or at high risk of developing these types of complications. In all cases DPP-4 inhibitors result in greater reductions in A1c compared to placebo. They are safe to use across the spectrum of renal dysfunction without the concern for any major adverse events, which cannot be said with any other classes of antihyperglycemic drugs. They offer some degree of protection and slow the progression renal disease, as evidenced by a reduction in micro and macro albuminuria.

Some currently available DPP-4 inhibitors their doses and routes of administration.

Name of the Drug	Dose(oral)
Saxagliptin	2.5 – 5 mg – 5mg/day
Sitagliptin	100mg/day once
Linagliption	5mg/day once
Vidagliption	25mg/day once
Teneligiption	20mg/day once

Conclusion

Given the increasing number of pharmacologic options for the treatment of diabetes, choosing an appropriate option for a given patient can be challenging. CV benefits have been demonstrated with some SGLT2 inhibitors (dapagliflozin, canagliflozin and empagliflozin), some GLP-1 receptor agonists(liraglutide and semaglutide) and Pioglitazone(known from earlier studies) with a mortality benefit seen in many observational studies. GLP-1 receptor agonist liraglutide is the only one in this class to demonstrate to lower the rate of nephropathy as evidenced by a reduction of new-onset macroalbuminuria. In the SGLT2 inhibitor class canagliflozin reduced the progression of albuminuria thereby arresting the progression to CKD. In the DPP-4 inhibitor class, all the agents have shown some degree of urine albumin reduction without any CV benefit. SGLT2 inhibitors and GLP-1 receptor agonists have all shown weight loss effects.

Those agents having considerable benefits in any class of drugs are worth considering for the effective management of diabetes with cardiovascular complications like heart failure and associated with mild to moderate renal failure.

14

Drug Therapy of Neuropathic Pain

Overview

Pain is an unpleasant sensory and emotional experience associated with, or resembling that associated with, actual or potential tissue damage. Pain is a warning about tissue damage signaled by specific receptors and fiber systems extending from the periphery to the brain. When the normal pathways are damaged, the immediate consequence is loss or reduction of function including pain. However, in some cases as a result of the lesion, pain develops, a condition termed as neuropathic pain.

Basic features of Neuropathic pain

Neuropathic pain (pain due to involvement of nerves) caused by a lesion (dysfunction) or disease of the somatosensory nervous system which provides information about body including skin, musculoskeletal, and visceral organs is a common chronic pain condition with major impact on quality of life. Examples include trigeminal neuralgia, painful polyneuropathy, post herpetic neuralgia, and central post stroke pain. Most patients complain of an ongoing or intermittent spontaneous pain of, for example, burning, pricking, and squeezing quality, which may be accompanied by evoked pain, particularly to light touch and cold. Ectopic activity in, for example, nerve-end neuroma, compressed nerves or nerve roots, dorsal root ganglia, and the thalamus may in different conditions underlie the spontaneous pain. Evoked pain (pain due to stimuli such as touch and cold) may spread to neighboring areas, and the underlying pathophysiology involves peripheral and central sensitization. Maladaptive structural changes and a number of cell-cell interactions and molecular signaling underlie the sensitization of nociceptive pathways. These include alteration in ion channels, activation of immune cells, glial-derived mediators, and epigenetic regulation. Neuropathic pain can be both central and peripheral in origin. Lesions of central nervous system are one of the well-known causes of neuropathic pain. Stroke or other lesions damaging somatosensory pathways from the spinal cord to the cortical structures may be accompanied by neuropathic pain. Peripheral types constitute the majority of neuropathic pain disorders. **Nociceptive pain (non-neuropathic pain) is the one that occurs due to injury to a particular part of the body that arises from actual or threatened damage to non-neuronal tissue and that results from over activation of nociceptors. Examples of nociceptive pain include pain due to burns, bruises, fractures, arthritis and sprains.**

Classification and types of neuropathic pain

Neuropathic pain is traditionally classified based on underlying disease. It is organized into peripheral and central types of pain based on the location or disease in the peripheral or central somatosensory nervous system.

1. **Peripheral neuropathic pain types**

   Peripheral neuropathic pain is multifactorol and involves many clinical conditions that include

   Trigeminal neuralgia, neuropathy following peripheral nerve injury, painful polyneuropathy due to diabetes mellitus; alcohol consumption; infections due to HIV, Lyme's disease, Epstein-Barr virus, Hepatitis c, Herpes Zoster, varicella Zoster, Covid-19 infection and leprosy; malignancy; Chemotherapy and chemotherapy medications; dug induced pain (INH and CV medications); post traumatic pain (stump or

Phantom pain); radiculopathy due to lesions involving cervical, thoracic, lumbar and sacral nerve roots caused by herniated disks and demyelisation in the spinal nerves; amylodosis; autoimmune diseases like rheumatoid arthritis, lupus erythematosus; Vasculitis; malnutrition due to deficiency of Vitamin B1, B6 and B12; toxins(heavy metals like lead): and non-freezing cold injury.

2. **Central neuropathic pain types**

Central post-stoke pain, spinal cord injury neuropathic pain, Multiple sclerosis, Guilain- Barre syndrome.

Clinical features of neuropathic pain

Pain may be the first symptom of neuropathy, but often is insidious in origin starting with parasthesia, and eventually dysesthesia or pain. The pain is usually ongoing squeezing, shooting, pricking, pins and needles or burning pain. The pain may be spontaneous or evoked due to touch or cold. Usually there would be allodynia (pain resulting due to stimulus that does not normally provoke pain) or hyperalgesia (increased pain from a stimulus that usually provokes pain). There might be decreased reflexes, weakness and autonomic changes. The most common form is a symmetric length-dependent polyneuropathy with symptoms in the feet, progressing proximally affecting lower legs and hands

Some examples and clinical manifestations of neuropathic pain

A) Trigeminal Neuralgia

It is a specific type of orofascial pain affecting one or more divisions of trigeminal nerve. Pain occurs due to pressure on the trigeminal nerve at the root entry zone by blood vessel which leads to demyelination of the nerve. Pain occurs in all the areas of supply by the trigeminal nerve, particularly in the lower part of the face and the pain is usually unilateral. The pain is described as stabbing, burning, shock-like, and feeling electrical and usually severe in nature. The pain attacks occur suddenly and provoked by light touch activities in the mouth, brushing the teeth, or face washing.

B) Diabetic Neuropathy

Diabetes mellitus with poorly controlled glycemic levels and persistent elevation of HbA1C levels over a period can cause peripheral nerve damage and dysfunction. Nerve damage is due to microvascular injury as a result of oxidative stress, inflammation and cell damage. There would be numbness, tingling, aching, burning sensation, and weakness of limbs with pain accompanied by allodynia and hyperalgesia. The features are present in the feet progressing proximally affecting lower legs and hands.

C) Radiculopathy

Radiculopathy encompasses several symptoms, such as pain, numbness, or weakness, in the neck, shoulders, upper back, arms and legs caused by compression of the nerve root either in the cervical, thoracic, or lumbar regions of the spinal cord. The symptoms are due to compression by herniated disks, degenerative changes, or spondylosis.

D) Carpal Tunnel Syndrome

It is the most prevalent focal mononeuropathy constituting 90% of all types of neuropathic pain. The pain occurs due to compression of median nerve as it travels through carpal tunnel, leading to entrapment neuropathy as manifested as pain, numbness, and parasthesias, within the median nerve distribution (wrist, hands, and fingers). It can further lead to loss of sensation if not treated early.

Treatment of Neuropathic Pain

Treatment of radiculopathy and carpal tunnel syndrome which are considered as non-neuropathic pain conditions consists of use of conservative measures and analgesics and if necessary surgical intervention. But the use of opioids is a common practice in both neuropathic pain and non-neuropathic pain types.

Drugs used in neuropathic pain may broadly classified as

1. Coanalgesics
2. Analgesics
3. Topical agents- Capsaicin 8% patch, Lidocaine 5% patch

Coanalgesics

Coanalgesic or adjuvant analgesic is a medication that is not primarily designed to control pain, but can be used for this purpose. They are the drugs of choice to treat neuropathic pain. They are of little use or of no use in the treatment of pain of musculoskeletal origin. They can be classified as

A) Selective Serotonin noradrenaline reuptake inhibitors (SSNRIs) –Duloxetine and Velnafaxine, Milnacipran
B) Tricyclic antideprssants- Amitryptiline, Nortryptiline
C) Anticonvulsants
   Lamotrigine, Gabapentine, pregabalin, Carbmazepine, oxcarbazine, topiramate

Analgesics

1. Opioids are the commonly used analgesic agents in combination with Coanalgesics for the effective control of neuropathic pain. They include tramadol, tapentadol, oxycodone, hydrocodone, dihydrocodeine,
2. Paracetamol and NSAIDS are of limited use in neuropathic pain when used alone , but may complement the actions of other agents used for the condition

Serotonin Noradrenaline reuptake inhibitors(SNRIs)

Duloxetine, Velnafaxine, milnacipran act by inhibiting the reuptake of serotonin and noradrenaline and increasing their levels at the post synaptic sites in the central nervous system. They are usually prescribed for various depressive disorders like major depression, generalized anxiety disorder, panic disorder and phobic disorder. However they are also useful in chronic pain disorders like peripheral diabetic neuropathy, painful peripheral neuropathy, central neuropathic pain secondary to multiple sclerosis, chemotherapy induced pain, pain due to malignancies and fibromyalgia. They are not of much use in other types of neuropathic pain. The pain relieving effect is independent of their antidepressant effect. Duloxetine is given in 20-120 mg/day, velnafaxine is given in doses of 100-150 mg/day

Tricyclic antidepressants

Tricyclic antidepressants relieve neuropathic pain by their unique ability to inhibit presynaptic reuptake of noradrenaline and serotonin, but other mechanism such as NMDA (N-methy-D-aspartate) receptor and channel blockade also play in their pain-relieving mechanism. In addition, they also block $\alpha 1$, H1, muscarinic cholinergic receptors which explains the adverse effects they cause such as orthostatic hypotension, sinus tachycardia, blurred vision, and urinary retention. Amitryptiline is given in doses of 10-25 mg 2 times a day, while nortryptiline is given in doses of 25mg 3 times a day. Imipramie the other drug most effective is given in 100 mg single dose/day.

Tricyclic compounds are the most effective first line drugs to treat peripheral neuropathy, postherpitic neuralgia, neuropathic pain post-spinal cord injury, chemotherapy induced pain and cancer pain

Gabapentine and Pregabilin

These drugs block α-2δ subunit of Ca^{2+} channels in the cerebral neocortex, hippocampus, and spinal cord inhibiting the release excitatory neurotransmitter NMDA (glutamate transmitter) and facilitate pain relief apart from having antiepileptic action. These drugs are most effective in diabetic neuropathy and postherpitic neuropathy. Gabapentine is given in doses of 300 mg 2 or 3 times a day, while pregabalin is given in doses of 75 mg 2 times a day.

Other antiepileptic drugs used in neuropathies

Carbamazepine, oxcarbazepine (**Na^+** Channel blockers) are most effective to treat trigeminal neuralgia, the respective daily doses of which being 600-1200mg and 1200-2400 mg. Lamotrigine (folate antagonist) is given in 50mg twice daily doses, and topiramte (glutamate inhibitor) given in twice daily doses of 25-200 mg are the other drugs used to treat trigeminal neuralgia.

Opioids used in neuropathic pain

The opioids used in neuropathic pain include tramdol 50-100 mg/day, Hydrocodone 2.5 mg+ acetaminpphen 325 mg, Oxycodone 10-40 mg/day, dihydrocodone 30 mg/day., oxymorphone 10-20/day and hydromorphone 2-4 mg/day. These preparations are used as adjutants to other drugs used for neuropathic pain

Topical agents used in neuropathic pain

These drugs include Capsaisin 8% cream or patch, Lidocaine 5% patch

1

Viva Voce

In the following chapters a series of probable, most likely and common questions usually asked in the viva voce are included. These equations and answers are of suggestive nature and cover all the essential theoretical aspects of the chapter/chapters concerned. The students are advised to follow them in principle to know the subject concerned and also to go through a standard text book for furthering their knowledge and even better prepared to excel themselves in the viva examination.

Chapter 1

General Pharmacology

1) What are the advantages of a sublingual drug preparation? Give suitable examples

Ans: This is the most preferred route of drug administration when rapid relief of symptoms is required. The drugs enter the systemic circulation directly bypassing any first-past metabolism, since the sublingual or buccal mucosa is highly vascular facilitating rapid absorption of the drugs.

Examples of the drugs given sublingually/buccally include glyceryl trinitrate or isosorbide dinitrate for rapid relief of pain in angina pectoris. The other example is buprenorphine for the relief of chronic pain or postoperative pain.

2) What is intrathecal drug administration? Give examples and their clinical uses

Ans: Intrathecal route of drug administration is a process of administering the drug into the spinal space/subarachnoid space to reach CSF bypassing blood brain barrier. Examples of the route include local anaesthetics for many lower lumbar surgeries, chemotherapeutic agents like methotrexate or cytarabine for cancer therapy, baclofen for muscular spasm due to cerebral palsy, and analgesics for the relief of postoperative pain, pain due to malignancy or other types of chronic pain and also for labor pain, caesarean section and back pain when they are administered epidurally.

3) What are transdermal patches? Give examples and their uses.

Ans: Transdermal patches are medicated adhesive patches formulated in layers and applied on the skin for the sustained release of the drug incorporated in the layers for a period of 12 – 24 hours. The drug enters the bloodstream directly and provides the desired therapeutic effect for the said duration. Examples include fentanyl for the relief of chronic pain, estrogen for menopausal syndrome, nitroglycerine for angina, clonidine for hypertension, scopolamine for travel sickness and rivastigmine for Alzheimer's disease.

4) What is endocytosis and exocytosis?

Ans: Endocytosis is a process wherein large substances or substances which are impermeable through the membrane are transported into the cell by binding to cell surface receptors which get converted into vesicles and then engulfed. The drugs that are transported by endoytosis include Vitamin B12, iron by binding to specific receptors (transferring receptors) on the cell surface.

Exocytosis is a process by which the stored particulate matter (transmitter) is released from the vesicles in the nerve endings into synaptic cleft or junction and the released transmitter binds to the postjunctional site. This process occurs for the release of acetylcholine, adrenaline, nor – adrenaline, dopamine, 5 – HT, GABA, and other neurotransmitters.

5) How can the drug action be prolonged? Give few examples

Ans: The duration of the drug action can be prolonged by making suitable modification with the addition of another drug, making changes in the formulation, by the addition of a suitable medium or by changing the pH.

Examples include

a) By the addition of adrenaline, non – adrenaline, phenylephrine (vasoconstrictor) to a local anaesthetic results in its slow absorption, prolonged duration of action and reduced systemic toxicity.
b) Penicillin – G is made poorly soluble by the addition of procaine that results in its slow absorption and prolonged action.
c) Esterification of steroid hormones like testosterone and medroxyprogesterone increases their solubility in oil that results in their slow absorption.
d) Regular insulin which has short duration of action can be converted either to a fine amorphous suspension that is rapidly absorbed (semilente insulin), or to a suspension of crystals from which insulin is released slowly by the addition of Zinc and modifying the pH (ultralente insulin). A mix of the two results in Lente Insulin which has sustained action.

6) What is first – pass metabolism, give examples and its significance

Ans: Usually the metabolism of a drug occurs in the liver after its desired therapeutic action is over. However, certain drugs undergo metabolism in the liver even before they are absorbed and the desired therapeutic effect sets in. Similarly, the drug may undergo presystemic metabolism in the intestines, lungs and other parts of the body. This results in reduced bioavailability of the drug given. The examples of drugs that undergo first-pass metabolism or presystemic metabolism include clonazepam, propranolol, morphine, pentazocine, meperidine, mercaptopurine, and isoproterenol.

7) What is half – life of a drug and how many half – lives are required to reach steady – state concentration, give few examples of drugs with lower half – lives.

Ans: A drug's half – life is an estimation of the time it takes for initial concentration in the plasma to get reduced by half (50%) of its original concentration. It is entirely based on first – order kinetics of the drug. **Steady – state concentration is state at which the plasma levels reach a peak or plateau** wherein the drug is administered at regular intervals and eliminated equally at fixed intervals (half – lives). Usually 5 half – lives are required to reach steady – state concentration. The example of drugs with lower half – lives include penicillin G, zidovudine, Amoxacillin, aspirin, morphine, and cephalexin.

8) What is bioavailability of a drug and what factors influence it?

Ans: Bioavailability of a drug is the extent and rate at which the active moiety of the drug enters the systemic circulation thereby gaining access to the site of action that results in drug's action. It is influenced by the route of administration, drug formulation, first – pass effect and rate of absorption.

9) What are the four types of receptors or binding sites for drugs action?

Ans: The four receptors or binding sites for drug's action include to ligand – gated ion channel, G – protein coupled receptor, kinase – linked receptor and nuclear receptor.

10) Give some examples of G – protein coupled receptors and related pharmacological actions?

Ans: Muscarinic Acetylcholine(mAch), α2, opioid, β – adrenergic, 5 – HT and histamine receptors, and also receptors for several hormones including glucagon are examples of G-protein coupled receptors. Muscarinic Acetylcholine receptor activation leads to contraction of the smooth muscle in different tissues, β – receptor activation leads to positive inotropic and chronotropic actions on the heart, relaxation of the vascular smooth muscle and breakdown of carbohydrates, triglycerides, glycogenolysis and gluconeogenesis; α2 receptor activation leads to inhibition of release non – adrenaline from the adrenergic nerve endings.

11) What is placebo effect?

Ans: Placebo is an inert and inactive substance used mainly as control in clinical trials to make a comparative study of an established drug with a newly introduced drug or to study the efficacy of a drug under investigation so as to make sure the drug affects are real or whether the effects are due to a psychological component displayed by the placebo.

12) What is drug synergism? give few examples

Ans: Drug synergism is a mechanism or a process by which combination of two drugs yields better than the arithmetic sum of the individual drugs and yields a better therapeutic effect. It is a quantitative effect. Here the mechanism of action of each drug may be different and acting at different sites.

Examples of synergism include

1. The combination of an ACE inhibitor and a thiazide results in better control of blood pressure
2. Levodopa and carbidopa are combined for a better therapeutic response in parkinsonism
3. Trimethoprim and sulfamethoxazole combination yield better antimicrobial effect.
4. INH, pyrazinamide, ethambutol combination yields better therapeutic effect to treat tuberculosis
5. Herceptin, paclitaxel, doxorubicin, combination for antimalignancy therapy(Breast cancer)

13) What are the advantages of drug synergism?

Ans: The advantages of drug synergism include maximizing the therapeutic effect, minimizing the adverse effects, shorter duration of drug therapy and allowing lower doses of drug combinations.

14) How do you define affinity and efficacy of a drug?

Ans: When a drug combines with a receptor, the intensity at which it takes place to activate the signalling system that results in a pharmacological response is known as affinity. Efficacy in the measure of the action of a drug once binding has occurred, that is the extent of action a drug can produce.

15) What is competitive antagonism? Give examples

Ans: When an agonist and antagonist act and compete for the same receptor site, the agonist shows both affinity and efficacy, while the antagonist exhibits only affinity but no efficacy. Here the actions of a agonist are blocked or nullified by the antagonist resulting in the reversal of pharmacological effect. The actions of antagonist can be overcome by increasing the concentration of the agonist and the feature is known as **competitive antagonism**.

Examples of competitive antagonism.

a) Ach and atropine at muscarinic receptors.
b) Ach and neostigmine at nicotinic receptors.
c) Histamine and diphenhydramine at H_1 receptors.
d) Histamine and ranitidine at H_2 receptors.

16) What is therapeutic monitoring of drugs? Give few examples?

Ans: Therapeutic monitoring of drugs is a process of estimating the plasma levels of a drug at periodical intervals to adjust the dose depending upon the therapeutic response particularly when it is given for extended periods, and when there is a possibility of fluctuations of plasma levels due to drug – drug interactions and with the possibility of developing adverse reactions. This is to avoid any possible organ damage likely to be caused by the drug, adjust the dose in the presence of any organ insufficiency and to be used in the case of such drugs which have low margin of safety and narrow therapeutic index.

Some drugs that require therapeutic drug monitoring include digoxin, lithium, gentamicin and other aminoglycosides, phenytoin, carbamazepine, methotrexate and theophylline.

17) Name some cardiotoxic drugs?

Ans: Inhalational general anesthetics (halothane), bleomycin, emetine, quinidine, terfenamide (H_1 blocker), celecoxib and rofecoxib (NSAIDS), INFα, D – penicillamine,

18) Name some drugs that can cause hepatotoxicity

Ans: INH, halothane, alcohol, paracetamol, rifampicin, methyltestosterone.

19) Name some drugs that cause nephrotoxicity

Ans: Aminoglycosides, vancomycin, aspirin, gold salts, cyclosporine, amphotericin-B, cidofovir (drug used to treat cytomegalovirus infection), INFα, D-penicillamine,

20) Name some teratogenic drugs

Ans: Thalidomide, cytotoxic drugs, antithyroid drugs, isotretinoin, alcohol, tetracylines, ACE inhibitors, phenytoin, valproic acid, warfarin, diethylstilbestrol.

21) Name some clinically significant drug – drug interactions

Ans:

a) Sulfamethoxazole/Trimethoprim interaction with warfarin with likely bleeding chances, and the dose of warfarin reduced by 25%. Metronidazole, Azole antifungals also necessitate the dose reduction of warfarin.

b) Cyclosporine/tacrolimus combination with pitavastatin is associated with high rate of muscular toxicity, hence combination of the two avoided.

c) Increased hypertensive response to the withdrawal of clonidine when a non-cardioselective β – blocker is being used. In the presence of β_2 receptor blockade (due to the use of non-cardioselective β-blocker), vasoconstrictor properties of catecholamines are unopposed, resulting in the exaggerated hypertensive response within 24-72 hours after discontinuing the use of clonidine. B-blockers should be tapered and discontinued several days before clonidine withdrawal to reduce the risk of rebound hypertension.

d) Combination of ACE inhibitors and potassium sparing diuretics (triamterene, amiloride, spiranolactone) can lead to hyperkalemia due to increased plasma level of potassium caused by both the group of drugs.

22) What is pharmacogenetics, give few examples

Ans: Drug responses may not be identical in all individuals and they are likely to vary in some individuals due to their genetic composition and it is a inherited genetic variation and the study of the variation in drug responses due to genetic variation of the individual is known as pharmacogenetics.

Examples:

a) In the treatment of tuberculosis INH may show different therapeutic responses due to its' varied metabolism in certain group of individuals. Some individuals with inherited autosomal trait show slow N – acetylation reaction resulting in increased plasma levels while others show fast acetylation resulting in decreased plasma levels and in both the cases the dose of INH has to be adjusted to avoid differences in drug response and its toxicity.

b) Succinylcholine a depolarizing skeletal muscle relaxant is metabolized by butyrlcholinesterase. Some patients hydrolyze a standard dose of succinylcholine more slowly, resulting in more prolonged muscle contraction and apnea. These patients have atypical butylrylcholinesterase resulting in slow acetylation of the drug with the resultant apnea (**succinylcholine apnea**).

c) Some persons receiving drugs like primaquine, chloroquine, PABA, Vitamin K analogs, nitrofuran derivatives are likely to develop hemolytic anemia. These persons are deficient in G_6PD (Glucose 6 – Phosphate dehydrogenase) which is responsible for oxidation, reduction reactions and deficiency of the same causes reduced reduction of glucose – 6 – phosphate to 6 – phosphogluconate and NADP to NADPH. NADPH in RBC is responsible for the maintenance of integrity of RBC and for the formation of reduced glutathione. In the absence of NADPH and glutathione, oxidative stress on the cells is increased resulting in haemolysis.

Chapter 2

Autonomic Nervous System

1) **What are the responses of Adrenaline, Non – adrenaline and isoprenaline on blood pressure and heart rate?**

Ans: **Adrenaline** by virtue of α – receptor action produces vasoconstriction, increases peripheral vascular resistance and raises the blood pressure instantly. This rise is also due to cardiac stimulation. This is followed by a fall of B.P due to β – receptor stimulation in the vasculature. Adrenaline increases the heart rate, force of contraction and an increase of conduction velocity.

Nor – adrenaline by virtue of its predominant action on α – receptor rises the blood pressure without producing a subsequent fall. It has a week β_1 stimulant action on the heart and does not cause any significant change in the heart rate.

Isoprenaline by virtue of its predominant action on β – receptors cause a fall of blood pressure due to peripheral vasodilation. It causes a reflux tachycardia which is also due to direct action on the cardiac β_1 – receptors.

2) **What is the action of sympathomimetic drugs on the respiratory system?**

Ans: Sympathominetic drugs like adrenaline, isoprenaline and other β_2 agonists cause relaxation of the bronchial smooth muscle followed by bronchodilation and the same effect is not effected by nor– adrenaline and other α – agonists.

3) **What are the metabolic effects of sympathomimetic drugs and why non-selective β – blockers are contraindicated while antidiabetic drugs are used concurrently?**

Ans: By virtue of α_2 – receptor activation in pancreatic cells, sympathomimetics decrease insulin release and increase blood sugar levels. They facilitate gluconeogenesis and glycogenolysis through α_1 and β_2 actions in the liver and skeletal muscle and hence increase the blood glucose levels. As β_2 action is predominant, non – selective β – blockers are likely to cause hypoglycemia with the use of antidiabetic drugs (a combination of β_2 receptor blockade and the action of an antidiabetic drug).

4) **What are the CVS effects of dopamine and dobutamine?**

Ans: Dopamine causes D_1 receptor activation and causes vasodilation in the renal, coronary, mesenteric vasculature and causes increased GFR, renal blood flow and natriuresis. In higher doses dopamine has predominant action on cardiac β_1 receptors and increases the force of contraction and a minimal to moderate increase in heart rate. In further higher doses it has predominant action on α_1 – receptors and increases the blood pressure.

Dobutamine has predominant action on the cardiac β_1 receptors and increases cardiac contractility and cardiac output and does not act on dopamine receptors to induce the release of NAD. **Dobutamine is less likely to produce hypertension, tachycardia, and arrhythmia. It is the preferred drug to treat acute decompensated heart failure.**

5) Mention the clinical uses of sympathomimetics

Ans: Sympathomimetic drugs are used in hypotensive states, anaphylactic shock, bronchial asthma, local vasoconstrictor action to arrest bleeding, to prolong the duration of local anesthetic action, to facilitate decongestion of the nasal mucosa, to produce mydriasis for funds examination, to facilitate uterine relaxation to prevent premature labor, to treat urinary incontinence, to treat attention – deficit hyperactivity disorder, treat narcolepsy and also to treat hypertension by the use of α_2 – agonist action which decreases the release of NAD from sympathetic nerve endings.

6) What are the uses of clonidine?

Ans: Clonidine is used mainly to treat hypertension by virtue of its central α2 receptor agonist action that inhibits the release of NAD. It is also used perioperatively for reducing stress responses to surgical procedures and investigations, to provide hemodynamic stability during operative procedures, to facilitate sedation and decreased requirements of volatile general anaesthetics. It also facilitates analgesic effects and can be used by parenteral, epidural, and intrathecal administration and can be used alone or combined with fentanyl or morphine to produce epidural analgesia in conditions of chronic pain including pain due to malignancy, lower back pain, neuropathic pain. It is a very useful analgesic for the relief of postoperative pain, labour pain, and pain during caesarean section.

7) What are the sedative drugs used in Intensive care units?

Ans: Sedative are used in critically ill patients in ICUS to reduce discomfort, increase tolerance of mechanical ventilation, prevent agitation – related harm, and reduce metabolic demands during cardiovascular and respiratory instability.

Benzodiazepine such as midazolam, lorazepam, and diazepam to a certain extent are the commonly used sedatives in the ICUs. Short acting IV general anaesthetics like propofol, are also used.. **Dexmedetomidine i**s a highly selective α2 – receptor agonist and used in ICUs to provide prolonged sedation and also to prevent emergent delirium following out – patient anesthesia. It is also used to provide procedural sedation and general anesthesia during diagnostic investigations and surgical procedures in combination with opioids, benzodiazepines and propofol.

8) What are the uses of α – receptor blockers?

Ans: α – receptor blockers are used in the treatment of pheochromocytoma followed by β – blockers to prevent the reflex stimulation of β – receptors that can cause cardiac effects. Further they are used in chronic hypertension, hypertensive emergencies, benign prostatic hyperplasia, erectile dysfunction in combination with papaverine.

9) What is the first – dose effect? How is it produced and what drugs produce it?

Ans: When α_1 –selective blockers are used to treat hypertension the first dose of the drug causes a greater degree of fall of blood pressure with a possible syncopal attack and hence the dose is given at bedtime when the patient is in a recumbent position in order to avoid orthostatic hypotension. The process of fall of blood pressure with the first dose itself is known as first dose effect. It is due to blockade of α_1 – receptors causing acute relaxation of vascular smooth muscle leading to vasodilation and fall of blood pressure. The drugs that produce first dose effect include prazocin, terazocin, doxazocin.

10) What is benign prostatic hyperplasia? Explain the role of α – blockers to treat the condition. What other drugs also used for the condition?

Ans: Benign prostatic hyperplasia (BPH) is non-malignant growth of prostate wherein there is enlargement of the gland and is manifested as urinary urgency, nocturnal urination, trouble in starting urination, weak urinary stream, dribbling of urine, and inability to empty the bladder fully. All the features are due to increased urinary outflow resistance.

The first line of drugs used to treat BPH include α_1– receptor blockers like alfuzocin, doxazocin, tamsulocin and silodosis. They block the contraction of smooth muscle of trigone and sphincter in the base of the urinary bladder and prostrate and help in decreasing the urinary outflow resistance and facilitate unobstructed urinary flow. Finasteride, a 5 – α reductase inhibitor that prevents the conversion of testosterone to dihydrotestosterone is also used to treat BPH.

11) What are the clinical or therapeutic uses of β - blockers?

Ans: Adrenergic β – receptor blockers are used in the treatment of hypertension, cardiac arrhythmias, ischemic heart disease, chronic stable angina, congestive heart failure, hypertrophic obstructive cardiomyopathy, alcohol withdrawal, prophylaxis of migraine, thyrotoxicosis to reduce sypraventricular tachycardia and consequent heart failure; in the treatment of glaucoma, pheochromocytoma along with α – receptor blockers, and for the reduction of portal hypertension.

12) What are the adverse effects of β - blockers?

Ans: β – blockers can cause heart – failure in susceptible individuals. They can cause or exacerbate heart failure in patients with compensated heart failures, acute MI or cardiomegaly. They can cause bradycardia, cold extremities, and withdrawal effects like tachycardia, angina, and ischemic episodes. Bronchoconstriction and hypoglycaemia when used in combination with antidiabetic drugs when non-selective beta blockers given.

13) What are the contraindications of β – blockers?

Ans: β – blockers are contraindicated in bronchial asthma and COPD, diabetes mellitus (when used in combination of non – selective β - blockers and antidiabetic drug), congestive heart failure and cardiomyopathy; Reynaud's or Burger's disease and non-healing ulcers.

14) What are cardioselective β – blockers? What are the advantages of their use in CVS condition?

Ans: Cardioselective betablockers like acebutolol, metoprolol, atenolol, bisoprolol, nebivolol, esmolol block the β1 receptors exclusively and selectively located in the heart and they do not have any significant action on the β_1 receptors situated at other locations, and also β_2 receptors located anywhere in the body. They are used to treat hypertension, chronic stable angina, supraventricular tachycardia (Esmolol), prevention of post MI angina, and congestive heart failure. Blockade of cardiac β_1 – receptors leads to decreased force of contraction, decreased heart rate, dcreased cardiac relaxation and decreased cardiac conduction time.

15) Name some choline esters and their uses?

Ans: Acetylcholine, methacholine, carbachol, bethanechol are the cholinesters. Bethanechol is the drug used to treat postoperative ileus (atony of stomach or intestines) and to increase the tone of the lower oesophageal sphincter in conditions of reflux esophagitis. Bethanechol is also used to relieve the postoperative, postpartum urinary retention and inadequate emptying of the bladder when organic obstruction is absent. It is also useful in urinary retention due to spinal injury and spinal anesthesia.

Carbachol and pilocarpine are used to treat glaucoma. Pilocarpine is also used to treat xerostomia that follows head and neck radiation.

16) What are anticholinesterase drugs? Mention their clinical uses

Ans: Anticholinesterases are the drugs which inhibit the enzymatic hydrolysis of cholinesterase enzymes, both AChE and Butyrlylcholinesterase with consequent increase in the levels of acetylcholine at the effector sites with more prolonged and intense action. Neostigmine in the drug of choice to treat paralyticus ileus and atony of the urinary bladder. Neostigmine, pyridostigmine, edrophonium, ambenonium, demecarium are used in the treatment of myasthenia gravis. Physostigmine, ecothiphate, demecarium, pilocarpine are used to treat glaucoma. **Physostigmine is the most effective drug to reverse the signs and symptoms of atropine poisoning.**

Rivastigmine, galantamine, donepezil are used to treat Alzheimer's disease.

17) What are organophosphorous compounds? How do you treat organophosphorus poisoning?

Ans: Organophosphorus compounds are irreversible cholinesterase inhibitors, and some of them include diisopropylfurophospate, parathion, malathion, chlorpyriphos, ecothiophate, and monocrotophos. They are used as insecticides and pesticides. Organophosphorus poisoning due to any reason can result in twitching, weakness, fatigability, tightness in the chest, respiratory paralysis, blurring of vision, miosis, ocular pain, sweating, diarrhea, abdominal pain and vomiting. There may be severe headache, confusion, slurred speech, ataxia and coma.

The lines of treatment consist of general supportive measures to maintain vital functions, termination of exposure to the compound by removing the patient from the area of contact, clearing and washing the entire area of exposure. Gastric lavage, endotracheal intubation to maintain the airway, endobronchial aspiration, and ventilator support if necessary are also instituted. Administration of oxygen is often required. Convulsions are controlled with the administration of diazepam and IV fluids given to maintain the body fluid balance.

Atropine is the antidote and should be given in large doses to antagonize both central and peripheral affects. Cholinesterase activators like pralidoxime, obidoxime are given to reactivate the cholinesterase enzyme and to facilitate rapid hydrolysis of the increased Ach levels.

18) What are the different groups of drugs used in glaucoma?

Ans: Cholinergic drugs like carbachol, physostigmine, demecarium and ecothiophate; adrenergic drugs like adrenaline, dipivefrin, apraclonidine, brimonidine, timolol, betoxalol, levobumalol; carbonic anhydrase inhibitor drugs like acetazolamide, doxazolamide, and ethoxazolamide; prostaglandin derivatives like latanoprost, brimatopost, unoprost.

19) What is motion sickness or travel sickness? What drugs are used to treat it?

Ans: Travel sickness or motion sickness is a condition caused when a person is making movements or experiences the movement of objects around him during a travel which may be a sea travel, road travel or space travel. Often the person experiences nausea and vomiting, dizziness sweating and a general feeling of discomfort. The drugs used to treat the condition include **scopolamine (anticholinergic drug)** used as transdermal patch, cyclizine, meclizine, promethazine, dimenhydrinate(H_1 antgonists) given orally or as a chewing gum.

Chapter 3

Cardiovascular System and Diuretics

1) Name some calcium channel blockers, what are their clinical uses

Ans: Nifedipine, amlodipine, felodipine, nicardipine, cilnidipine, diltiazem, bepredil and mibefradil are some of the calcium channel blockers. They are used for the treatment of hypertension, variant angina, exertional angina, cardiac arrhythmias, prophylaxis of migraine, preterm labor, vestibular disturbances, hypertrophic cardiomyopathy and Raynaud phenomenon (Peripheral vascular disease).

2) Name some ACE – inhibitors, what are their clinical uses?

Ans: Enalapril, lisinopril, ramipril, trandolapril, fosinopril, benazepril are some of the ACE inhibitors. They are used mainly to treat hypertension, systolic heart failure, congestive heart failure, diabetic nephropathy, left ventricular dysfunction after MI, chronic kidney disease (CKD) associated with hypertension.

3) Explain the cardiovascular effects of ACE inhibitors

Ans: They reduce the afterload which results in increased cardiac output, cardiac index, stroke volume, and a reduction systolic blood pressure without increasing the heart rate. All the effects are due to a decrease of peripheral vascular resistance. They also decrease venous capacitance with a decrease of venous return to the heart which in turn leads to a decrease of preload. All the beneficial effects are due to a reduction of rennin-angiotensin- aldosterone activity.

4) Name some important adverse effects with ACE inhibitors

Ans: Hypotension, hyperkalemia, renal insufficiency in the presence of renal artery stenosis or renal stones, pregnancy fctopathy, dry unproductive cough, angioedema, dysgeusia are some of the adverse effects of ACE inhibitors.

5) Name some angiotensin receptor blockers, what are their indications?

Ans: Losartan, valsartan, telmisarton, candesartan, olmesartanare some of the angiotensin receptor blockers. They are mainly used in the treatment of hypertension and congestive heart failure in combination with diuretics.

6) How do you explain the antihypertensive action of β – blockers?

Ans: β – blockers reduce the blood pressure by virtue of blockade of cardiac β1 receptors, inhibition of release of noradrenaline presynaptically, inhibition of release of rennin from JG (Juxaglomerular) apparatus in the kidney, a decrease of peripheral vascular resistance over a period of drug treatment, α - receptor blockade as found with carvedilol and lebetalol which block both α – and β – receptors and causing vasodilatation with drugs like celiprolol.

7) Name some directly acting arteriodilators, what are their uses and adverse effects?

Ans: Hydralazine, minoxidil, diazoxide, fenoldopam are some of the atreriodilators. They are used to treat severe hypertension in combination with diuretics; Minoxidil is used to treat androgenic alopecia as a topical cream, and scarring alopecia. The adverse effects of arteriodilators include retention of salt and water, reflex tachycardia with a possible anginal episodes, and immunological responses produced by hydralazine. Minoxidil can produce increased cardiac output; pericardial effusion and 'T' wave changes in the ECG.

8) What are the drugs useful to treat hypertensive emergency?

Ans: The drugs used in hypertensive emergencies include sodium nitroprusside, fenoldopam, esmolol, nitroglycerine, clevidipine, nicardipine, labetalol and hydralazine.

9) What is glyceryl trinitrate? What are its pharmacological responses and uses?

Ans: Glyceryl trinitrate or nitroglycerine is a directly acting arteriovenodilator having predominant action on the coronary vasculature.

They produce an increase of coronary blood flow, cause redistribution of coronary blood from non-ischemic areas to ischemic areas, decrease myocardial oxygen requirements, and increase cardiac output due to reduced afterload.

It is mainly indicated in typical angina or angina of effort, unstable angina, acute left ventricular failure, vasospastic angina, cyanide poisoning, and to produce uterine relaxation in obstetric practices such as manual extraction of retained placenta after caesarean section, emergency treatment of uterine inversion, and pregnancy associated hypertension. Glyceryl trinitrate is also useful to treat chronic anal fissures to increase local circulation as rectal ointment.

10) What are different drugs used to treat Angina?

Ans: Nitrates, β – blockers, calcium channel blockers, potassium channel openers like nicorandil, fatty acid oxidation inhibitors like ranolazine.

11) What are the adverse effects of nitrates?

Ans: Orthostatic hypotension, headache, flushing of the face, dizziness, weakness, nausea, and development of tolerance after prolonged use.

12) How do you treat myocardial infarction in an emergency department?

Ans:

- Immediate cardiopulmonary resuscitation if cardiac arrest is found.
- Nitroglycerine given sublingually/ IV or as spray.
- Restoration of the balance of oxygen supply and demand by monitoring oxygen saturation and pulse oximetry.
- Continuous oxygen supplementation
- Electric cardioversion by using quick, low – energy shocks to restore a regular heart rhythm if there are cardiac arrhythmias.
- Analgesics – non-enteric coated chewable aspirin to be followed by morphine given IV.
- Reperfusion of the blocked coronary blood vessels by giving thrombolytic drugs alterplase, tenecteplase, streptokinase, anistreplase, urokinase.

- Unfractioned heparins like enoxaparin, fondaparinux for the prevention of a possible reinfarction.
- Nitroglycerine drip if the pain persists or recurs.
- Percutaneous reperfusion intervention if earlier fibrinolytic/thrombolytic treatment not given and done by the placement of drug – eluting or bare metal stents.
- Post MI management is followed by the use of β – blockers, Calcium – channel blockers, antiplatelet drugs (aspirin, clopidogral)

13) Name the drugs used to treat congestive heart failure

Ans: Cardiac glycosides like digoxin, renin – angiotensin antagonists like ACE inhibitors, AT1 receptor blockers; β – blockers like metoprolol, carvedilol, and bisoprolol; diuretics like frusemide, potassium sparing diuretics like eplerenone, canrenone, finerenone; vasodilators like sodium nitroprusside and glyceryltrinitrate, inodilators like levosimendon, sympathomimetic inotropic drugs like dopamine and dobutamine and sacubitril – valsartan combination preparation are the drugs used to treat congestive heart failure depending on the stage and severity of the failure.

14) Name the important cardiac actions of digoxin

Ans: Digoxin is a cardiac glycoside and exhibits a positive inotropic (force of contraction), negative chronotropic (heart rate) and dromotropic (conduction) effects without any effect on cardiac excitation. It increases the force of contraction by its direct action on the cardiac muscle. It decreases heart rate by an increase of vagal activity; increases cardiac output and cardiac index by an increase of stroke volume and stroke work. It decreases AV-nodal conduction and increases effective refractory period causing bradycardia. It decreases preload and end – diastolic filling pressures.

15) What are the adverse effects of digoxin?

Ans: Digoxin in higher doses produces bradycardia, extrasystoles, pulsus bigeminus, heart block, ventricular arrhythmia. It also produces gastro – intestinal adverse effects like anorexia nausea, and vomiting and neurological disturbances such as disorientation, visual disturbances, confusion, and disturbances of color perception.

16) Name sympathetic positive inotropic drugs and their clinical uses

Ans: Dopamine and dobutamine are the sympathetic positive inotropic drugs. They are given by IV route and used to treat acute congestive heart failure as they increase cardiac contractility and cardiac output.

17) Name the phosphodiesterase inhibitors used in acute congestive heart failure due to systolic dysfunction

Ans: Inamrinone, milrinone, vesnarinone, enoximone are the phosphodiesterase inhibitors used to treat heart failure due to systolic dysfunction.

18) Name the drugs affecting renin – angiotensin system?

Ans: ACE inhibitors like lisinopril, ramipril, fosinopril, AT_1 receptor blockers like Valsartan, telmisartan.

19) Name the vasodilators used in acute decompensated cardiac failure

Ans: Sodium nitroprusside and glyceryltrinitrate are the drugs used to treat acute decompensated heart failure and given IV along with loop diuretics like frusemide.

20) What is valsartan, sacubitril combination and what for it is used?

Ans: Valsartan is a AT_1 receptor blocker and sacubitril is a neprilysin inhibitor. Valsartan blocks the effects of rennin – angiotensin on cardiovascular system causing a fall of blood pressure, regression of left ventricular hypertrophy. Sacubitril is a neprilysin inhibitor that increases the levels of natriuretic peptides (ANP,BNP) thereby causing natriuresis, increased myocardial force of contraction and peripheral vasodilatation. The combination of the drugs is used to treat congestive heart failure and hypertension.

21) Name some aldosterone antagonists and their uses

Ans: Spiranolactone, eplerenone, canrenone, finerenone are the aldosterone antagonists. They are used to treat hypertension, congestive heart failure, chronic kidney disease associated with Type – 2 diabetes mellitus.

22) Name the drugs used to treat atrial fibrillation

Ans: Calcium channel blockers like verapamil, diltiazem, and β – blockers like metoprolol, esmolol, bisoprolol are the commonly used drugs to control atrial fibrillation.

23) What is amiodarone and what for it is used?

Ans: Amiodarone is a multichannel blocker having action on cardiac Na+, Ca+, K+ channels. It is used to treat both atrial and ventricular arrhythmias.

24) What is the most effective drug for the rapid control of ventricular arrhythmias?

Ans: Lidocaine given IV.

25) What drugs are given to control supraventricular arrhythmias?

Ans: Propranolol, metoprolol, adenosine, verapamil, diltiazem are the drugs given to control supraventicular arrhythmias.

26) What are loop diuretics? Why they are called high ceiling diuretics?

Ans: Loop diuretics act at the thick ascending limb of loop of Henle and reduce the reabsorption of Nacl by binding to **NKCC2 transporter** which facilitates reabsortion of Na+ and Cl- at the site. As they facilitate the maximum capacity or highest natriuresis and diuresis when compared to the effect produced by other groups of diuretics they are called high ceiling diuretics. Examples of loop diuretics include frusemide, ethacrinic acid, torsemide and bumetanide.

27) Mention the clinical uses of diuretics

Ans: Diuretics are used in the treatment of edema associated with congestive heart failure, hepatic cirrhosis, and nephrotic syndrome to offload the extracellular fluid volume. They are also used in pulmonary edema, and hypertension when used alone or in combination with any other class of antihypertensive drugs. They are further used to treat calcium nephrolithiosis, hypercalcemic states such as hyperparathyroidism or parathyroid malignancy. Loop diuretics are used to counteract hyperkalemia caused by potassium – retaining diuretics or ACE inhibitors. They are also used to induce forced diuresis to facilitate rapid removal of toxic substances form the circulation.

28) What are the adverse effects of loop diuretics?

Ans: Volume and electrolyte depletion which may cause hyponatremia, hypokalemia leading to metabolic acidosis and further to hypotension, reduced GFR and circulatory collapse and susceptibility to develop cardiac arrhythmias. Loop diuretics can also cause ototoxicity, hyperuricemia and increased levels of LDL – C and triglyceride levels.

29) What are osmotic diuretics and their clinical uses?

Ans: Osmotic diuretics like mannitol, urea, glycerol and isosorbide produce osmosis secondary to an increase in osmotic pressure in the proximal tubular fluid and in the descending limb of loop of Henle thereby retarding reabsorption of water. They do not facilitate the loss of salts. They are used to induce diuresis while preventing or treating the oliguric phase of acute renal failure before irreversible kidney damage occurs. They are also used to reduce intracranial pressure, intraocular pressure (glaucoma), as adjuvant therapy for treatment of poisoning to excrete the toxic products from the body.

30) What are carbonic anhydrase inhibitors, what are their clinical uses?

Ans: Carbonic anydrase inhibitors like acetazolamide, ethoxazolamide, methazolamide decrease the activity of carbonic anhydrase that catalyzes the interaction of carbon dioxide and water to produce carbonic acid and eventually to bicarbonate. By inhibiting the enzyme, the bicarbonate reabsorption from the proximal tubule in the kidney is inhibited, resulting in increased elimination of bicarbonate in the urine.

They are used in the treatment of glaucoma; as adjuvant therapy while treating oedema due to congestive heart failure, epilepsy, acute mountain sickness and urinary alkalinisation in the condition of hyperuricemia seen in gout.

Chapter 4

Central Nervous System

1) **Name the inhibitory neurotransmitters in the CNS?**

Ans: GABA, glycine, dopamine and opioids are the major inhibitory transmitters in the CNS. 5 – HT is both an inhibitory and excitatory transmitter.

2) **Name the excitatory neurotransmitters in the CNS?**

Ans: Acetylcholine, nor-adrenaline, glutamate (NMDA), histamine and 5 –HT (partially) are the inhibitory neurotransmitters in CNS.

3) **Name some barbiturates, what is their mechanism of action?**

Ans: Phenobarbitone, secobarbitone, thiopentone and methohexitone. They act by binding to GABA receptors at a specific site facilitating intracellular Cl^- influx leading to hyperpolarization of the neuronal membrane which in turns results inhibitory transmission.

4) **What are the pharmacological actions of barbiturates on CNS?**

Ans: Barbiturates produce sedation and hypnosis and decrease anxiety. They also have anticonvulsant action. They produce dose dependant CNS depression and may cause respiratory and cardiovascular depression in higher doses.

5) **What are the uses of barbiturates?**

Ans: Barbiturate are used to treat insomnia due to primary anxiety states, anxiety associated with clinical conditions like hypertension, angina, stress induced ulcers, and physical and mental exhaustion due to any cause, to provide preoperative sedation, to facilitate for induction of general anesthesia with thiopental, methohexitol; countering the convulsions associated with tetanus, eclampsia, and status epilecticus and drug induced convulsions. They are also used to treat grandmal epilepsy (tonic-clonic seizures) and hyperbilirubinemia and kerniecterus in neonates.

6) **How do you treat barbiturate poisoning?**

Ans: Barbiturate poisoning due to drugs' accumulation should be treated conservatively as there is **no specific antidote.** Initial measures include suctioning and endotracheal intubation to facilitate cardiopulmonary resuscitation. This is followed by correction of dehydration by giving IV fluids and plasma expanders. Gastric lavage in done early if poisoning has occurred in less than two hours. Activated charcoal is given through nasogastric tube to facilitate adsorbent action and for binding the unabsorbed drug. Forced diuresis with furosemide or mannitol along with alkalinisation of urine facilitates rapid removal of the drug from the body. Hemodialysis may also be considered to increase the rate of removal of the barbiturate from the body.

7) **What are the common pharmacological effects of benzodiazepines?**

Ans: Benzodiazepines have antianxiety and sedative effects, cause impairment of psychomotor skills, induce hypnosis, have anticonvulsant and muscle relaxant actions. All are due to GABA agonist action at a specific site (benzodiazepine site on the GABA receptor)

8) Mention the clinical uses of benzodiazepine?

Ans: Benzodiazepines are used in anxiety disorders, panic disorders, sleep disorders such as insomnia resulting from anxiety, psychological disturbances, organic disease, age – related factors and during surgical procedures. Benzodiazepine can also be used as anticonvulsants including convulsive emergencies such as status epilepticus or tetanus spasms (diazepam, lorazepam)), myoclonic jerks, absence seizures and infantile spasms (clonazepam, clobazam), to relieve skeletal muscle spasticity associated with multiple sclerosis and paraplegia resulting from spinal trauma. They are used for preanesthetic medication, induction and maintenance of anesthesia(midazolam), alcohol withdrawal symptoms, to control CNS manifestations like agitation, excitability, disorientation and hyperexcitability of central nervous system such as caused by atropine, phencyclidine. Further they can be used in delirium and hallucinations commonly associated with overdose of organophosphorous poisoning.

9) What is the drug used to treat benzodiazepine overdose?

Ans: Fumazenil is the benzodiazepine antagonist used in self – poisoning due to benzodiazepines.

10) What is preanesthetic medication and what drugs are used for it?

Ans: Preanesthetic medication is the use of drugs to improve intraoperative status of the patient and the postoperative recovery from anesthesia. It is aimed to decrease anxiety and produce sedation, improve postoperative analgesia, improve amnesia, decrease postoperative nausea and vomiting, decrease acid secretion, and postoperative eructation and to decrease aspirations. The drugs used as preanesthetic mediation include alprazolam, midazolam or diazepam to relieve anxiety and to produce sedation preferably given the night before surgery or in the early morning of the surgery; morphine 1 hour before surgery to provide analgesia, mild sedation; pantoprazole or any protonpump inhibitor to decrease acid secretions; metoclopramide or ondonsetron to prevent acid regurgitation and nausea and vomiting, and atropine or glycopyrolate to reduce tacheobronchial secretions.

11) What are the properties of an ideal general anaesthetic?

Ans: An ideal general anesthetic should produce rapid induction and recovery, should not produce any cardiac irregularities, should not cause any organ damage, should not cause respiratory, cardiovascular and renal dysfunction, should provide good analgesia, and adequate skeletal muscle relaxation.

12) Name some inhalational general anesthetics?

Ans: Liquids like halothane, enflurane, isoflurane, desflurane, sevoflurane, and gases like nitrous oxide.

13) What are the advantages and disadvantages of nitrous oxide as of general anesthetic?

Ans: Because of its poor solubility, nitrous oxide passes very quickly from the inspired gas oxygen mixture and quickly attains alveolar concentrations and reach equilibrium is all compartments quickly and thereby produces rapid induction and onset of anesthesia.

However it is more an analgesic than a potent anesthetic and requires higher concentrations for induction of anesthesia. It can increase cerebral blood flow and raise intracranial pressure. It does not produce required skeletal muscle relaxation. It may get deposited in air pockets in the lungs, middle ear, intestines and may rise the pressure in the said locations.

14) Name some intravenous general anesthetics and what for they are used?

Ans: Thiopental, methohexitol, etomidate, propofol, ketamine, midazolam, fentanyl are some of the commonly used intravenous general anesthetics. They are used for the induction of general anesthesia followed by the use of a potent general anesthetic for maintenance.

15) What is dissociative anesthesia? What drugs produce it?

Ans: Dissociative anesthesia is characterized by catalepsy, catatonia, analgesia, amnesia without loss of consciousness. Ketamine is the general anesthetic that produces dissociative general anesthesia.

16) Name non – depolarizing skeletal muscle relaxants. What is their mechanism of action? How do you antagonize their action

Ans: D – tubocurarine, atracurium, mivacurium, pancuroneum, rapacuronium, rocuronium, vecuronium are some of the non – depolarizing skeletal muscle relaxants used in surgical procedures.

They block the acetylcholine nicotinic receptors(nAch) at the motor endplate thereby preventing the action of acetylcholine at the site that results in relaxation of the skeletal muscle.

17) How do you block the actions of non – depolarizing drugs?

Ans: The actions of non – depolarizing agents can be blocked or antagonized by giving cholinesterase inhibitors like neostigmine. **Sugammadex** blocks the actions of rocuronium, vecuronium and unlike neostigmine it is not a cholinesterase inhibitor and does not produce cholinergic effects seen with neostigmine.

18) What is Succinylcholine? What is its mechanism of action? How is its actions blocked in case of overdose?

Ans: Succinylcholine in a short acting depolarizing skeletal muscle relaxant and causes persistent depolarization of the motor endplate and because of the sustained depolarization, the muscle gets unexcitable and fatigued and gets relaxed. It produces initial spastic state followed by flaccid state that follows relaxation of the muscle. Its actions are reversed by the administration of fresh plasma containing cholinesterase enzyme as It has no specific reversal agent.

19) What are the indications of succinylcholine?

Ans: Succinylcholine is a rapid acting and short duration skeletal muscle relaxant and is used mainly as adjuvant to general anesthesia, to facilitate endotracheal intubation and mechanical ventilation and for short investigative procedures. It is also commonly used as a muscle relaxant during electroconvulsive therapy.

20) What are the possible adverse effects of succinylcholine?

Ans: Succinylcholine can cause apnea due to the presence of atypical pseudocholinestercase which normally hydrolyses succinylcholine. This results in accumulation of acetylcholine that causes contraction of the respiratory muscles resulting in respiratory distress. It is due to the presence of a genetic disorder of the hydrolyzing enzyme. Succinylcholine can also produce hyperkalemia, malignant hyperthermia, and respiratory paralysis that can occur during general anesthesia. It can also cause increased intraocular pressure.

21) Name some centrally acting skeletal muscle relaxants?

Ans: Diazepam baclofen, tizanidine, dantrolene, gabapentine, pregabalin and botulinum toxin are the centrally acting skeletal muscle relaxants.

22) What are the uses of centrally acting skeletal muscle relaxants?

Ans: They are used in spastic disorders associated with central nervous system in conditions like cerebral palsy, multiple sclerosis and cerebral stroke.

23) What is the mechanism of action of local anesthetics?

Ans: Local anesthetics cause blockade of the voltage-gated sodium channels which contain the receptor site of action for the agents, thereby preventing the permeability of Na^+ into the excitable membranes. This results in a decrease of depolarization preventing the impulse transmission along the neuronal pathway leading to aesthesia in a localized area.

24) Why vasoconstrictors are used along with local anesthetics?

Ans: Vasoconstrictors like adrenaline, nor-adrenaline and phenylephrine are combined with local anesthetics to induce local vasoconstriction and facilitate slow absorption at the site and prevent systemic absorption and to increase the duration of action of the local anesthetic.

25) Name some commonly used local anesthetics?

Ans: Lidocaine, etidocaine, prilocaine, bupivacaine, ropivacaine and mepivacaine are some of the commonly used local anesthetics.

26) Which local anesthetic is used to treat digitalis-induced ventricular arrhythmia? How do you explain the mechanism?

Ans: Lidocaine is the local anesthetic used to treat digitalis- induces ventricular arrhythmia. It acts by blocking the cardiac Na^+ channels and depresses the abnormal pace maker activity, excitability, and conduction.

27) What are the different types of local anesthesia?

Ans: Surface anesthesia, infiltration anesthesia, nerve block anesthesia, epidural anesthesia, spinal anesthesia and intravenous anesthesia are the commonly employed types of local anesthesia.

28) What is spinal anesthesia and what for it is used?

Ans: Spinal anesthesia is a procedure where a local anesthetic is injected into the lumbar subarachnoid space and the anesthetic agent in taken up rapidly to produce anesthesia at the areas below the level of site of injection in the lumbar region. The listed site is L1 to L3 of lumbar spine. It is a very commonly employed procedure in surgical practices involving lower abdomen, pelvis, perineal areas and lower extremities. It is largely beneficial for procedures done below the umbilicus. Bupivacaine, lidocaine, mepivacaine, ropivacaine are some of the commonly used local anesthetics for this purpose.

29) What is epidural anesthesia and what for it is used?

Ans: Epidural anesthesia is a procedure where a local anesthetic agent is injected into epidural space between the dura matter and the periosteal lining in the vertebral canal. Through this route analgesics like fentanyl can also be given using a catheter to provide continuous supply of the drug in conditions of chronic pain. Onset of anesthesia or analgesia occurs within 10 to 20 minutes. The site of injection can be anywhere into the epidural space of the spinal cord as per the need. It is indicated in major hip and knee surgery, pelvic fractures, caesarean delivery, for labor analgesia, hepatic, gastric or colonic surgeries, thoracotomy, nephrectomy, prostatectomy, amputations of lower extremities, trauma and rib fractures.

30) What are levodopa and carbidopa? What for they are used and why they are combined for therapeutic use?

Ans: Levodapa is the precursor of dopa and is used to treat bradykinasea associated with Parkinson's disease. As dopamine cannot cross the blood brain barrier to reach the central sites of action – $\mathbf{D_2}$ receptors, its precursor levodopa (L – dopa) is given which can pass the blood:brain barrier. However, It gets decarboxylated peripherally to the extent of 90% and 10% only crosses the blood - brain barrier. Carbidopa is a pripheral decarboxylase inhibitor and hence a combination of levodopa and carbidopa in the ratio 100mg and 25mg can increase the levels of L – dopa peripherally which crosses the blood-brain barrier easily and gets converted to dopamine which in turn acts on central D_2 for the control of symptoms of the condition.

31) What are the adverse effects of levodopa?

Ans: The adverse effects of levodopa include GI symptoms like anorexia, nausea and vomiting, CVS symptoms like cardiac irregularities, CNS effects like dyskinasia, behavioral effects and fluctuations in response.

32) What is bromocriptine? What are its issues?

Ans: Bromocriptine is an ergot derivative and acts on $\mathbf{D_2}$ receptors and used as adjuvant to levodopa to treat Parkinson's disease. It is also used to treat hyperprolactinenia in men to correct prolactin – related hypogonadism manifested as oligospermia, loss of libido, impotence and galactorrhea, prolactinomas, acromegaly and for inhibition of lactation after stillbirth or to suppress puerperal lactation. It is also used as a supplemental drug for adults with type 2 diabetes mellitus as an add-on therapy with metformin as it increases endogenous insulin sensitivity.

33) What is end – of – dose or wearing off reaction? What drugs are used to control the condition?

Ans: End – of – dose or wearing off reaction is the fluctuations in drug response with levodopa use after the end of successful treatment for 3 – 5 years. It is manifested mainly as akinasia (loss of spontaneous voluntary muscle movement) due to gradual depletion of dopamine stores. These motor fluctuations are alterations between periods of positive response to levodopa **("on"),** and periods of re-emergence of parkinsonian symptom **("off")** as the response to levodopa wears off. It can be managed by the administration of dopamine agonists apomorphine, pramipexole, ropinirole or COMT inhibitors like tolcapone. The adjutants are given after proper adjustments of levodopa dose to prevent any excess dopaminergic effects.

34) What drugs are given to treat Alzheimer's disease?

Ans: Cholinesterase inhibitors like donepezil, galantamine, rivastigmine or NMDA antagonist memantine are the drugs useful to treat Alzheimer's disease.

35) Name some selective 5 – HT reuptake inhibitors and their therapeutic uses?

Ans: Citalopram, escitalopram, fluoxetine, fluoxamine, paroxamine and sertaline are the selective 5-HT reuptake inhibitors. They are used to treat major depressive disorder, anxiety disorders, such as social anxiety disorder, generalized anxiety disorders, obsessive – compulsive disorder, chronic pain and also for posttraumatic disorder.

36) What is haloperidol? What for it is used?

Ans: Haloperidol is an antipsychotic drug and used to manage positive symptoms of schizophrenia like delusions, hallucinations; reality disorders, hyperactivity disorder and severe behavioural disorder in children.

37) What are the uses of antipsychotic drugs other than their use in schizophrenia?

Ans: Chlorpromazine, promethazine, prochlorperazine are used to control nausea and vomiting of any origin, particularly due to morning sickness and hyperemesis gravidarum. They are also used for preanaesthetic medication to produce sedation and usually combined with meperidine (for analgesia) and atropine (to dry up secretions). They are also used as antipruretic agents. Droperidol is used to produce **neurolept anaesthesia** (a state of CNS depression and analgesia and consists of profound sedation, immobilization, and intense analgesia, without loss of consciousness) in combination with fentanyl. They are also useful to control alcohol hallucinations.

38) What is phenytoin? What is it's mechanism of action and uses?

Ans: Phenytoin is an antiepileptic drug. It acts by blockade of use – dependent Na+ channels reducing the repetitive firing of neurons. It prolongs the inactivated state of Na^+ channel or delays the recovery from the inactivated state. It also blocks Ca+ channels inhibiting voltage dependent neurotransmission at the level of synapse. It decreases the excitatory glutamate release and increases the action of GABA at the synaptic junctions.

It is used to treat partial and tonic – clonic seizures. It can also be used to control seizures due to status epilecticus.

39) What are the adverse effects of phenytoin?

Ans: Phenytoin can cause GI distress, nystagmus, diplopia, ataxia, gingival hyperplasia, hirsutism, osteomalasia, and megaloblastic anemia. If it is given during pregnancy to treat epilepsies it is likely to produce a group of symptoms known as fetal hydantoin syndrome consisting of congenital malformations of children born to them

40) What is ethosuximide? What is it's mechanism of action and uses?

Ans: Ethosuximide is an antiepileptic drug. It abolishes low threshold Ca+ currents ('T' currents) thereby suppressing spike wave activity seen typically in absence seizures. It is the drug of choice to treat absence seizures.

41) Name the benzodiazepines used in epileptic disorders?

Ans: Clonazepam is used in acute management of epilepsy and acute treatment of non – convulsive status epilecticus, infantile spasms, absence seizures, myoclonic seizures, panic disorders, Lennox – Gastaut syndrome and for sedation in sleep disorders. Diazepam is used to control convulsions in status epilepticus. Clobazam and clorazepate are used in partial seizures.

42) What is carbamazepine? What are its uses?

Ans: Carbamazepine is a voltage – gated Na+ channel blocker, abolishes repetitive neuronal firing in the cortical areas of the brain thereby abolishing sustained depolarisations and spread of seizure activity.

It is mainly used to treat partial seizures particularly psychomotor and temporal lobe epilepsy and generalized tonic seizures (grandmal epilepsy). It is also used to treat trigeminal neuralgia, pain associated with multiple sclerosis, tabes dorsalis and postherpetic neuralgia and also for bipolar disease.

43) What is valproic acid, How does it act and what are it's uses?

Ans: Valproic acid is an antiepileptic drug. It acts by blocking Na^+ channels, inhibition of transaminase enzyme responsible for degradation of GABA, thereby increasing its levels, and also increasing the synthesis of GABA, the principle inhibitory neurotransmitter. It also modulates Ca^+ channels. It is mainly used to treat complex partial seizures, absence seizures, migraine prophylaxis, and bipolar mania.

44) What are Gabapentine and pregabalin? What are their uses?

Ans: Gabapentine is an anticonvulsive drug and a GABA agonist binding to a different site on the GABA receptor. It is indicated to treat partial seizures as adjuvant drug. It is also used to treat postherpetic neuralgia, diabetic neuropathy, restless leg syndrome, fibromyalgia, bipolar disorder, postmenopausal hot flashes, anxiety states, various types of neuropathies including diabetic neuropathy, spastic disorders of skeletal muscles of central origin.

Pregabalin has similar actions and uses as that of gabapentine.

45) What are the drugs used to treat status epilecticus?

Ans: Lorazepam is the preferred drug to rapidly control the seizures associated with status epilepticus since it has rapid onset of action. Diazepam is also preferred if lorazepam is not available. Antiepileptic drugs like fosphenytoin, phenytoin, levetiracetam and valporic acid are also useful for simultaneous administration along with other anticonvulsants.

46) What are the important pharmacological actions of morphine?

Ans: Morphine is a centrally acting opioid analgesic. It produces analgesia, drowsiness, changes in the mood, and mental clouding. It causes euphoria, sedation, nausea and vomiting, produces respiratory depression, miosis, trunkal rigidity, decreased GI motility and constipation, biliary tract spasm, and histamine release.

47) What are the uses of morphine?

Ans: Morphine is used as analgesic in acute conditions like MI, postoperative pain, pain associated with biliary spasm along with atropine; It is also used for pre – anaesthetic medication, as adjuvant to general anaesthesia, epidural and intrathecal analgesia in chronic pain conditions, and acute pulmonary edema.

48) What are the contraindications for morphine use?

Ans: Morphine use is contraindicated in conditions like head injury, in elderly people or debilitated patients, patients with renal or hepatic dysfunction, Addison's disease, prostatic hypertrophy or urethral stricture, children, hypoxia states, atrial flutter and supraventricular tachycardia, acute abdomen, hypotensive state, convulsive disorders, bronchial asthma, COPD and hypersensitivity reactions.

49) How are morphine withdrawal symptoms treated?

Ans: Drugs like buprenorphine, methadone (morphine substitutes) are more effective for managing morphine withdrawal in terms of severity of withdrawal and duration of withdrawal treatment. Other drugs that can be used include clonidine and lofexidine both being alpha-2 adrenergic agonists which lower nor-adrenaline levels that are responsible for the withdrawal symptoms.

50) How do you treat morphine or opioid overdosage?

Ans: Opioid antagonists like naloxone which can be given intravenously or intranasally is effective in controlling the respiratory and CNS depression produced by overdose of opioids. The other opioid antagonists that can be used for opioid overdose include naltrexone with longer duration of action and nalmephene.

51) What are fentanyl, sufentanyl and alfentanyl?

Ans: Fentanyl and sufentanyl are potent opioids and are used as anesthetic adjuvants during perioperative period in reducing painful stimuli due to endotracheal intubation and surgical incision. They are combined with droperidol to produce neurolept anesthesia. They are also used to provide preemptive (analgesic intervention given before noxious stimulus such as surgical incision takes place) analgesia and for the control of postoperative pain, and labor pain in combination with local anaesthetic, in caesarean section, to relive chronic pain due to malignancy when given epidurally or intrathecally, or as trandermal patches and transmucosal lozenzes.

52) Name some nonsteroidal anti-inflammatory drugs and their indications?

Ans: Aspirin, paracetamol, ibuprofen, diclofenac, aceclofenac, mefenamic acid, piroxicam, meloxicam and nabumetone are some of the commonly used non-steroidal anti-inflammatory drugs.

They are mainly used as analgesic, anti-inflammatory and antipyretic drugs. Salicylates are used in rheumatic fever, rheumatic arthritis, and other arthritic conditions. Aspirin is used as antiplatelet drug for the prevention of thrombotic disorders in conditions like stable angina, unstable angina, MI, stroke, deep vein thrombosis, and transient ischemic disorders. Aspirin is also used for prevention of colon cancer, migraine pain, inflammatory bowel disease, ulcerative colitis. The common indications for all non – steroidal drugs include osteoarthritis ankylosing spondylosis, rheumatoid arthritis, tendinitis, bursitis, postoperative pain, and pain due to many musculoskeletal disorders. Paracetamol is mainly used as antipyretic and analgesic drug.

53) What are the adverse effects of Non – steroidal anti-inflammatory drugs?

Ans: NSAIDS produce moderate to severe gastric irritation and erosion, gastric ulceration, activation of peptic ulcer, epigastric distress and gastritis.

They also more likely to produce hyperkalemia, retension of sodium and water, acute kidney injury, nephritic syndrome and chronic kidney disease.

54) What are selective COX2 inhibitors and why some of them withdrawn from clinical use?

Ans: Celecoxib, Rofecoxib, Etoricoxib, Veldecoxib are some of the COX_2 inhibitors. Rofecoxib has been withdrawn from clinical because of its potent cardiovascular damage and likely to produce peripheral oedema, an increase of blood pressure, renal dysfunction and cardiac arrhythmias.

55) What are the advantages and disadvantages of selective COX2 inhibitors?

Ans: Selective COX_2 inhibitors inhibit – COX_2 selectively sparing the inhibition of COX_1 expressed predominantly in the stomach. As COX_1 is responsible for the synthesis of cytoproteitive prostaglandins

PGI_2, PGE_2 and as they are not inhibited by selective COX_2 inhibitors, GI adverse effects that are usually present with non – selective inhibitors are absent with the use of selective COX2 inhibitors. However COX_2 selective inhibitors like rofecoxibib is more likely to produce CV adverse effects and since withdrawn from clinical use.

56) Name disease – modifying antirheumatic drugs. Why they are preferred over the conventional antirheumatic drugs?

Ans: Methotrexate, chlorambucil, cyclophosphamide, azathioprine, hydroxychloroquine, D- Penicillamine, and leflunomide are some of the disease – modifying drugs used to treat chronic rheumatoid arthritis to prevent its rapid progression and to provide sustained relief from the symptoms of the disease.

57) What is gouty arthritis? What drugs are used to treat the conditions?

Ans: Gouty arthritis is a condition that develops due to deposits of monosodium urate crystals in the joints bringing about a pathological reaction that leads to the development of arthritis.

The drugs used to treat gouty arthritis include uricosuric drugs like probenecid and sulfinpyrazone that block the reabsorption of urate in the proximal renal tubule and enhance its eliminations from the body lowering the uric acid levels. Allopurinol, febuxostat are xanthine oxidase inhibitors that inhibit the synthesis of uric acid and lower the serum uric acid levels.

58) Define alcohol tolerance, physical and psychological dependence?

Ans: Alcohol tolerance is a state of reduced behavioral or physiological response to the same dose of alcohol that occurs on extended periods of alcohol consumption. Physical dependence is elicited as withdrawal syndrome when alcohol consumption is terminated abruptly and occurs after about 8 hours and lasts for 24 hours. Psychological dependence on alcohol is characterized by a compulsive desire or craving to posses the drink and to experience the pleasure of its consumption.

59) How do you characterize and treat alcohol withdrawal syndrome?

Ans: Alcohol withdrawal syndrome is characterized by autonomic dysfunction resulting from the excitation of CNS and manifested as elevated blood pressure, tachycardia, palpitations, insomnia, tremulousness, hyperreflexia, anxiety, headache, hallucinations, agitation, alcohol withdrawal seizures, altered sensorium, hyperthermia, diaphoresis and a final state of delirium tremens.

Alcohol withdrawal syndrome is treated by substituting with a drug having similar effects like sedatives, tranquilizers, hypnotics gradually reducing the dose and then tapering of. Long acting benzodiazepine like diazepam, chlordiazepoxide, clorazepate are effective in controlling the anxiety, agitation, insomnia, tremors and sympathomimetic effects due to alcohol withdrawal. Similarly, β – blockers are effective in controlling sympathomimetic effects. Clonidine also has the similar effects.

60) How do you treat chronic alcoholism or alcohol addiction?

Ans: Detoxification is usually first initiated which consists of stopping the intake of alcohol gradually over a period. This is followed by psychosocial therapy consisting of counseling and rehabilitation. This is followed by medical management which consists of administering opioid antagonists like naltrexone which reduces alcohol consumption and carving. It reduces the urge to drink. The other drugs that are effective for the said purpose include nalmefere and acomprosate which reduce drinking frequency and relapse drinking in abstinent alcoholics.

61) What is disulfiram? What are its uses?

Ans: Disulfiram is a drug used to treat chronic alcoholism by causing an aversion to drink or consume alcohol. It acts by inhibiting aldehyde dehydrosenase which is responsible for the breakdown of acetaldehyde which is in turn formed by the metabolism of alcohol by alcohol dehydrosenase. This results in increased levels of acetaldehyde causing flushing of the face, throbbing headache, nausea and vomiting, sweating, thirst, chest pain, hypotension, mild syncope, vertigo, blurred vision and confusion. All these effects make the person to be averse to the consumption of alcohol.

62) How do treat methanol poisoning?

Ans: The treatment of methanol poisoning is aimed to provide life support to maintain vital functions, halt the metabolism of methanol to formic acid which is responsible for all the adverse effects by methanol and to facilitate the rapid removal of methanol from the body and to correct acidosis.

Administration of ethanol which shares the common metabolic pathway by the same enzyme systems facilitates the diversion of metabolism of methanol and thus prevents the formation of the toxic formic acid. 4 – methylpyrazole and fomepizole are inhibitors of alcohol dehydrogenase (ADH) and have similar use and prevent the formation of toxic formic acid. Folinic acid is given to counter the folate deficiency.

63) Name some drugs of misuse?

Ans: Opioids like morphine, diacetylmorphine (heroin), codeine, oxycodone, meperidine used as euphoritic drugs; amphetamine derives like methylenedioxy–amphetamine (MDA), methylene dioxymethamphetamine(MDMA) are psychostimulant drugs; barbiturates, benzodiazepines are sedative and antianxiety drugs; LSD, mescaline, psilocybin, ketamine, cannabis are hallucinogenic drugs.

Chapter 5

Autacoids, Ergot Alkaloids, Eicosanoids

1) Name some commonly used H_1 antagonists?

Ans: Pheniramine, chlorpheneramine, diphenhydramine, dimenhydrinate, cyclizine, meclizine, promethazine, loratadine, desloratadine, cetrizine, levocetrizine are some commonly used H_1 antagonists.

2) What are the clinical uses of H_1 antagonists?

Ans: They are used in many allergic, hypersensitivity disorders like common cold, hay fever, rhinitis, utricaria, conjunctivitis, purities and drug reactions. They are also used for motion or travel sickness and vestibular disturbances.

3) Name some 2nd generation H_1 antagonists and their advantages over 1st generation H_1 antagonists?

Ans: Loratadine, desloratadine, cetrizine, levocetrizine, ebastine, rupatadine. Being hydrophilic polar compounds, they do not cross blood – brain barrier and hence do not cause sedation or drowsiness. They have long half-life and hence single dose per day in sufficient for clinical use. They do not have autonomic effects and hence do not produce adverse anitcholinergic effects like dryness of the mouth and also they do not cause ventricular arrhythmias.

4) Name the drugs used in migraine?

Ans: Acute episodes of migraine is treated with aspirin which is usually combined with an antiemetic like domperidone; Alternatively ergotamine and caffeine combination is also used in the acute episodes of migraine.

For prophylactic treatment of migraine drugs like propranolol and amitryptiline are quite effective. Similarly valproic acid, topiramate, calcium channel blockers like verapamil or flunarizine are also used for the similar purpose. Tryptans like sumatryptan, zolmitryptan are used to treat moderate to serve attacks of migraine.

5) Name some tryptans, mention their uses and adverse effects?

Ans: Sumatryptan, almotryptam, naratryptan, zolmitryptan, rizatryptan are some tryptans used to treat moderate to serve attacks of migraine and also to treat migraine earlier at the onset of attack, when the headache in still mild to moderate. Tryptans can also be used for preventing migraine headaches and cluster headaches.The adverse effects of tryptans include coronary artery spasm, transient myocardial ischemia, and arrhythmias, nausea, fatigue, numbness or tingling of the feet.

6) What are the definite contraindications of tryptans?

Ans: Uncontrolled hypertension, ischemic heart disease, primzmetal angina, cardiac arrhythmias, atherosclerotic vascular disease are the definite contraindications of tryptans.

7) Name some 5-HT antagonists and their clinical uses

Ans: Ondansetron and its derivatives are used as antiemetics given for prevention and control of nausea and vomiting associated with radiation therapy, malignancy, and for postoperative vomiting. Clozapine another 5-HT antagonist is used for schizophrenia; methysergide is used for prophylaxis of migraine

8) What are the uses of ergot alkaloids?

Ans: Ergot alkaloids are useful to treat acute attacks of migraine, to control postpartum hemorrhage, hyperprolactinemia, and senile dementia.

Ergonovine or methylergonovine are the ergot preparations given to control postpartum hemorrhage. Bromocryptine is the effective ergot preparation to control hyperprolactinemia caused by pituitary tumours.

9) Mention the therapeutic uses of prostaglandins?

Ans: Prostaglandins like dinoprostone (PGE_2) and carboprostone $PGF_{2\alpha}$), misoprostal (PGE_1 derivative) are used in combination with mifepristone to induce medical termination of pregnancy. alprostadil (PGE_1) is used to treat erectile dysfunction; alprostadil is also used for the maintenance of ductus arteriosus; Misoprostol is used to treat drug induced duodenal ulcer; brimatoprost, latanoprost ($PGF_{2\alpha}$derivatives) are used to treat glaucoma; epoprostenol, iloprost (PGI_2 derivatives) are used to treat pulmonary hypertension.

Chapter 6

Antibiotics

1) What are the sites of action of antimicrobials on the bacteria?

Ans: Penicillins, cephalosporins, carbapenems, cycloserine, vancomycin and bacitracin inhibit the cell wall synthesis of bacteria, polymyxin, nystatin and amphotericin–B increase the bacterial cell wall permeability and cause leakage of intracellular contents, tetracyclines, chloramphenicol, aminoglycosides, clindamycin and macrolides inhibit 30s or 50s ribosomal unit and inhibit bacterial protein synthesis, rifampicin acts by inhibiting DNA dependant RNA polymerase, and Quinolones act by inhibiting DNA gyrase, Sulfonamides, sulfones, and trimethoprim act by inhibiting folic acid synthesis, Antiviral drugs act by inhibiting DNA polymerase and HIV drugs act by inhibiting HIV reverse transcriptase.

2) What is antimicrobial resistance? How does it occur?

Ans: Antimicrobial resistance is a condition when microbial organisms evolve mechanisms that protect them from the effects of antimicrobial agents. All microbial organisms such as bacteria, viruses, fungi and parasites can exhibit resistance to the corresponding antimicrobial agents. As a result of resistance the use of antimicrobial agents becomes ineffective that needs frequent change of antibiotics and invention of new antimicrobial agents to effectively control the infections. This happens usually due to misuse of antibiotics.

Resistance can occur due to impermeability of the antibiotic through the outer membrane of the organism, inactivation of or destruction of the drug by enzymes produced by the organism, inactivation of or destruction of the drug by enzymes produced by the organisms (betalactamases), mutations in the target site of action (DNA,RNA, Ribosomal units and others), efflux of the antimicrobial from the cell, or due to altered binding site for the drug in the organism.

3) What are the organisms that exhibit resistance to the effective use of antibiotics?

Ans: Pseudomonas, klebsiella pneumonia, enterobacter, e.coli, and candida.

4) What is the need for combination of antimicrobial agents?

Ans: Antimicrobial combinations are used for empirical therapy in acute severe infections in which causative organism cannot be identified immediately. This is particularly useful while treating nosocomial (hospital acquired) infections. It is also used for the treatment of polymicrobial infections associated with intra – abdominal, hepatic, pelvic and brain abscesses. The combination of antibiotics is useful to enhance the antimicrobial activity and to prevent bacterial resistance.

5) Give some examples of antimicrobial combinations and the associated clinical conditions for their use

Ans: A combination of penicillin and streptomycin or gentamicin is useful to treat bacterial endocarditis caused by enterococci or viridance streptococci. A combination of antipseudomonal betalactam antibiotic like carbenicillin and gentamicin is effective to treat recurrent urinary tract infections caused by pseudomonas aeruginosa.

A combination of three or four drugs like INH, ethambutol, pyrazinamide and rifampicin is used to prevent bacterial resistance and to enhance therapeutic effect while treating mycobacterium tuberculosis.

6) What is prophylactic use of antibiotic? Give some examples

Ans: The use of an antibiotic before a potential exposure and after exposure to a microbial infection is called prophylactic use of antibiotics or chemoprophylaxis.

Examples of chemoprophylaxis include use of rifampicin to prevent meningococcal meningitis, use of penicillin for the prevention of gonococcal infection before contact, use of antibiotics in patients of rheumatic valvular conditions before any surgical or dental procedures to prevent the development of bacteremia. Combination of antibiotics is also used in patients undergoing organ transplantation, to prevent wound infection before surgical procedures, to prevent recurrent urinary tract infections, to prevent malarial attacks before a person enters endemic areas of prevalence of malaria.

7) Name the therapeutic uses of sulphonamides

Ans: Sulphonamides are used to treat urinary tract infections, toxoplasmosis, malaria (sulfadoxine in combination with pyrimethamine), nocardiosis, and mild systemic bacterial infections.

8) What is cotrimoxazole? What are its uses?

Ans: Cotrimoxazole is a combination of sulfamethoxazole and trimethoprim in the ratio of 5:1 usually 400mg + 80mg respectively. The combination provides better antimicrobial action on a range of microorganisms and the action is known as synergistic effect.

It is used to treat urinary tract infections, bacterial and respiratory infections, gastrointestinal infections, infection caused by pneumocystis jirovecii both for treatment and prevention, and in patients of neutropenia to protect against any possible bacterial infections.

9) Name some fluoroquinolones and their clinical uses

Ans: Ciprofloxacin, ofloxacin, sparfloxacin, levofloxacin, gatifloxacin, moxifloxacin, lomefloxacin are some of the fluoroquinolones.

Fluoroquinolones are used to treat urinary tract infections, prostatitis, respiratory tract infections, sexually transmitted diseases (gonococcal urethritis caused by H.ducrei or Chlamydia trachomattis), gastrointestinal infections, typhoid fever, bone, joint and soft tissue infections.

10) Name the drugs most effective to treat typhoid fever

Ans: Fluroquinolones mostly ciprofloxacin is the most effective drug to treat typhoid fever. In ciprofloxacin resistant cases. Azithromycin, ceftriaxone, cefotaxime, cefepine oral are the other effective drugs to treat typhoid fever. The other lesser choices are cotrimoxazole, and amoxacillin.

11) Name some penicillinase resistant penicillins and their clinical use

Ans: Cloxacillin, dicloxacillin, methicillin, nafacillin, oxacillin are some penicillinase resistant penicillins. They are used mainly in infections caused by penicillinase producing organisms, particularly, staphylococci, not responding to Penicillin – G.

12) Name the aminopenicillins, mention their advantages and clinical uses

Ans: Ampicillin, amoxicillin are the commonly used aminopencillins. They are acid – resistant, hence effective when used orally unlike natural penicillins. They are combined usually with β–lactamase inhibitors clavulanic acid and sulbactam and used to treat bacterial infections such as bronchitis, bronchiectasis, otitis media, sinusitis, urinary tract infections and bacterial diarrhea.

13) Name the antibiotics used to treat pseudomonas infections

Ans: Infections caused by pseudomonas aureginosa can be treated with extended spectrum penicillins like carbenicillin, indanyl carbenicillin, ticarcillin, ureidopenicillins like azlocillin, mezlocillin; carbapenems like imipenem, meropenem; cephalosporins like cefepime, ceftazidime and fluroquinolones like trovafloxacin.

14) Name the antibiotics used to treat anaerobic infections

Ans: Anaerobic infections that include oral, abdominal, pelvic cavities and head and neck infections can be treated with metronidazole, clindamycin, IV amoxicillin and sulbactam, piperacillin and tazobactam, cefoxitin, cefotetan, meropenem, levofloxacin and moxifloxacin.

15) Name the clinical uses of 2nd generation cephalosporins

Ans: Second generation cephalosporins are used to treat bone and joint infections, pneumonia, septicemia, skin and soft tissue infections, burn wound infections, urinary tract infections and meningitis caused by S.pneumoniae, H.influenzae, N.meningitidis, bronchitis, otitis media, phyringitis and sinusitis.

16) Name some third generation cephalosporins and their clinical uses

Ans: Cefotaxime, ceftizoxime, ceftazidime, ceftriaxone, cefoperazime, cefixine are some of the 3rd generation cephalosporins.

They are used to treat gonococcal infections, meningitis, bone and joint infections, female pelvic infections, intra – abdominal infections, pneumonia, septicaemia, soft tissue infections, burn infections and complicated urinary tract infections.

17) Name some betalactamase inhibitors and their clinical uses

Ans: Clavulanic acid, sulbactam, tazobactam and avibactam are the commonly used betalactamase inhibitors. They inhibit the actions of many β – lactamases which are responsible for the inactivation of β – lactam antibiotics. In combination with certain antibiotics in fixed doses they are able to facilitate unhindered antimicrobial activity of the antibiotic. The common combinations are clavulanic acid and amoxicillin, sulbactam and ampicillin; piperacillin and tazobactam, and avibactam combined with ceftazidime.

18) What are the clinical uses of vanacomycin?

Ans: Vancomycin is a lifesaving drug used to treat staphylococcal endocarditis, and other infections caused by Staphylococci such as septicaemia, osteomyelitis, lower respiratory tract infections, and cellulitis, virindans induced endocarditits, meningitis caused by highly resistant strains of pneumococci, and antibiotic associated pseudomembranous colitis.

19) What are the common properties of aminoglycosides?

Ans: They are effective against Gram negative infections only, administered parenterally and given as once daily doses. They have concentration – dependent bactericidal action, and have postantibiotic effect and continue to kill the bacteria even after their plasma levels fall below the minimum inhibitory concentration. They cause ototoxicity and nephrotoxicity. They are all useful in acute fulminating conditions like bacterial endocarditis, urinary tract infections, septicemias and pulmonary tuberculosis.

20) Name the clinical uses of gentamicin

Ans: Gentamicin is useful in serious, life – threatening Gram – negative infections such as bacteremia and sepsis, infected burns, osteomyelitis, pneumonia, peritonitis produced by pseudomonas, enterobacter, klebsiella, serratia and proteus.

It is also useful to treat bacterial endocarditis caused by enterococci, viridians streptococci, and streptococcus pneumonia, in urinary tract infections, nosocomial pneumonia and for topical use in infections of eye, ear and skin.

21) Name the adverse effects of aminoglycosides

Ans: Aminoglycosides can cause cochlear toxicity seen as tinnitus, vestibular disturbances causing vertigo, loss of equilibrium and posture, nystagmus, and ataxia. Aminoglycosides can also cause nephrotoxicity, and neuromuscular blockade.

22) Name the clinical uses of tetracyclines

Ans: Tetracyclines are useful to treat mycoplasma infections, Rickettsial infections, sexually transmitted diseases caused by H.ducrei, chlamydia trachomatis; psittacosis, chlamydia pneumoniae, uncomplicated gonococcal urethritis. Tetracyclines are also used to treat infections caused by granuloma inguinale, lumphogranuloma venerium; brucellosis, tularaemia, cholera, plague, acne, amebiasis, prophylaxis of malaria, upper respiratory tract infections and meningitis caused by N.meningitidis and in H.Pylori infection.

23) What are the adverse effects of tetracyclines?

Ans: Tetracyclines can cause GI adverse effects such as GI irritation, nausea and vomiting, abdominal discomfort, diarrhoea and pseudomembranous colitis due to toxins produced by clostridium difficile and vaginal candidiasis.

Tetracyclines can cause discolouration of teeth, retardation of bone growth, photosensitivity, hepatotoxicity, and renal toxicity. They are contraindicated for use during pregnancy as they are likely to cause teratogenic effects.

24) Name the macrolides and their clinical uses

Ans: Erythromycin, clarithromycin, azithromycin, roxithromycin are the commonly employed macrolides.

They are used in many streptococcal infections like pharyngitis, scarlet fever, pneumococcal pneumonia, otitis media and periodontal and oral cavity infections.

They are also employed to treat Chlamydial and sexually transmitted diseases, diphtheria, pertusis, campylobacter jejuni infections, H.pylori infection, prophylaxis of endocarditis, and mycobacterial infections, enteric fever, toxoplasmosis, clostridicum difficile infection, and pelvic inflammatory disease.

25) Name the clinical uses of clindamycin

Ans: Clindamycin can be used in skin and soft tissue infections, serious infections caused by anaerobic bacteria, particularly B.fragilis, serious staphylococcal, pneumococcal, and streptococcal respiratorytract infections, for prophylaxis of endocarditis with valvular disease, pneumocystis jiroveci pneumonia in HIV –infected patients, AIDS related toxoplasmosis, acne (used as gel for topical application), and for treating falciparum malaria given in combination with chloroquine

26) What do you understand by nosocomial and community acquired infections?

Ans: Nosocominal infection is a hospital acquired infection originating from impatient department, ICUs, operation theatres, nursing homes, rehabilitation centers, and diagnostics laboratories. Nosocomial infections can cause severe pneumonia, urinary tract infections, blood stream infections including septicaemia, puerperal fever, and catheter associated infections and mechanical ventilation induced infections.

Community acquired infections are the infections acquired from the nearby community areas and the infections include influenza, bacterial pneumonia, legionellosis, botulism, asymptomatic bacteriurea, antimicrobial – resistant infections, HIV, viral hepatitis, and Corona virus infection.

27) What are the antibiotics used to treat nosocomial pneumonia?

Ans: As a good range of microorganisms that might be involved in nosocomial infections, a combination of antibiotics with good coverage of both Gram positive and Gram-Negative organisms is preferred for rapid control of the infection. Usually a third generation of cephalosporin ceftazidime and avibactam along with daptomycin and linezolid is the most preferred initial antimicrobial therapy. Alternatively, a combination of meropenem and amikacin along with daptomycin can also be used.

28) Name the first line drugs used to treat mycobacterium tuberculosis infection

Ans: INH, rifampicin, pyrazinamide and ethambutol are the first line drugs to treat Mycobacterium tuberculosis.

29) What are the adverse effects of INH?

Ans Hepatotoxicity is potentially the most serious side effect produced by INH and its toxicity is increased in the presence of underlying liver disease or when it is co administered with other hepatotoxic drugs like pyrazinamide or rifampicin.

The other adverse effect produced by INH is peripheral neuropathy which can be reversed by the use of pyridoxine.

30) What are the second – and – third line drugs for tuberculosis?

Ans: Streptomycin, ethionamide, prothionamide, cycloserine, fluroquinolones, linezolid, kanamycin and amikacin, capremoycin, terizidone, imipenem – cilastatin, amoxacillin and clavulanate are some of the 2nd and 3rd generation drugs used to treat tuberculosis mostly for multidrug resistant cases.

31) What is multidrug resistant tuberculosis and what drug combinations are used for the same?

Ans: Multidrug resistant tuberculosis is the one in which organisms gain resistance and clinical response to at least two of the most powerful anti TB drugs INH and refampicin is not seen. Extremely drug-resistant TB is the one in which resistance develops to at least three of six classes of second line drugs.

The usual combination of drugs given for multidrug resistant or extremely drug resistant TB cases include Streptomycin/Kanamycin/Amikacin/Clarithromycin+Fluoroquinolone+ Ehionamide/prothionamide for a period of at least 6 months. The other drugs most effective in extremely drug resistant TB include Bedaquiline, delamanid, pretomanid in combination with at least 3 other drugs earlier mentioned.

32) What is directly observed therapy (DOT) for tuberculosis? What are its advantages?

Ans: Directly observed therapy in a WHO – sponsored programme for achieving effective cure rates in tuberculosis. It consists of the use of sputum smear microscopy for diagnosis of TB, a standard 6 – 9 months treatment that is directly observed by a community health worker at least for the first 2 months period, a regular and uninterrupted supply of medicines and reporting of the progress of treatment to government officials.

33) What is a kit of drugs for tuberculosis?

Ans: AKT-4 is a kit used for the treatment of tuberculosis consists of first – line drugs 800mg of ethambutol and 300mg of INH, 750mg of pyrazinamide and 450mg of rifampicin. The patient is asked to take contents of one kit per day.

34) What is the role INH in the treatment of tuberculosis?

Ans: INH is the most potent drug for killing rapidly multiplying mycobacteria

35) What is the role of pyrazinamide and rifampicin in the treatment of tuberculosis?

Ans: Pyrazinamide and rifampicin have sterilizing activity and the ability to kill bacilli which are in dormant (not active) state. This action persists beyond the early months of therapy, thus decreasing the risk of relapse.

36) What are the phases of treatment in a patient of TB?

Ans: There are two phases of treatment with TB – The initial intensive first phase of 2 months and later a continuous phase of 4 months.

37) What are the drugs given in the two phases of drug treatment for TB?

Ans: The initial intensive first phase is started with four drugs consisting of INH, rifampicin, pyrazinamide and ethambutol given for two months. In phase 2 given for 4 months continuously consists of the use of rifampicin, INH and ethambutol discontinuing pyrazinamide. The total period of treatment is for 6 months.

38) What are the drugs used to treat leprosy?

Ans: Sulfones like diaminodiphenyl sulfone (DDS) and its derivatives, clofazimine, rifampicin are the first line drugs and, ofloxacin, minocycline and clarithromycin are the second line drugs used to treat leprosy.

39) What is the WHO recommendation for treating leprosy

Ans: Paucibacillary leprosy is treated with dapsone 100 mg/day+ rifampicin 600 mg once monthly+ clofazamine 300 mg once monthly given for six months and the same drug regimen is given for 12 months in multibacillary leprosy.

40) What is lepra reaction? How do you treat it?

Ans: Lepra reaction is exacerbation of lepromatous leprosy while the treatment for leprosy in continuing. It is a type – 2 reaction known as Erythema Nodosum Leprosum or may be a delayed hypersensitivity reaction of type – 1. Both the conditions can be treated with corticosteroids and thalidomide.

41) What is the mechanism of action of chloroquine in malaria?

Ans: Chloroquine is a weak base that in its neutral form freely diffuses into food vacuole of the parasite and gets protonated with a rise of internal pH. The accumulated protonated chloroquine binds to the toxic heme in the food vacuoles of the parasite and prevents its conversion to hemozoin, a nontoxic product. Thus the accumulation of toxic heme in the parasite results in its disintegration and lysis.

42) What are uses of chloroquine?

Ans: Chloroquine is used in acute clinical attack of malaria caused by P.Vivax, P.malariae, and P.ovale and sensitive forms of P.falciparum. It is also used as a suppressive chemoprophylactic agent in endemic areas of falciparum malaria; Further it is used to treat hepatic amebiasis, chronic progressive rheumatoid arthritis, systemic lupus erythematosus, and lepra reaction.

43) What are the antimalarial drugs used to treat hypnotic or dormant forms of P.Vivax and P.Ovale?

Ans: Primaquine and tafenoquine are the two drugs most effective to treat dormant (hypnotic) hepatic forms of P.Vivax and P.Ovale thereby preventing the relapse of malaria. Primaquine is given for a period of two weeks and tafenoquine given as a single dose which is more effective than the former.

44) What are the uses of mefloquine?

Ans: It is most effective to treat acute clinical attacks of falciparum and vivax malaria.

45) What are the uses of Quinine?

Ans: Quinine is useful in treating chloroquine, mefloquine, sulfadoxine – pyrimethamine combination resistant cases of falciparum malaria. It is also used in severe fulminating acute malarial attack such as cerebral malaria. It is also used to treat nocturnal muscle cramps.

46) What is proguanil and with what other drug it is combined? What for the combination used ?

Ans: Proguanil is a biguanide and is combined with atovaquone and the combination drug is most effective for treating both acute clinical attack of falciparum malaria and also for its prophylaxis.

47) What for pyrimethamine sulfadoxine combination used?

Ans: Pyrimethamine sulfadoxine fixed dose combination is used to treat chloroquine resistant cases of falciparum malaria, toxoplasmosis and pneumocystis jeroveci induced pneumonia.

48) What for artemisinin derivatives used?

Ans: Artemisinin, artemether and artesunate are used to treat an acute attack of falciparum malaria, including chloroquine – resistant, multidrug resistant falciparum malaria, and cerebral malaria. They are combined with lumifantrine or amodioquine.

49) What drugs are used for chemoprophylaxis of malaria?

Ans: Malarial chemoprophylaxis is aimed at eradicating liver schizont (hypnozoites) and, blood schizonts of the plasmorium falciparum, vivax and ovale parasites. The medications are used before, during and after the travel to the endemic areas of malaria. The drugs are used to prevent, or suppress and relapse of the malarial infection.

The drugs that are used for chemoprophylaxis include combinations of ***chloroquine and proguanil***, and ***atovaquone and proguani***l; ***proguanil with mefloquine or doxycycline in chloroquine – resistant malarial*** attacks and primaquine in multidrug – resistant P.Vivax and P.Ovale infections to provide terminal prophylaxis wherein it is effective to eliminate dormant hypozoities (hepatic forms) and hence provide radical cure of relapsing malaria.

50) What are the drugs used to treat intestinal amebiasis?

Ans: Metronidazole and its derivatives such as tinidazole; diloxanide furoate, paramomycin, tetracyclines, iodoquinol and clioquinal are the drugs commonly used to treat intestinal or luminal amebiasis.

51) What are the drugs used to treat extraintestinal amebiasis?

Ans: Chloroquine, dehydroemetine, metronidazole and its derivatives are the drugs given for extraintestinal (hepatic) amebiasis.

52) What are the different uses of metronidazole?

Ans: Metromidazole can be used to treat both intestinal and extraintestinal amebiasis, giardiasis, trichomomiasis, anaerobic infections, dracumculiasis, ulcerative gingivitis and H.Pylori infections.

53) What are the drugs used for leishmaniasis?

Ans: Sodium stibogluconate, meglumine antimoniate, pentamidine, amphotericin B, miltifosine and Paramomycin are the drugs used to treat both visceral and cutaneous leishmaniasis.

54) What is Gancyclovir and what are its uses?

Ans: Gancyclover is used to treat and to arrest progression of cytomegalovirus – induced retinitis, colitis, esophagitis and for the prevention of cytomegalovirus infection in organ transplant patients.

55) What drugs are used in combination therapy to treat HIV infection and what for the combination drugs employed?

Ans: As a single drug is not effective in suppressing HIV on its own, a combination of three drugs belonging to three different classes are used to effectively treat HIV infection.

Each class of drugs acts by different mechanisms and provide a synergistic effect thus reducing the resistance and facilitating a rapid suppression of viral load and clinical cure rates.

The combination usually consists of two nucleoside reverse transcriptase inhibitors like tenofovir, abacavir, lamivudine, zidovudine and one or two belonging to other class like efavirenz, delavirdine and saquinavir.

56) What are the treatment guidelines to HIV infection?

Ans: The guidelines to treat HIV include to effectively suppress viral load, restore CD_4+ counts, improve survival rates, and to minimize the adverse effects and also to prevent transmission of the HIV infection.

57) What are the uses of Ketoconazole?

Ans: Ketoconazole is used to treat cutaneous fungal infections, ringworm, tenia pedis, (Athelete's food), tenia corporis (fungal infections of the body), tenea cruris (ringworm of groin), seborrheic dermatitis (dandruff), tena versicolor, pityriasis versicolor.

58) What is Amphotericin-B and what for it is used?

Ans: Amphotericin-B is a antifungal drug given IV to treat systemic fungal infections like systemic candidiasis, invasive aspergillus, cryptococcus meningitis, histoplasmosis, blastomycosis, and coccidioidomycosis.

59) What are the adverse effects of Amphotericn-B?

Ans: The adverse effects caused by amphotericin-B include infusion related effects like fever, chills, rigor, headache, nausea, and hypotension. It can cause renal toxicity, and normochromic normocytic anemia

60) What for mebendazole used?

Ans: Mebendazole is used to treat pinworm infestation, ascariasis, trichinosis, ankylostomiasis, Trichuris trichuria and echinococcus infestations.

61) What are the uses of Ivermectin?

Ans: Ivermectin is used for the treatment of onchosersiasis, strongyloidosis, cutaneous larva migrance, lymphatic filariasis, scabies,and Loa Loa infestations.

62) What are the uses of methotrexate?

Ans: Methotrexate is used for childhood leukemias, chorioepithelioma, hydatiform mole, breast cancer and solid tumours such as osteogenic carcinoma, squamous cell carcinoma of lungs, rheumatoid arthritis, and psoriasis.

63) What are the uses of vinka alkaloids?

Ans: Vinka alkaloids are used to treat metastatic testicular tumours, Hodgkin's disease, lymphocytic lymphomas, kaposisarcoma, breast cancer, Wilms' tumor and ovarian cancer.

64) What are the common adverse effects of anti-malignancy drugs?

Ans: Damage to gastrointestinal epithelium including oral mucous membrane causing anorexia, nausea, vomiting and diarrhoea, loss of hair, bone marrow suppression leading to leucopoenia, secondary bacterial and fungal infections due to immunosuppression, impaired wound healing and teratogenicity and mutagenicity.

Chapter 7

Hormones

1) **What are the uses of GnRH and its analogs?**

Ans: GnRH and its analogs like Leuprolide are used to treat endometriosis, assisted pregnancies, uterine fibroids, central precocious puberty in children, and advanced prostatic cancer.

2) **What are the uses of Oxytocin?**

Ans: Oxytocin is used for induction of labor, augmentation of labor, control of postpartum hemorrhage, and for treatment of incomplete, inevitable or elective abortion to induce uterine contractions after a suction curettage.

3) **Name the drugs used to induce therapeutic abortion or medical termination of pregnancy?**

Ans: Dinoprostone (PGE_2), carboprost ($PGF2_{\alpha}$) and mesoprostal (PGE_1) are used in combination with mifepristone, a progesterone antagonist to induce medical termination of pregnancy.

4) **What are the uses of vasopressin and its derivatives?**

Ans: Vasopressin is useful to treat diabetes insipidus (DI) of central origin. Its derivative desmopressin is used to treat nocturnal enuresis also apart for its use in DI for which it is given via mucous membrane of the nose. It is also used in esophageal varicies and portal varicies. Its derivative terlipressin is used as vasopressor to rise the blood pressure in conditions of a fall in conditions like septic shock

5) **Name the uses of glucocorticoids?**

Ans: Glucocorticoids are used to treat Addison's disease, rheumatic fever, arthritis, ankylosing spondylitis, rheumatoid arthritis, nephrotic syndrome, allergic diseases including anaphylactic shock, bronchial asthma and COPD, various allergic skin conditions, for immuno suppression in organ transplants, GI disease like inflammatory bowel diseases, malignancies such as acute lymphatic leukaemia in children; cerebral edema, ocular conditions like iritis, iridocyclitis and fetal congenital anomalies.

6) **What are the adverse effects of glucocorticoids?**

Ans: Glucocorticoids can cause hyperglycemia and insulin resistance, myopathy and muscle wasting, secondary fungal, viral and bacterial infections due to immunosuppressant action, growth retardation in children, osteoporosis and spontaneous fractures, cataract and neuropsychiatric disorders.

7) **Name some commonly used glucocorticoids in clinical practice?**

Ans: Prednisolone, methyl prednisolone, triamcinolone, Dexamethasone, Betamethasone, beclomethasone and hydrocortisone, clobetasol, fluticasone, budesonide are some of the commonly used glucocorticoids in clinical practice.

8) Name some thyroid preparations and their clinical uses?

Ans: Sodium levothyroxine, liothyronine, liotrix and thyroid extract are some of the thyroid hormone preparations.

They are used to treat hypothyroidism due to iodine deficiency, autoimmune thyroid disease, Hashimoto thyroiditis, drug induced hypothyroidism, thyroidectomy, radiation induced hypothyroidism, surgical removal of thyroid gland and drug induced hypothyroidism.

9) Name some thioamide antithyroid drugs and their mechanism of action?

Ans: Propylthiouracil, methimazole, carbimazole, are the commonly used thioamide antithyroid drugs. They inhibit thyroid peroxidase induced reactions in the synthesis of thyroxine hormone. Thus they inhibit iodination of tyrosyl residues in thyroglobulin, coupling of iodotyrosyl groups (monoiodotyrosine and diiodotyrosin) and formation of T3 and T4 and inhibit their release. Propylthiouracil also inhibits peripheral conversion of T4 to T3.

10) What is Lugol's iodine and what are its indications?

Ans: The combination of elemental iodine and potassium iodide is known as Lugol's iodine. It is used in combination with propylthiouracil in the immediate preoperative preparation of a patient about to undergo thyroid surgery. It is also used in the management of thyrotoxic crisis to rapidly inhibit thyroid hormones secretion. It also decrease the vascularity, and sponginess of thyroid gland required before surgery.

11) How do you treat thyrotoxic crisis or thyroid storm?

Ans: Thyrotoxic crisis or thyroid storm is a sudden increase of hyperthyroid state due to inadequate treatment of hypethyroidism or sudden withdrawal of antithyroid drugs. The treatment consists of administration of propylthiouracil, Lugol's iodine combination, a β – blocker like propranolol to control sympathomimetic effects, and hydrocortisone to prevent the person from going into a state of shock and to antagonize the immunological responses that are likely to occur during the thyroid crisis.

12) Name some commonly used estrogen preparations?

Ans: Ethinyl estradiol, conjugated estrogens, synthetic estradiol, estrone sulfate, quinestrol and tibolone are some of the commonly available estrogens for clinical use.

13) What are the uses of estrogens?

Ans: Estrogens are used for hormone replacement therapy at the onset of menopause, female hypogonadism, primary ovarian insufficiency, symptoms associated with menopause including vulvovaginal atrophy, dyspareunia, hot flashes, and night sweats, and for prevention of osteoporosis. They are also used for oral contraception in combination with progesterones, moderate acne vulgaris, and in prostate cancer for palliative therapy.

14) What are the adverse effects of estrogens?

Ans: Estrogen can cause breast tenderness, nausea, vomiting, bloating of stomach, headaches, weight gain, hyperpigmentation of the skin, hair loss, vaginal itching, abnormal uterine bleeding or breakthrough bleeding while being used along with progestins as oral contraceptives, thrombophebitis or thromboembolism, retention of water and salts and hypertension.

15) Name some commonly used progesterone preparations

Ans: Hydroxyprogesterone, medroxyprogesterone, dimethestirone, norethindrone, lynestrenol, levonorgestril, norethsterone are some of the commonly used progesterone preparations

16) What are the uses of progesterone preparations?

Ans: Progestins are used for menopausal syndrome, oral contraception in combination with estrogens, for contraception without oestrogen combination, abnormal uterine bleeding(AUB) and endometriosis related pain, recurrent or habitual abortions or miscarriages, dysmenorrhoea, suppression of ovarian cysts including polycystic ovarian syndrome, and for hormone replacement therapy in combination with estrogens.

17) What is oral contraception and what preparations are used for it?

Ans: Oral contraception is a method used to prevent pregnancy to take place. It consists of the use of combination of estrogen and progesterone preparations for a fixed period or as a continuous progesterone alone therapy. The combination preparations may be monophasic, biphasic or triphasic in nature. In monophasic forms there is a fixed dosage of hormones during the cycles. In biphasic or triphasic forms there is variation of dosage of either or both the hormones once or twice during the cycle.

18) How are oral contraceptives used?

Ans: Oral contraceptives are available in two types of package forms, one containing the 28 tablets and the other containing 21 tablets. Both packs contain estrogen and progesterone preparations for a 21 - day cycle. In the 28 – day pack, the last 7 tablets contain a placebo (vitamin) and taken serially for 28 days. In the case of 21 - day pack, one tablet is taken each day for 21 days with a break of 7 days at the end of the cycle. In both the cases one tablet is taken starting on day 5 of the menstrual bleeding and continued for 21 days or 28 days as the case may be. Withdrawal bleeding occurs in both the cases at the end of the 21 day active medication.

19) What is progestin – only emergency contraceptive pill?

Ans: Progestin – only oral contraceptive pill also known as postcoital pill in aimed at reducing the rates of unwanted pregnancy after unprotected sexual intercourse. This is also referred to as morning after contraception. In this, two tablets of levonorgestrel (0.75mg) are taken any time before 72 hours after unprotected sex and the second 12 hours later. Mifepristone, the progesterone antagonist is also used for the similar purpose.

20) What are the advantages and disadvantages of progestin only contraceptive?

Ans: Progestin – only preparations do not contain estrogen, thereby decreasing the complications attributed to estrogens such as thrombophlebitis, CV risk and pulmonary embolism and also reduced incidence of endometrial and ovarian cancer, potential improvement of pain associated with endometriosis and also suppression of pain with ovulation. The main disadvantage in breakthrough bleeding it often produces.

21) What are the other forms of delivery of progesterone preparations for contraception?

Ans: Progestins can also be delivered as injecatables such as medroxyprogesterone as a depot preparation given IM, subdermal implants (Norplast implantation), and as transdermal patches along with estrogens.

22) What is the mechanism of action of oral contraceptives?

Ans: The combination of estrogens and progestins present in the oral contraceptive tablets inhibit the anterior pituitary and prevent the release of FSH and LH thereby preventing ovulation and corpus luteum formation. They also bring about a change in the cervical mucus which becomes viscid and scanty thus inhibiting sperm penetration and motility, bringing about changes in the endometrium and secretions in the uterine tubes, all of which prevent fertilization and a possible implantation.

23) What are the adverse effects of oral contraceptives?

Ans: The adverse effects of oral contraceptives include GI effects like anorexia, nausea, vomiting, headache, and worsened migraine episodes. Breakthrough bleeding is very common with progesterone only preparations. The other adverse effects include breast tenderness, weight gain (more common with progestins with androgenic activity). The serious vascular disorders include thrombophlebitis, venous thromboembolism, increased risk of MI and strokes.

24) What is clomiphene? What for it is used?

Ans: Clomiphene a selective estrogen receptor modulator (SERM) is a partial estrogen receptor agonist. It has dual action on the estrogen receptors, one that binds the receptors (antagonist action) and blocks the negative feedback inhibition of release of pituitary gonadotropins (FSH,LH) by oestrogen and facilitates the release of FSH and LH during midcycle. Hence, it acts as an ovulation inducing agent. It is used in ovulatory dysfunction (Polycystic ovarian syndrome) to facilitate conception. It is often given to induce ovulation in anovulatory, or oligo-ovulatory infertility.

25) What is Tamoxifen and what for it is used?

Ans: Tamoxifen is a first generation selective estrogen receptor modulator and is used to treat breast cancer and also as a prophylactic drug for the prevention of breast cancer, particularly after the patient undergoes surgery and radiation therapy. It has both agonist and antagonist activity on the estrogen receptors. Thus it has antagonist action on the breast tumor cells and hence used for breast cancer. It has agonist action on the bone and prevents osteoporosis in postmenopausal women. It has a similar agonist action on the uterine tissue thus causing uterine hyperplasia.

26) What are the advantages of raloxifene?

Ans: Raloxifene is a second generation selective estrogen receptor modulator having agonist action on the bone and hence used to treat osteoporosis in postmenopausal women. It acts as an antagonist on the breast tumor cells and hence used for prophylaxis of breast cancer in postmenopausal women. It has no agonist action on the uterine tissue and hence does not cause uterine hyperplasia unlike tamoxifen.

27) What are the clinical uses of anabolic steroids?

Ans: Androgen steroids are used for delayed puberty in boys, hypogonadotropic hypogonadism, GnRH release deficiency, bone marrow stimulation in leukemia, aplastic anemia, kidney failure, and hereditary angioedema, and for anabolic effects to increase muscle mass in conditions of muscle wasting and protein loss associated with AIDS, chronic illness, in elderly patients in tuberculosis, malignancy, surgery, trauma and chronic immobilization.

28) What is danazol? What are its uses?

Ans: Danazol is a synthetic hormone derived from ethisterone with weak progestational, androgenic and glucocorticoid activities and is used to suppress ovarian function.

It is used to treat endometriosis and menorrhagia uterine fibroids fibrocystic breast disease, hereditary angioedema, autoimmune hemolytic anemia, and immune thrombocytopenia.

29) Name some androgen receptor antagonists and their clinical uses

Ans: Cyproterone, flutamide, nilutamide, bicalutamide and apalutamide are some of the androgen receptor antagonists.

They are used in the treatment of prostatic cancer either alone or as adjuvant therapy. They are combined with a GnRH analogue which is started 8 weeks before they are administered for the condition.

30) Name some 5α – reductase inhibitors and their clinical uses

Ans: Finasteride, dutasteride are the commonly used 5α – reductase inhibitors used to treat benign prostatic hyperplasia. They can be combined with α_1 – receptor antagonists for better therapeutic effect.

31) Name some rapid acting insulin analogues

Ans: Lispro, aspart, glulisine are the rapid acting insulin preparations.

32) Name the short – acting insulin preparation.

Ans: Regular insulin or soluble insulin /crystalline insulin is the short – acting insulin preparation

33) Name the intermediate – acting insulin preparations

Ans: NPH human and Lente insulins are intermediate – acting insulins.

34) Name the long – acting insulin preparations.

Ans: Detemir, glargine, degludec, icodec ultralente insulin, PZI insulin are the long acting insulin preparations.

35) Name the various forms of administration of insulin preparations.

Ans: Insulin is usually administered subcutaneously and given as insulin pen injector devices, insulin pumps and also as inhaled insulin. In treating the emergency conditions like diabetic ketoacidosis it is given intravenously.

36) What are the target sites of insulin action and what type of a receptor insulin is?

Ans: Insulin acts through insulin receptors located in liver, skeletal muscle and adipose tissue. It is a tyrosine–kinase receptor.

37) How does insulin act?

Ans: Insulin increases glucokinase activity in the liver and traps glucose in the hepatocytes and converts it into glycogen for storage. Insulin also inhibits the breakdown of glycogen, proteins and fatty acids and their conversion to glucose (inhibitionof glycogenolysis and gluconeogenesis): In both skeletal muscle and adipose tissue, insulin facilitates the movement of glucose into the cell through a specific transporter. Insulin also facilitates glycogen synthesis and storage in the liver. In the adipose tissue insulin facilitates glucose uptake into the fat cells and also activates lipoprotein lipase which hydrolyzes triglycerides from lipoproteins and subsequent storage of triglycerides and fatty acids in the adipose tissue.

38) What are insulin secretogogues? Name them

Ans: Insulin secretogogues are those drugs which increase insulin release by acting on the pancreatic β – cells. They are sulfonylureas like glibenclamide, glipizide, glimepiride and gliclazide. They also include non-sulfonylurea derivatives nateglinide and repaglinide.

39) How do sulfonylureas act?

Ans: Sulfonylureas bind to sulfonylurea receptor(SUR_1) present on the pancreatic β – cells and cause closure of K+ channels preventing the efflux of K^+ that leads to depolarization which is triggered by the entry of Ca+ inside the pancreatic β – cell. The influx of Ca+ triggers insulin release.

40) How does metformin act?

Ans: Metformin acts by inhibiting glucose production in the liver, slowing glucose absorption from GI tract, enhancing insulin sensitivity, suppressing fatty acid oxidation, and causing a reduction of hypertriglyceridemia thereby preventing their conversion to glucose, stimulating anaerobic glycolysis in tissues with increased glucose removal from the blood and by facilitating peripheral glucose uptake and utilization.

41) What are the indications of metformin?

Ans: Metformin is indicated as a monotherapy or in combination with other antidiabetic drugs to effectively lower the blood glucose levels and to treat and control type – 2 diabetic mellitus. It is the first – line drug for treating type-2 diabetes particularly in patients who are obese and insulin- resistant and those who are in a prediabetic state. It exerts antihyperglycemic effect and does not cause hypoglycemia unlike sulfonylureas.

42) What are GLP-1 analogues? Name some of them

Ans: GLP-1 analogues are the derivatives of an incretin hormone GLP-1 (glucagon – like peptide – 1) produced in the endocrine cells of epithelium of small intestine. They act on the β – cells of the pancreas and stimulate the release of insulin. The example of GLP-1 analogues includes exenatide, liraglutide, dulaglutide and semaglutide and they are used to treat type – 2 diabetic mellitus.

43) What are Sodium – glucose co–transporter – 2 (SGLT – 2) inhibitors? What for they are used?

Ans: SGLT – 2 inhibitors are the drugs used to treat Type – 2 diabetes. They inhibit SGLT – 2 transporter across the proximal renal tubule which is responsible for the reabsorption of glucose from the site and thereby preventing glucose reabsorption leading to its elimination in the urine and lowering the blood glucose levels. Dapagliflozin, empagliflozin, canagliflozin are few examples of SGLT – 2 inhibitors. Apart from their use to treat Type – 2 Diabetes, they also used to treat decompensated congestive heart failure.

44) How do you treat Diabetic Ketoacidosis?

Ans: The treatment of diabetic Ketoacidosis consists of administering IV fluids to correct hypovolemia, restore tissue perfusion and clear ketone which is also useful to improve glycemic control. This is continued along with the administration of insulin preferably short – acting soluble insulin at regular intervals at the rate of 0.1 units/kg body weight. Potassium replacement is done if the serum potassium levels are below the normal. Sodium bicarbonate should also be given when the patients are severely acidotic with lower values of blood pH.

45) What is glucagon and what for it is used?

Ans: Glucagon is a hormone secreted by α – cells of the Pancreatic islet cells. It is used to treat hypoglycemia to increase the blood glucose levels when they are at the very lower levels. It is also used to slow GI motility in radiographic studies. It is also used to counter the actions of the beta – blockers and calcium channel blockers when given in excess doses.

46) What are the various forms of Vitamin D and what for they are used?

Ans: Vitamin D is available as cholecalciferol (Vitamin D3) and ergocalciferol (Vitamin D2). The commonly available Vitamin D derivatives include 25 – hydroxy vitamin D3 – (Calcifediol) 1, 25 – dihydroxy Vitamin D3 (calcitriol) and dihydroxy tachysterol.

They are useful to treat osteomalacia, osteoporosis, rickets, and treatment of other Vitamin D deficiency conditions, secondary hypoparathyroidism, and in renal dialysis patients.

47) What are the various drugs used in the treatment of osteoporosis?

Ans: Osteoporosis can be treated with Vitamin D derivatives, bisphosphonates like alendronate, etidronate and Zoledronate, selective oestrogen modulations like raloxifene and lasoxifene and parathyroid hormone and fragments of parathyroid hormone.

Chapter 8

Anemias and Blood Coagulation Disorders

1) How do you diagnose iron deficiency anemia?

Ans: Pallor is the most important clinical sign, followed by fatigue, a decreased ability to work, sore tongue, and brittle spoon – shaped nails, shortness of breath or worsening of congestive heart failure, and increased susceptibility to infections.

Blood examination shows microcytosis, hypochromia, and anisocytosis. The other features include decreased hemoglobin level, a low mean corpuscular hemoglobin and hemoglobin volume, decreased ferritin and iron levels, and an increase of transferrin levels, and total iron – binding capacity.

2) Name the commonly used oral iron preparations

Ans: Ferrous sulfate, ferrous fumarate, ferrous gluconate, carbonyl iron, feostat chewable tablets, are some of the example of oral iron preparations

3) Name the commonly used parenteral iron preparations

Ans: Iron dextran complex, iron – sorbitol – citric acid complex, iron – sucrose complex, sodium ferric gluconate, ferric carboxy maltose are some of the examples of parenteral iron preparations.

4) What are the side effects of oral iron preparations? How are they managed?

Ans: Nausea, vomiting, abdominal cramps and constipation are some of the side effects of oral iron preparations. These side effects can be minimized with their administration along with food and also making them available as enteric coated preparations.

5) What are the adverse effects of parenteral iron preparations?

Ans: Hypersensitivity or anaphylactic reactions are likely to occur with parenteral iron preparations. Intramuscular preparations can cause local induration, pain and sterile abscess. They can also cause discoloration of the overlying skin when given IM.

6) How do you treat iron toxicity?

Ans: Iron toxicity can be treated by administrating the chelating agent desferrioxamine.

7) What is megaloblastic anemia? How do you treat it?

Ans: Megaloblastic anemia is a condition due to impaired DNA synthesis which inhibits nuclear division, while cytoplasmic maturation which in dependent of RNA and protein synthesis is less impaired that leads to asynchronous maturation of nucleus and cytoplasm in the RBC which is the reason for large size of the megaloblasts. This condition is due to the deficiency of Vitamin B12 and folic acid through the dietary resources and other causes.

8) How do you treat megaloblastic anemia?

Ans: Vitamin B12 available as hydroxycobalamine, cyanocobalamine or methyl cobalamine and folic acid are taken together in the treatment of megaloblastic anaemia.

9) What is erythropoietin and what for it is used?

Ans: Erythropoietin is the erythropoiesis growth factor produced in the kidney that stimulates erythroid proliferation and differentiation by interacting with specific erythropoietin receptors on red cell progenerators. It stimulates red blood cell production. Epoetin alfa, darbepoetin are the erythropoietin derivatives.

Erythropoietin is used in the treatment of anemia secondary to chronic renal failure, cancer related anemia, anemia in AIDS patients, and in postoperative anemia.

10) Name some low molecular weight heparins , what is their mechanism of action

Ans: Enoxaparin, dalteparin and tinzaparin are some of the low molecular weight heparins. They bind to and potentiate the endogenous antithrombin III which inactivates factor Xa(prevents conversion of prothrombin to thrombin), and IIa. Inhibition of thrombin (Factor IIa) leads to inhibition of conversion of fibrinogen to fibrin thus prevents the coagulation.

11) What are the advantages of low molecular weight heparins?

Ans: Low molecular weight heparins provide predictable anticoagulant activity, have a better safety profile, have more bioavailability due to lesser plasma and endothelial binding, longer half – lives, less frequent administration and lesser antigenic reactions, less activation of osteoclastic activity thus causing lesser bone loss, safety of use during pregnancy, and do not cause thrombocytopenia.

12) What are the uses of heparins? What is the antagonist for the heparin?

Ans: Heparin preparations are used for both prophylaxis and treatment of thromboembolic disorders such as deep vein thrombosis, pulmonary embolism, peripheral arterial embolism, treatment of embolization associated with atrial fibrillation and/or prosthetic heart valve replacement, in hip replacement surgery, abdominal surgery, knee replacement surgery, patients with longer periods of immobility, in the dialysis procedures, and as adjuvant therapy in the treatment of unstable angina or non – ST segment elevation of MI. Protamine is the antagonist of heparin that reverses its effects.

13) Name some oral anticoagulants and how do they act?

Ans: Warfarin, acenocoumarol, dicoumarol, phenprocoumon are some of the commonly used oral anticoagulants. They act by antagonizing Vitamin K which is essential for the synthesis of coagulation factors II, VII, IX and X.

14) What are the uses of warfarin?

Ans: Warfarin is used for prophylaxis and treatment of venous thromboembolism including deep vein thrombosis, pulmonary embolism, prophylaxis and treatment of thromboembolic complications from atrial fibrillation or cardiac valve replacement, reduction in the risk of death, recurrent myocardial infarction and thrombotic events like stroke, and systemic embolization. It is also used for secondary prevention of recurrent stroke and transient ischemic attacks.

15) What are the adverse effects of warfarin?

Ans: Warfarin is a drug of low margin of safety and slight variation of dose on the upper scale can cause hemorrhage, most commonly intracranial hemorrhage, GI hemorrhage, intraocular bleeding and epistaxis. Warfarin is contraindicated during pregnancy as it can easily pass through the placental barrier and can cause hemorrhagic disorder in the fetus and birth disorders. Warfarin can cause many drug interactions. It can increase bleeding chance with the simultaneous use of antiplatelet drugs, other anticoagulants, NSAIDs, serotonin-reuptake inhibitors (SSRIs). Due to inhibition of CYP_{50} enzyme system antibiotics like metronidazole, co-rtrimoxazole, ciprofloxacin can increase bleeding with their simultaneous use with warfarin, hence avoided during the combined therapy. Amiodarone use with warfarin can also increase the chances of bleeding.

16) What is INR test and what for it is used?

Ans: INR (International normalized ratio) test in done in patients taking Vitamin K antagonists. It is used to assess the risk of bleeding or the coagulation status of the patient and to adjust the dose of Vitamin K antagonists.

17) How do you reverse the action of warfarin?

Ans: Warfarin action can be reversed by the administration of Vitamin K, that is required for the formation of coagulation factors 11 (factor 2),V11, IX, and X.

18) What are the new – generation oral anticoagulants? How do they act?

Ans: Rivaroxaban, Apixaban, edoxaban are some of the new – generation oral anticoagulants. They act by directly inhibiting factor Xa, blocking the propagation phase of the coagulation cascade preventing conversion of prothrombin to thrombin.

19) What are fibrinolytic drugs ? Mention their clinical uses.

Ans: Streptokinase, urokinase, alteplase, tenecteplase are some of the fibrinolytic drug used clinically. They dissolve intravascular clots to prevent ischemic damage followed by restoration of the blood flow through the blood vessel. They are the life – saving drugs in acute thrombotic conditions like myocardial infarction, deep vein thrombosis, pulmonary embolism, acute ischemic stroke, and acute peripheral arterial occlusion, occlusion of indwelling catheters, intracardiac thrombus formation and severe frostbite

20) Name the contraindications for the use of fibrinolytic drugs.

Ans: Fibrinolytic drugs are absolutely contraindicated in conditions like active internal bleeding from any source, history of any cerebrovascular accident, intracranial neoplasm, arteriovenous malformations or aneurysm, recent (of two months duration and less) intracranial or intraspinal surgery, past or present bleeding disorder, uncontrolled hypertension, pregnancy, elderly people particularly associated with multiple disease, previous thrombolytic therapy, and patients receiving oral anticoagulants.

21) Name some antiplatelet drugs and mention their clinical uses?

Ans: Aspirin in low doses, clopidogrel, prasugrel, ticagrelor, eptifibatide and vorapaxor are some of the antiplatelet drugs used clinically. All of them belong to different classes and prevent platelet aggregation by different mechanisms and thrombus formation.

Aspirin and clopidogrel are available as a combination preparation and given for prophylactic prevention of formation of thrombi and used for secondary prevention of MI who have had a recent ischemic episode. They are used similarly as prophylactic drugs for the secondary prevention of cerebral ischemic stroke. Apciximab, eptifibatide, are used as adjuvant to percutaneous coronary intervention (PCI) during coronary angiography and stent placement.

Chapter 9

Drugs for Respiratory Disorders

1) Name some sympathomimetic drugs used in the treatment of bronchial asthma. How do they act?

Ans: Salbutamol, terbutaline, salmeterol, metaproterenol, pirbuterol and formoterol are some of the sympathomimetic drugs used to treat bronchial asthma. They act as agonists of β_2 receptors in the bronchioles and cause relaxation of the bronchial smooth muscle and relieve the symptoms of asthma.

2) Name anticholinergic agents used to treat bronchial asthma. How do they act?

Ans: Ipratropium, tiotropium are the anticholinergic drugs used in bronchial asthma. They act by blocking the M_3 receptors in the bronchial smooth muscle, relieving the bronchoconstriction followed by relaxation of the bronchial smooth musculature and thus relieving the symptoms of bronchial asthma.

3) Name the leukotriene inhibitors used in the treatment of bronchial asthma. How do they act?

Ans: Leukotriene synthesis inhibitors like zileuton; leukotriene receptor antagonists like zafirlukast, montelukast are some of the leukotriene inhibitors used in bronchial asthma. They act either by inhibiting the synthesis of leukotrienes LTB_4, LTC_4, LTD_4 and LTE_4 (Zileuton) or by blocking their receptors (Montelukast, Zafirlukast). Thus they relieve the bronchospasm produced by the leukotrienes and cause relaxation of the bronchial smooth muscle and relieve the symptoms.

4) Name the corticosteroids used in the treatment of bronchial asthma. How do they act?

Ans: Beclomethasone, budesonide, fluticasone, flunisolide, mometasone arc some of the corticosteroids used in the treatment of bronchial asthma. They act by inhibiting the airway inflammation which is responsible for bronchoconstriction. They act by suppressing many inflammatory mediators, including cytokines, chemokines and inflammatory enzymes.

5) Name the mast cell stabilizing agents used in the treatment of bronchial asthma. How do they act?

Ans: Cromolyn sodium, nedocromil are the two commonly employed mast cell stabilizing drugs used in bronchial asthma and given by inhalation. They act by stabilizing the mast cells thereby preventing the release of inflammatory mediators upon an antigen attack. Thus they relieve bronchoconstriction and cause relaxation of the bronchial smooth muscle.

6) Name the theophylline derivatives and mention their mechanism of action.

Ans: Theophylline, Etophylline, aminophylline are some of the theophylline derivatives used in the treatment of bronchial asthma. They are xanthine derivatives and cause inhibition of phosphodiesterase enzyme causing accumulation of cyclic AMP that causes relaxation of the bronchial smooth muscle. They can be given both by oral and IV routes.

7) What is omalizumab? How is it useful in bronchial asthma?

Ans: Omalizumab is a monoclonal antibody used in the treatment of bronchial asthma. It acts by blocking the IgE receptor, which is bound on the mast cells. By blocking the IgE receptors, it prevents the release of inflammatory medicators from the mast cells thus inhibiting their bronchoconstrictor activity followed by relaxation of bronchial smooth muscle.

8) How do you treat an acute case of bronchial asthma?

Ans: In acute status of asthma, immediate oxygen administration is provided to relieve the patient of symptoms of hypoxia if any present. This is followed by the administration of short – acting inhaled β_2 – agonists like salbutamol through nebulization or through metered dose inhaler with spacer. Alternatively methyl prednisolone or hydrocortisone can be given intravenously along with salbutamol if the patient is in a state of severe hypoxemia with tachypnea, breathlessness, cough and the presence of wheeze. Thereafter, anticholinergic drugs like ipratropium along with fenoterol are given by inhalation continuously for sustaining the bronchodilation and betterment of the clinical features.

9) What is COPD? How do you treat it?

Ans: COPD is chronic obstructive pulmonary disease which is characterised by chronic bronchitis and emphysema, persistent cough, and breathlessness. It is a chronic inflammatory disease of lungs with irreversible airflow obstruction commonly seen in chronic smokers. It is treated with short acting β_2 agonists like salbutamol in combination with anticholinergic drugs like ipratropium or tiotropium by inhalation in the presence of mild to moderate dyspnoea. But in cases of severe dyspnoea a combination of long-acting β_2 agonists like salmeterol and formoterol and anticholinergics are used to provide sustained relief from symptoms.

10) Name some commonly used antitussives

Ans: Codeine phosphate, noscapine, dextromethorphan, pipazethate, pholcodeine are some of the commonly used antitussives.

11) Name some commonly used mucolytic drugs

Ans: N-acetylcysteine, carbocysteine, ambroxol, bromhexine and guanfascine are some of the commonly used mucolytic drugs.

Chapter 10

Drugs for Gastrointestinal Disorders

1) What are H_2 receptor antagonists, Name some of them, how do they act?

Ans: H_2 receptor antagonists are the drugs used in the treatment of all types of acid – peptic disorders like gastric and peptic ulcers, gastroesophageal reflux disease (GERD), stress induced ulcers. They inhibit acid production by reversibly competing with histamine for binding to H_2 receptors on the basolateral membrane of parietal cells. Famotidine, Ranitidine, Nizatidine are some of the examples H_2 receptor antagonists.

2) What are Proton Pump inhibitors, name them, how do they act?

Ans: Proton Pump inhibitors are the drugs used in the treatment of peptic ulcer disease, gastroesophageal reflux disease, reduction of risk of upper GI bleeding in critically ill patients with high – risk ulcers, and NSAID – associated gastric and duodenal ulcers and H. Pyloric infection. Omeprazole, Lansoprazole, Pantoprazole, Rabeprazole, and Esomeprazole are few examples of Proton Pump inhibitors.

They act by binding to H+/K+ATPase **(Proton pump)** which is the final common pathway of H^+ secretion and formation of HCl thereby inhibiting the synthesis and release of the acid into the gastric lumen.

3) Name some commonly used antacids and their indications?

Ans: Aluminum hydroxide, Magnesium hydroxide, Magnesium trisilicate and Calcium carbonate are some of the commonly used antacid preparations.

They are used for the symptomatic relief of symptoms of gastritis that include heartburn, epigastric distress, dyspepsia, nausea and abdominal discomfort within few minutes of oral administration. They can also control the symptoms of GERD initially.

4) Name the prostaglandin analogue used in the treatment of gastric disorders and how does it act?

Ans: Misoprostol, a derivative of prostaglandian E_1 is used for the prevention of NSAID or aspirin induced peptic ulcers. It acts as an agonist at the PGE_1 receptors and inhibits basal and stimulated gastric acid secretion mediated by PGE_1.

5) Name some colloidal Bismuth Compounds and their indications

Ans: Bismuth subsalicylate, Bismuth subcitrate, Bismuth subnitrate, and tripotassium dicitrate – bismuthate are some of the bismuth compounds used in the treatment of dyspepsia and acute diarrhea.

6) How do you treat H. Pylori infection?

Ans: For eradication of H. Pylori infection, triple therapy is commonly given in which one proton pump inhibitor and two antibiotics are added. The usual combination consists of omeprazole or any other proton pump inhibitor and clarithromycin and amoxacillin. The other antibiotic that can be used in combination is metronidazole. The duration of therapy is for a period of 10 to 14 days.

7) Name the 5 – HT_3 receptor antagonists used as antiemetic drugs, and mention their clinical uses

Ans: Ondansetron, granisetron, tropisetron and dolasetron are some of the 5– HT_3 receptor antagonists used as antiemetic drugs.

They are used to control nausea and vomiting associated with cancer chemotherapy, radiation therapy and surgery(for the post operative nausea and vomiting).

8) Name the Dopamine receptor antagonists used as antiemetic drugs. Mention their clinical uses

Ans: Metoclopramide and domperidone, droperidol, chlorpromazines are some of the dopamine receptor antagonists used as antiemetic drugs.

They are used as antiemetic and prokinetic drugs in the management of gut motility disorders, GERD and in conditions like dyspepsia, for control of nausea and vomiting of central and local origin, nausea and vomiting associated with chemotherapy and radiation therapy, acute attacks of migraine and in post surgical period.

9) Name the osmotic purgatives, how do they act?

Ans: Magnesium hydroxide, magnesium sulphate, sodium phosphate, and sodium – potassium tartarate are some of the commonly used osmotic or saline purgatives.

They are poorly absorbed and retained in the intestine and increase the water content and bulk of the fecal mass exerting osmotic action, facilitating easy evacuation due to increased peristaltic activity.

10) Name the commonly used purgatives to treat constipation

Ans: Vegetable fibers like Plantago, ispaghula husk, polycarbophil, lactulose, lactitol, methylcellulose bisacodyl and agar-agar are some of the commonly used drugs to treat constipation working by different mechanisms.

11) Name the therapeutic indications of purgatives and laxatives

Ans: They are used before surgery on large bowel and rectum for evacuation of bowels, for radiographic examinations like sigmoidoscopy, colonoscopy of the large gut, as adjuvant therapy for hemorrhoids and anal fissures to facilitate softening of the stool thereby preventing hemorrhage, to releive constipation induced by drugs like opioids, diabetic gastroparesis, habitual constipation is elderly populations, in helminthic infestations, and before parturition and abdominal surgery.

12) Name some commonly used antidiarrheal drugs

Ans: Opioid agonists like loperamide, diphenoxylate, bismuth salts, kaolin, and pectin are the commonly used antidiarrheal drugs for treating nonspecific diarrhea, and traveler's diarrhea due to food poisoning

13) What drugs are used to treat diarrhea due to suspected bacterial infections?

Ans: Campylobacter jejuni, salmonella, Shigella, E – coli, entamoeba histolytica, giardiasis, clostridium difficile are likely to cause diarrhoea of bacterial origin. The antibiotics that can be used in such condition include fluoroquinolones, metronidazole, tetracyclines and orally administered neomycin.

Chapter 11

Drugs for Lipid Disorders, IV Fluid Therapy, and Immunology

1) What are statins? Name some of them, what for they are used?

Ans: Statins are HMG – COA reductase inhibitors which inhibit the HMG – COA reductase enzyme preventing the conversion of HMG – COA to mevalonic acid and its further conversion to cholesterol in the hepatic cells thereby lowering LDL – C levels. Atorvastatin, lovastatin, pravastatin and rosuvastatin are few examples of HMG – COA reductase inhibitors.

They are used to decrease the plasma LDL levels and to prevent cardiovascular events in patients with cardiac risk factors. They are useful for primary prevention to prevent a possible MI, stroke, revascularization procedures and angina. They are also useful in secondary prevention of coronary heart disease to reduce the risk of fatal MI and stroke, and hospitalizations for congestive heart failure and angina.

2) What are the guidelines to treat hypercholesterolemia?

Ans: Hypercholesterolemia can be treated or managed with a healthy lifestyle, an optimum body weight, abstinence from smoking, and a diet low in saturated and trans–fatty acids and enriched in fiber, fruit, and vegetables and fatty fish for non – vegetarians or omega – 3 contained dried fruits for vegetarians. The class of drugs that can be used to decrease LDL – C levels by 22-50% include statins. The next group of drugs that can be used include **Ezetimibe**, which decrease absorption of cholesterol, and to further decrease LDL – C levels, that arc particularly needed in patients with atherosclerotic cardiovascular disease. Nicotinic acid(Niacin) is used in combined hyperlipidemia and is the most effective drug to increase HDL- cholesterol and combined with statins to have a better reduction of LDL-C and elevation of HDL-C. A new class of drugs PCSK-9 inhibitors namely monoclonal antibodies like evolocumab, alirocumab and evinocumab may lower LDL – C levels up to 60% in combination with statins.

3) What are the adverse effects of statins?

Ans: Statins are likely to cause myopathy due to increased creatinine kinase activity

4) What are the indications for Dextrose 5% solution?

Ans: Dextrose 5% solution is used to treat hypoglycemia in condition of insulin shock. It is also used in dehydration and to provide blood glucose balance during perioperative and postoperative periods. It is combined with 0.9% NaCl and used in starvation, dehydration, and all phases of surgical procedures to provide electrolyte and glucose requirements; heat – related disorders; fresh – water drowning and peritonitis.

5) What are plasma expanders? Name some of them and their clinical uses

Ans: Plasma expanders are colloid solutions and exert colloidal pressure, do not pass through membranes and remain in the intravascular compartment and attract extravascular fluid into the circulation thereby increasing plasma volume.

Human albumin, Dextran, degraded gelatine polymer, hydroxyethyl starch and polyvinyl pyrrolidone are the commonly used plasma expanders. They are used in conditions where blood or plasma has been lost or has moved to extra vascular compartments as seen in burns, hypovolemic shock, severe trauma, endotoxin shock, and extensive tissue damage.

6) What are the various methods of IV administration?

Ans: IV fluids can be given as bolus or a single dose at a time, as intermittent administration or as continuous infusion through a peripheral IV line placed in a peripheral vein. They can also be given through a peripherally inserted central catheter (Central venous catheter), with its tip terminating in the superior vena cava. This provides IV access that can used for a prolonged period of time in conditions of chemotherapy regimen, extended antibiotic use, for the administration of pain relief medication or for total parenteral nutrition. The catheter may also be placed into a vein in the neck, chest, or groin and passed through a central vein, most commonly the internal jugular, subclavian, or femoral until the tip of the catheter resides within the superior vena cava, inferior vena cava, or right atrium.

7) Name some immunosuppressive drugs and their uses

Ans: Cyclosporin, tacrolimus, sirolimus, cyclophosphamide, azathioprine, methyl prednisolone and dexamethasone are some of the commonly used immunosuppressive drugs. They are used clinically in solid organ transplantation for the prevention of organ rejection of allograft kidney, liver, and heart transplantations and also for prophylaxis of post – transplant organ rejection.

8) What are the vaccines given for a child at birth?

Ans: The vaccines given for a child at birth include BCG vaccination, Hepatitis B vaccine, and oral polio vaccine.

9) What is pentavalent vaccine and when is it given for a child?

Ans: Pentavalent vaccine in the vaccine given to a child to protect against diphtheria, pertussis, tetanus, Hib, and Hepatitis B infections. It is given at 6, 10 and 14 weeks of childhood.

10) At what periods of paediatric life oral Polio vaccine given?

Ans: Oral polio vaccine is given at the ages of birth, 6, 10 and 14 weeks with a booster dose at 16 – 24 weeks of life.

11) When is Rotavirus vaccine given and for what for it is given?

Ans: The vaccine is given to children to protect against a possible measles, mumps and rubella (German measles) infections. It is given to children around 9 months to 15 months of age, with a second dose at 15 months to six years of age, with at least four weeks gap between the doses.

12) What is DPT vaccine and when is it given as a booster dose?

Ans: DPT vaccine gives protection against diphtheria, pertussis and tetanus. After primary vaccination given as pentavalent vaccine earlier, booster doses are given at the age of 16 – 24 months and 5 – 6 years.

13) What is pneumococcal conjugate vaccine and when is it administered?

Ans: Pneumococcal conjugate (PCV) is given to protect the children against a possible pneumococcal pneumonia and given at the ages of 6 weeks, 14 weeks and 9 months.

14) What is Hib vaccine and when is it given to the child?

Ans: Hib vaccine is given to the child to prevent any possible infection with Hemophilus influenza virus as a component of pentavalent vaccine before six months of age, the first dose being given at 4 weeks of age followed by one or two further doses with 4 weeks interval.

15) What is HPV vaccine, when is it given and what for it is given?

Ans: HPV vaccine is Human papilloma virus vaccine. It is given to girls aged between 9-11 years before they get used to sexual activity. It is given in two doses with 12 months apart between the doses. It gives protection to girls against developing genital warts and cancer of vagina, vulva, and most importantly protection against cervical cancer.

16) What are the various types of vaccines available for corona-19 infection?

Ans: The vaccines available for vaccination against corona virus-19 include Covax, covisheild, Moderna (m-RNA type), Novavax (protein subunit vaccine), PfizerrBioNTech, Oxford/AstraZeneca(Viral vector type)

Chapter 12

Treatment of Toxic Disorders and Drugs Acting on the Uterus

1) What are the general principals of emergency management of a case of poisoning?

Ans: As soon as the patient in brought to the emergency department of a suspected case of poisoning, a quick study has to be done by obtaining the information from the attendants regarding the history and sequence of events preceding the reporting of the case, which may help to identify the toxic agent and to initiate the appropriate therapy.

The first step in the management of a case of poisoning is to induce vomiting to empty the stomach of the suspected poisonous substance by lavage. This is followed by administering activated charcoal to bind the poisonous substance to prevent its absorption. If the nature of the poison is known the respective antidote is given to neutralize the effects of the poison. Supportive measures that include maintenance of vital functions like blood pressure, heart rate, respiration, body fluid balance and electrolytes are initiated at the earliest. Endotracheal intubation may be needed if the patient is unconscious and not able to breath on his own. It maintains airway and helps prevent suffocation and supply oxygen. Renal elimination of the poison is felicitated by giving osmotic diuretics like mannitol. Dialysis may also be needed for the rapid removal of the poison from the body.

2) Name some commonly used antidotes and their indications for cases of poisoning or overdose

Ans: Naltrexone is used to treat opioid overdose, flumazenil is used to antagonize benzodiazepine overdose, Atropine is used to treat organo – phosphorus poisoning, Vitamin K is used to antagonize coumarin anticoagulants, D – penicillamine is used to antagonize the copper poisoning, Dimercaprol is used in lead and arsenic poisoning, ethyl alcohol is used to antagonize the effects of methanol toxicity.

3) What is chelation? Name some chelating agents used for certain heavy metal poisoning cases

Ans: Chelation is a unique chemical reaction in which complex organic molecule (chelating agents) combines with a metal to form a complex ring structure known as chelate in which a metal atom is held or trapped by electron donors by like oxygen, nitrogen and sulfur. Dimercaprol binds lead, arsenic and mercury, Desferrioxamine binds iron, calcium EDTA binds lead, D – Penicillamine binds copper.

4) What are the uses of oxytocin?

Ans: Oxytocin is used to induce or augment labor in women whose pregnancy is continued and delayed beyond the expected period of pregnancy that is likely to lead to maternal and fetal morbidity and mortality. It is used for induction of labor for women who have preeclampsia, maternal diabetes, premature rupture of membranes, women with incomplete abortion in the 2nd trimester of pregnancy. Oxytocin is also used for the control of postpartum hemorrhage, promotion of involution of the uterus, uterine inertia and for inefficient milk ejection soon after delivery.

5) Name the prostaglandins used for medical termination of pregnancy

Ans: Dinoprostone which is a derivative of PGE_2, carboprost a derivative of $PGF_2\ \alpha$ and misoprostol, a PGE_1 derivative are the prostaglandins used for the medical termination of pregnancy in combination with mifepristone, a progesterone antagonist.

6) Name the ergot alkaloids and their uses during pregnancy

Ans: Ergonovine and methylergonovine are the ergot alkaloids used to control postpartum hemorrhage.

7) What are tocolytic drugs? Name some of them.

Ans: Tocolytic drugs are the agents which cause relaxation of the uterine smooth muscle contractions and used to delay the onset of labor during specified indications and guidelines. They are used to arrest the preterm labor which is most likely to occur during the gestation period of 20 to 37 weeks. β_2 agonists like ritodrine, terbutaline, isoxsuprine, salbutamol and calcium channel blockers like nifedipine and glyceryl trinitrate and magnesium sulphate are some of the agents used as tocolytic drugs.

Prescription Writing

A drug prescription is a written order given by a qualified medical practitioner to a pharmacist in charge of a pharmacy or drug store to compound and dispense a required medication for an individual patient. It consists of

1. **Superscription** wherein the name and address of the prescribing physician is given along with his qualifications, address, medical registration number, telephone number, e – mail address and the date of the prescription. All the details are usually present in the prescription pad.

   It also contains the name and address of the patient along with age, and gender. It further contains the provisional diagnosis or the diagnosis of the case. It also contains the symbol ℞, the abbreviation of which means "recipe or taken thou".

2. **Inscription** contains name or names of the drugs, its format (tablet, ointment, injection, powder), the strength of the drug expressed as g (gram), mg (milligram), mcg (microgram) U (units), or ml (milliliters). Usually the generic name of the drug should be mentioned.

3. **Subscription** provides information to the pharmacist about the quantity and dosage form of the drug to the dispensed.

4. **Transcription** in the prescriber's direction to the patient about amount of the drug, time and frequency of doses to be taken.

   The internationally accepted symbols for dosage forms include **stratum** (straight away);

   SOS (if necessary); **OD** (once daily); **bid** (two times a day); **tid** (three times a day); **qid** (four times a day); **qd** (every day). Usually the frequency is mentioned in hourly intervals for convenience and better understanding of the patient.

   The route of administration should be written in clear terms and abbreviations can be used such as **PO** (oral); IM (intramuscular); IV (intravenous); **SC** (subcutaneous); **IN** (intranasal); **TP** (topical); **SL** (sublingual); **IP** (intraperitoneal).

5. **Refill information** is with regard to how many times the patient is allowed to use the current prescription before it can be reviewed or modified according to the progress of the treatment. **Prescription format is the same for any specific clinical condition. One can change name and particulars of the physician or prescriber and that of the patient also. However, one has to adopt a correct procedure in order to avoid errors.**

6. **Signature** contains the signature of the physician.

   Prescription errors

   Medication error is common in general practice and in hospitals. Both errors in the act of writing (prescription errors) and prescribing faults can result in harm to the patient. The errors can occur due to the following conditions

   1) Faulty medical diagnosis due to inadequate or incomplete knowledge about the clinical condition due to poor academic knowledge of the prescribing physician. This usually occurs when a prescription is given by an unqualified person

2) Any step in the prescribing process can generate errors for example irrational, inappropriate prescribing, under prescribing, over prescribing, faulty drug selection, faulty dose selection, faulty route of administration, faulty directions for the use of the prescribed medications that include the frequency of the drug administration in the day,
3) The prescription errors also include failure to address the adverse drug reactions, drug interactions, and drug incompatibilities while prescribing the drug. Errors also can also occur when consideration of the age, gender, and the associated comorbidities of the patient are not taken into consideration.
4) Errors can take place while compounding and dispensing the drug by the pharmacist that includes calculation errors.
5) Inaccuracy in writing and poor legibility of hand writing, use of abbreviations or incomplete writing of a prescription, incomplete directions to the pharmacist often led to prescription errors.
6) Among doctors a heavy work load, stressful conditions, difficult work environment, insufficient communication within the team and not being in good physical and mental condition are among the primary causes of prescribing faults and prescription errors.
7) Inadequate communication between the doctors, nursing staff also contribute to prescription errors
8) Improper Interpretation of the hand writing in the prescription is most likely to cause a severe harm to the patient. For example faulty interpretation of the name of the drug diltiazem to diazepam can cause alarming effects in a patient.

One can give one or two prescriptions for a clinical condition as per the requirements, suitability, and convenience

1. **Prescribe drugs for a case of community acquired pneumonia**

   A)

Name of the patient : Jayaram
Age of the patient : 35 years, Male
Address : No.3, Keerthi Apts, Sainikpuri, Hyderabad

Name of the doctor : Dr. Balaram, MD
No.8, Balaji Colony, UPPAL, Hyderabad.
Registration No : ——
Date : 08/08/2018
Diagnosis : Community acquired pneumonia

℞
Tablet – Amoxacillin 500mg
Clavulanic acid 125mg

One tablet to be taken twice a day orally
Dispense 10 tablets for 5 day use

Signature of the physician

B) The same prescription format can be used and the following alternative drugs can be used for the condition.

℞x.

Tab. Azithromycin 500mg

One tablet to be taken once daily for 3 – 5 days

2. Prescribe drugs for a case of bacterial meningitis in a child aged 8 years.

a. ℞

Inj. ceftriaxone 1g IV

One dose (1g) to be given intravenously twice a day for 7 to 14 days.

b. Alternatively the following prescription can also be given

Inj. Vancomycin 250 mg IV/1mL

1mL to be given 6th hourly

Cefotaxime 500 mg/mL IV

1mL to be given 6th hourly

3. Prescribe drugs for a case of rheumatoid arthritis in a female patient aged 58 years with a associated history of acid peptic disorder

℞

Tab. Etoricoxib 60mg one tablet to be taken once daily

Tab. Rabiprazole 20mg 1 tablet to be taken orally daily in the morning

Comment

Etoricoxib is a selective COX – 2 inhibitor and better tolerated than non – selective COX inhibitors like diclofenac, indomethacin and other drugs of the category which are likely to cause moderate to severe GI distress. Hence etoricoxib is preferred as it has a long half – life of 22 hours and can be given once daily. Rabeprazole is added to cover underlying acid peptic disorder.

4. Prescribe drugs for a case of chronic progressive degenerative rheumatoid arthritis not responding to non steroidal antiinflammatory drugs

℞

Tab. Hydroxychloroquine 200mg

1 tablet to be taken once daily

Tab. Methotrexate – 7.5mg

1 tablet to be taken once weekly

Tab Folic acid 400mcg

1 tablet to be taken once daily

Comment

Hydroxychloroquine is a better tolerated drug than the ones in other categories. It is a disease modifying drug used in chronic rheumatoid arthritis. Methotrexate, a folic acid antagonist and has mild adverse effects in low doses and can be used safely for 2 to 3 weeks. Folic acid is added to supplement folate deficiency that is likely to occur with methotrexate.

5. Prescribe drugs for a case of multidrug resistant tuberculosis

℞

Tab. Moxifloxacin 400mg

1 tablet taken once daily

Tab. Linezolid – 600mg

1 tablet to taken once daily

Tab. Bedaquiline 400mg

1 tablet to be taken once a day for 2 weeks and then

Inj Amikacin 300mg IM

One injection to be given IM once daily

All the drugs to be taken for a period of 6 to 9 months.

Comment

Multidrug – Resistant tuberculosis is a condition in which the microbe (TB bacillus) is extremely resistant to at least two of the most powerful first – line anti – TB drugs – namely INH and rifampicin. It should be treated aggressively. The injectables (Amikacin usually as it is less toxic than the other aminoglycosides) and fluoroquinolones are usually given in this condition. Moxifloxacin in the fluoroquinolone selected. Linezolid is the most effective drug used to treat extremely drug resistant tuberculosis. Bedaquiline or Delamanid is the most preferred drug in the combination along with linezolid as it achieves high intracellular concentrations.

6. Prescribe drugs for a case of an acute case of falciparum malaria

A)

℞

Tab. Chloroquine phosphate 600mg given as a loading dose, followed by 300mg at 6, 24, 48 hours.

B)

℞

Tab. Artemisinin 1.5g given on the first day followed by 0.75g/day for the next 6 days

7. Prescribe drugs for a case of multidrug – resistant falciparum malaria and also useful for the treatment and prophylaxis of the condition

℞

Tab. Atovaquone – 250mg

+

Tab. Proguanil – 100mg

4 tablets are given as a single daily dose on 3 consecutive days for multidrug – resistant malaria. One tablet is given daily starting two days before travelling to a malarial area and continued till 7 days after leaving if for prophylactic use.

8. Prescribe drugs for a case HIV infection

℞

Tab. Zidovudine 300mg

1 tablet given twice daily

Tab. Abacavir 300mg

1 tablet given twice daily

Tab. Lamivudine 150mg

1 tablet given twice daily

The treatment should be continued indefinitely in order to arrest progression of HIV to a full blown AIDS.

Comment

The drugs used to treat HIV infection include two or more drugs from one or more drug class (nucleoside reverse transcriptase inhibitors, nucleotide reverse transcriptase inhibitors, protease inhibitors)

The aim for the combination of drugs is to provide more safety, greater durability, decreased risk of drug resistance, improved pharmacokinetics, and longer duration of action. Now with the newer developments just two drugs are given once daily or twice daily unlike earlier use of 3 drugs or more per day. The other drugs that could be prescribed include elvitegravir (600 mg), tenofovir(300mg), cobicistat(150mg), disoproxil(300mg) and others.

Some newer drugs given once or twice daily include

1. Emtricitabine 200mg+ Tenofovir 25mg
2. Ziagen 600mg+ Empivir 300 mg
3. Lopinavir 200 mg+ Norvir 50 mg twice daily
4. Retovir 300 mg+ Repivir 150 mg twice daily

9. Prescribe drugs for a case of gastroesophageal reflux disease

℞

Tab. Pantoprazole 40mg

Tab. Domperidone 10mg

One tablet each to be taken on empty stomach for a period of 14 days

10. Prescribe drugs for a case of chemotherapy induced nausea and vomiting

℞

Tab. Ondansetron 8mg

1 tablet taken orally twice a daily, with the first dose administered 30 minutes before the start of chemotherapy and the subsequent dose 8 hours later; then 8mg twice daily for 1 to 2 days

Inj. Dexamethasone 10mg IV

One dose before and two doses later to chemotherapy given along with ondansetron

11. Prescribe drugs for a case of type – 2 diabetes mellitus in adult patient aged 62 years

℞

Tab. Glipizide 5mg

+

Tab. Metformin 500mg

1 tablet each to be taken orally twice a daily.

12. Prescribe drugs for a case of type – 2 diabetes in an adult patient aged 65 years who is obese and overweight

℞

Tab. Semaglutide 7mg

1 tablet taken once daily

Comment

Semaglutide is a GLP – 1 (glucagon – like peptide 1) analog used to treat type – 2 diabetes in obese and overweight individuals as it causes weight loss in addition to its antidiabetic action. It decreases $HbA1_c$levels quickly, does increase risk of vascular events and may reduce all-cause mortality and has a high safety profile. Semaglutide can be used as monotherapy in addition to other requirements for the control of overweight and diabetes (diet and exercise). It can also be given in dose range of 0.5 to 2 mg **once weekly IM**. Usually it is stated on a dose of 3 mg per day given orally and gradually increased to 7 mg/day and later to 14 mg/day. It is the most preferred drug to control diabetes and obesity associated diabetes.

13. Prescribe drugs for a case of osteoporosis in a post menopausal woman

℞

Tab. Alendronate 10mg

1 tablet to be taken once daily in an upright posture to avoid esophageal regurgitation and a possible other esophageal complications

Tab. Cholecalciferol 1000u

1 tablet taken orally per day

Tab. Calcium carbonate 1g

1 tablet to be taken once daily

14. Prescribe drugs for a case of primary hypertension in a person aged 65 years with early manifestations of congestive heart failure

℞

Tab. Amlodipine 5mg

1 tablet to be taken once daily

Tab. Torsemide 5mg

1 tablet to be taken per day in the morning

Comment

In this case amlodipine can be replaced with ACE inhibitor lisinopril to be taken in 10mg daily doses and continuing torsemide in the same dose.

15. Prescribe drugs for a case of chronic resistant hypertension associated with left ventricular failure in a person aged 65 years.

℞

Tab. Telmisartan 40mg

1 tablet to be taken once daily

Tab. Amlodipine 5mg

1 tablet to be taken once daily

Tab. Eplerenone 25mg

1 tablet to be taken once daily

Comment

In chronic resistant hypertension associated with left ventricular failure a combination of 3 drugs is given each of which belongs to different category to effectively control the blood pressure and also to prevent further progression of heart failure. Here AT1 receptor blocker (telmisartan), amlodipine (calcium channel blocker) and eplerenone, an aldosterone antagonist have synergistic action to effectively control hypertension.

16. Prescribe drugs for a case of Parkinsonism in a geriatric patient aged 70 years

℞

Tab. Levodopa 100mg + Tab. Carbidopa 25mg (combination preparation)

1 tablet to be taken 3 times a day 30 to 60 minutes before meals and the dose to be increased with a frequency of 4 times a day over a period.

17. Prescribe drugs for a case of depression in a patient diagnosed with personality disorder

℞

Tab. Fluoxetine – 20mg

1 tablet to be taken once daily

Comment

Fluoxetine can be replaced with or substituted with sertraline given in a daily dose of 100mg

18. Prescribe drugs for a case of hypotension due to septic shock

℞

Inj. Noradrenaline 4mg/50ml for IV infusion.

8 mcg/minute till the blood pressure increases adequately, then 2 – 4 mcg/minute as maintenance dose given as continuous infusion with 5% dextrose solution.

19. Prescribe drugs for a case of atrial fibrillation due to rheumatic valvular disease

℞

Tab. Diltiazem 120mg (Sustained release/modified release)

1 tablet to be taken once daily

Tab. Apixaban 5mg

1 tablet to be given twice daily

Comment

Diltiazem is a calcium channel blocker and is the most preferred drug for the rate control in a trial fibrillation. However, it can be substituted with metoprolol 50mg given twice daily. Apixaban is an oral anticoagulant and acts by inhibiting factor Xa. It is given to prevent any possible intravascular coagulation and to prevent the development of stroke or MI or peripheral thromboembolism.

20. Prescribe drugs for a case of chronic bronchial asthma in an adult with acute exacerbations

℞

Iratropium inhalation 500mcg (metered dose)given as a nebulizer repeated 3 to 4 times a day or 20 mcg/puff, two puffs to be taken at a time repeated 2or 3 times a day

Or

Salmeterol (powder) 50mcg taken by inhalation, twice daily.

21. Prescribe drugs for a case of cardiogenic shock

℞

Inj. Dobutamine 2.0 mcg/Kg/min to be increased to 5mcg/Kg/min

Given as IV infusion

Inj. Frusemide 40-80 mg given as IV

Comment: Dobutamine is a preferred drug to improve the cardiac function in this case because of its ionotropic action with minimal chronotropic effect. It has predominant action on cardiac β_1 receptors though it is a dopaminergic drug and has no action on α_1 receptors which is in contrast to dopamine which has action on both the types of receptors which explains tachycardia and rise of blood pressure produced by it.

22. Prescribe drugs for a case of Acne vulgaris

℞

Benzoyl peroxide 5%+ erythromycin 3% cream

Small quantities to be applied over the affected areas

Cap. Minocycline 100 mg

1 capsule to be taken orally along with the cream for considerable periods.

Comment

Acne velgaris can be treated with a wide variety of drugs that include topical retinoids like retinol, tretinoin, isotretinoin, acetretin, and adapalene which is the most effective topical retinoid. It can also be treated with topical antibiotics like clindamycin, erythromycin, metronidazole, and azelaic acid. The systemic antibiotics that could be effective include doxycycline and minocycline. Hence any of the individual or combination drugs (systemic and topical agents) could be used to have effective cure rates though recurrence rate is high.

23. Prescribe drugs for a case of scabies

℞

A) Permethrin 5% cream for topical use

Small quantities to be applied over the affected areas

B) Gamma benzene hexachloride 1% cream for topical use

Small quantities to be applied over the affected areas

C) Tab. Ivermectin 1.5g PO

1 tablet to be taken orally as a single dose

24. Prescribe drugs for a case of primary dysmenorrhea in a young adult woman

℞

Tab. Meclofenamic acid 50 mg

1 tablet to be taken orally 3 times a day for a period not exceeding 6 days.

Comment:

Primary dysmenorrhea that occurs in women of menstrual age is manifested as recurrent, crampy, lower abdominal pain that occurs during monthly periods. The drugs most effective to treat the condition include fenamates like meclofenamic acid, bromphenamic acid, flufenamic acid, and tolfenamic acid. They are most effective than other agents (propionic acid derivatives and aspirin) because they not only inhibit prostaglandin synthesis but also inhibit their action on the uterine smooth muscle thus causing immediate relief from symptoms.

25. Prescribe drugs for a case of preeclampsia in a woman gravid 2 and para1 and with a BP reading of 160 /90 mmHg and history of recurrent seizures

℞

Inj. Labetalol 10 mg/mL IV

1 mL to be given as IV push with repeat bolus every 10 min until systolic BP comes to normal range.

Inj. Magnesium sulfate 4g/mL

1 mL to be given by infusion pump over 5-10 minutes followed by an infusion of 1g/hour maintained for 24 hours till seizures last.

Comment: While treating preeclampsia or eclampsia the first step would be to control the elevated blood pressure for which a good number of drugs are available such as **labetalol, hydralazine** (5-10 mg given IV slowly over 2 minutes followed by similar dose 20 minutes later), **nifedipine** (10 mg immediate release preparation given orally, repeated 30 minutes with similar dose or sustained release preparation 30 mg/ day), **methyldopa** (250 mg given orally 3 times a day or 250-500 mg given IV over a period of 30-60 minutes). For controlling seizures in preeclampsia magnesium sulfate is the only agent to be effective.

Critical Evaluation of a Prescription

Evaluation of prescription is a necessary process of evaluating and auditing the appropriateness of drug usage, discovering existing errors and formulating solutions and rewrite the correct prescription in correct order. It comprises to check the format namely, if all the contents of the format like superscription, inscription, subscription, transcription, signature and refill information are included or not. It also emphases the mention of correct diagnosis and appropriateness of the drugs prescribed according to the diagnosis. It is also essential to check for inclusion of unnecessary, irrational and harmful drugs and also for any irrational combination of drugs. It is very essential to check the doses prescribed and make corrections if necessary, to check the route and frequency of the drug administration and to make suitable modifications if necessary. It is also essential to be able to decipher or understand the prescribers' hand writing which should be legible to avoid misreading and misinterpreting it and to avoid any prescription error. It is very essential to make a note of any possible drug – drug interaction in the prescribed drugs. Usually generic names of the drugs are to be mentioned with few exceptions here and there where brand names also could also be made.

1. **Critically analyze and rewrite the following prescription given for a patient of atrial fibrillation who is also associated with tuberculosis and receives one of the drugs in the combination therapy and with associated sleep disturbances.**

℞

Tab. Warfarin 1.5mg

Cap. Rifampicin 300mg

Tab. Phenobarbitone 100mg

1 tablet to be given once a day

Critical evaluation of the prescription

Here the usual subscription in the prescription not given. In the inscription the dose of warfarin (vitamin K antagonist) is low. Rifampicin and phenobarbitone induce hepatic microsomal enzymes and enhance the metabolism of warfarin and a reduction of its action. In the presence of a lower dose of warfarin and the use of rifampicin and phenobarbitone, the dose of warfarin is ineffective and INR is lowered with a chance of clot formation. Hence the dose of the warfarin is to be increased to 2.5 to 3.5mg/day and alternative drugs for tuberculosis and sedation should be given. Warfarin is a drug of narrow margin of safety and can produce a number of drug interactions. It can be replaced with newer anticoagulants like Apixaban, Edoxaban which are direct factor X_a inhibitors

The correct prescription

Name of the patient: RajaRam
Age of the patient : 38 years, Male
Address : No.4, Lalith Apts, Sainikpuri, Hyderabad - 500094

Name of the doctor: Dr. Vijaya Gopal, MD
No.46, Balaji Colony,
Hyderabad - 500094.
Registration No : ——
Date : 10/10/2018
Diagnosis : Atrial fibrillation

℞
Tab. Warfarin 3.5mg
1 tablet to taken per day
Tab. INH 300mg
1 tablet to be taken per day along with other anti – TB drugs
Tab. Alprazolam 0.5mg/ 1 tablet to be taken at bedtime.

Signature of the physician

2. **Critically analyze and rewrite the following prescription of a male person aged 50 years and weighing 60kg and reported for peritonitis. He has an underlying renal dysfunction with creatinine clearance of 40ml/min.**

Tab. Gentamicin 100mg PO

1 tablet to be taken 3 times a day for 7 days

Critical evaluation of the prescription

Here the usual subscription in the prescription not given. In the inscription route of administration of gentamicin is given as oral. Gentamicin is always given IM/IV route only. The normal initial parenteral dose of gentamicin is 300mg. The frequency of dosing and timing of gentamicin depends on patient's renal function. In this case as the creatinine clearance is 40ml/min and as the patient has underlying renal impairment, the dose of gentamicin would be 180 mg every 48 hours A third generation cephalosporin can also be added to have an extended coverage of microorganisms..

The correct prescription

Inj. Gentamicin 300mg/5mL vial

3mL is given IV/every 48 hours

Inj. Cefotaxime 2g/mL

1mL to be given every 6 hours

3. **Critically analyze and rewrite the following prescription for a patient aged 53 years diagnosed with partial seizure for the past 2 years.**

℞

Tab. Ethosuximide 250mg

1 tablet to be taken once daily

Tab. Clonazepam 10mg

1 tablet to be taken once daily

Critical evaluation of the prescription

Apart from filling all the features of an ideal prescription, the following corrections need to be made.

Ethosuximide is used in absence seizures only, hence it is not given in this case and its usual dose is 500mg/day when given for the absence seizures and infantile spasms and not recommended for partial seizures. The dose of clonazepam is 0.5 – 1.0mg/day when it is used for the absence seizures.

The correct prescription

℞

Tab. Carbamazepine 400mg

1 tablet to be taken 2 times a day

Tab. Gabapentine 300mg

1 tablet to be taken twice daily

4. **Critically analyze and rewrite the following prescription for a patient aged 48 years diagnosed with hypertension with a BP reading of 190/100 Hg and associated rheumatoid arthritis.**

℞

Tab. Ramipril 1mg

1 tablet to be taken once daily

Tab. Ibuprofen 400mg

1 tablet to be taken 3 time a day

Critical evaluation of the prescription

Apart from filling all the feature of an ideal prescription, the following corrections need to be made.

Ramipril(ACE inhibitor) dose is low and need to be increased to 10mg/day. When it is used with NSAIDS (Ibuprofen) there would be a reduction of its blood pressure lowering effect. The mechanism is via a reduction in glomerular filtration through a reduction of local prostaglandin E2 synthesis with corresponding reactive secretion of renin. NSAIDs can also cause a reduction of the effects of diuretics and β- blockers acting through different mechanisms. While treating the patients of rheumatoid arthritis with associated hypertension, better approaches could be made to relieve the arthritic pain by giving paracetamol, tramdol and topical analgesics

The correct prescription.

℞

Tab. Ramipril 10mg

1 tablet to be taken orally once daily

Tab Paracetamol 500 mg twice a day

Ibuprofen topical gel (10% w/v) to be applied as per the need

5. Critically analyze and rewrite the following prescription for a person of known alcoholic addiction suffering from amoebic dysentery

℞

Tab. Metronidazole 200 mg

1 tablet to be given twice daily for 10 days

Tab. Ciprofloxacin 500 mg

1 tablet to taken twice daily for 10 days

Critical evaluation of the prescription

The drugs used for amoebic dysentery include metronidazole and others like tinidazole, ornidazole, and tetracyclines. Ciprofloxacin has no action against Entamoeba histolytica. In the prescription the dose of metronidazole is low and it should be increased to 400 mg 3 times a day. Metronidazole causes disulfiram-like action and causes nausea and vomiting if given to an alcoholic person. Ornidazole can be given instead of metronidazole. If necessary a tetracycline can be added.

The correct prescription

℞

Tab. Ornidazole 500 mg

1 tablet to taken twice daily for 5 days

Cap. Doxycycline 100 mg

1 capsule to be given twice a day for 5 days

6. Critically analyze the following prescription for a case of typhoid fever

℞

Cap. Chloramphenicol 1g

One capsule to be taken 6th hourly for a period of 7 days

Inj. Cefoxitin 1g IM/2mL ampoule

2 mL to be given every 6 hours for a period of 7 days

Critical evaluation of the prescription

Chloramphenicol was once the drug of choice to treat typhoid fever. But its use was discontinued because of adverse effects like bone marrow suppression leading to anemia, leucopenia, thrombocytopenia, and to pancytopenia. More over many species of salmonella species developed resistance to chloramphenicol. It has been replaced with ceftriaxone, a third generation cephalosporin. The other drugs that could be effective include azithromycin, carbapenems(Imipenem, meropenem, doripenem), tigicycline (tetracycline). Earlier trimethoprim, ampicillin were also effective. Cefoxitin is a second generation cephalosporin mostly used for anaerobic infections but not effective in typhoid fever.

The correct prescription

℞

Inj. Ceftriaxone 1g IV/mL

1 mL to be given IV two times a day for 5 days

List of Spotters

1) Receptor families
2) Drug antagonism (Interaction between agonists and antagonists)
3) Time concentration curve
4) Blood pressure changes of sympathomimetic drugs
5) Tachyphylaxis
6) AUC and AUC segment (Linear plot of plasma concentration and time of drugs)
7) Routes of drug administration
8) Vasomotor reversal (Dale's vasomotor reversal)
9) Motor end plate –Site of action of skeletal muscle relaxants
10) Metered dose inhaler
11) Osteoporosis
12) Transdermal patch
13) Straub's test-Action of Morphine on mice tail
14) SGLT-2 inhibitors
15) Cardiac action potential
16) Bacteria- structure
17) Iron deficiency anaemia
18) Megaloblastic anaemia
19) Foxglove plant- Source of digitalis
20) Tenia unguam- Fungal infection of nails
21) Myasthenia gravis
22) Gingival hyperplasia
23) Exophthalmus (Grave's disease)
24) Atherosclerosis
25) Leprosy
26) Acromegaly
27) Scabies

Identification of the Spotters

1)

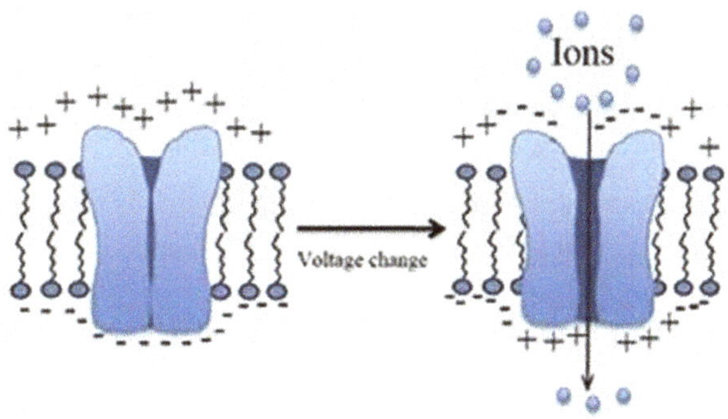

a) Identify the channel shown in the diagram
b) What changes take place through the transit of ions in the channel?
c) Name the drugs that act through the channel

2)

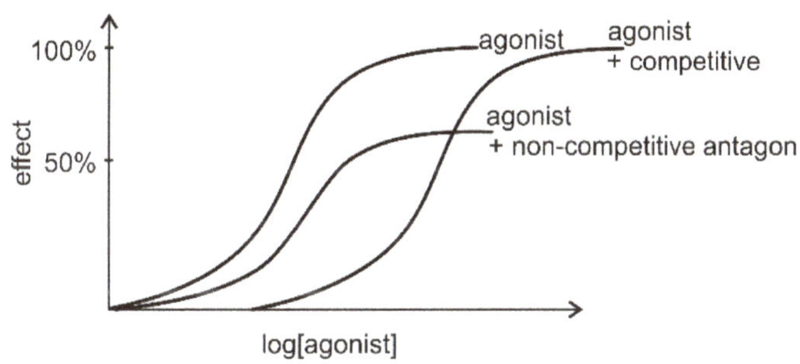

a) Identify the interaction between the drugs shown in the graph and how does it operate?
b) Mention two examples of interaction between drugs as per the above shown mechanism

3)

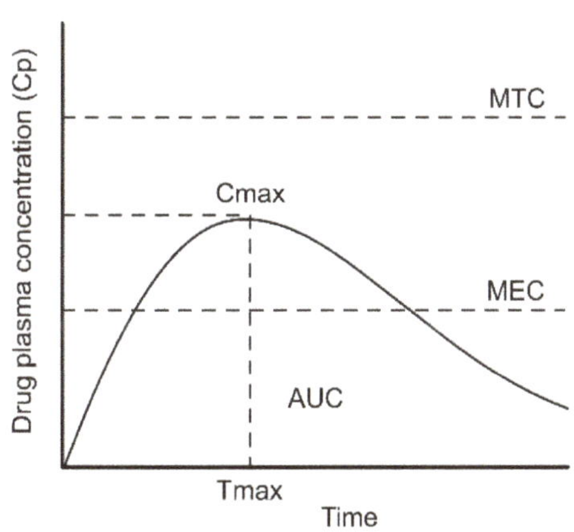

a) Identify the graph shown above and what does it explain?
b) What do Cmax, MTC, MEC mean?

4)

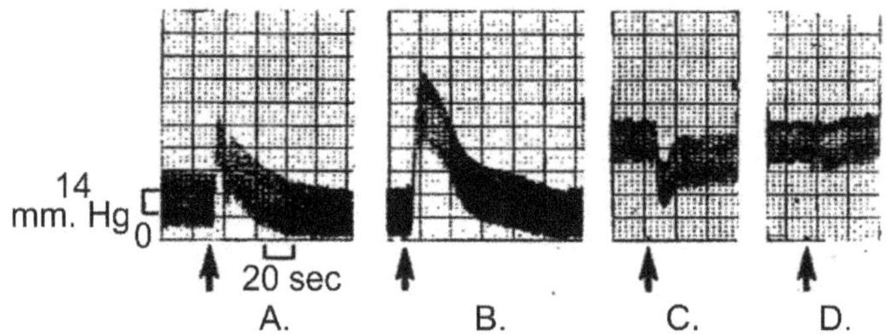

a) Identify the responses of drugs A, B, C, D shown above shown graph
b) Name the drugs that affect the changes in the respective graphs

5)

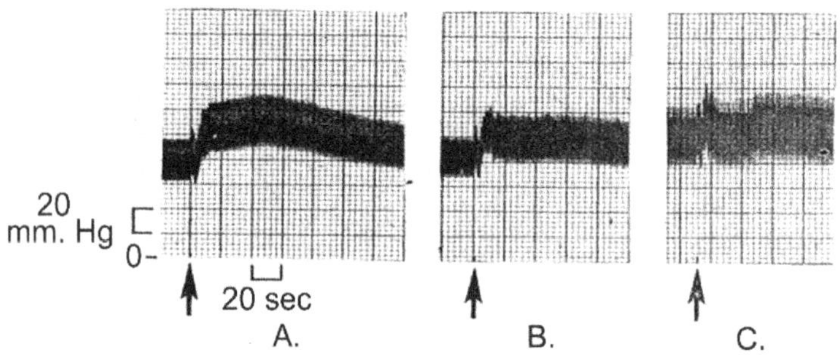

a) Identify the responses shown in the graph in an experimental presentation and explain the mechanism for the effect
b) Mention two drugs which can cause the effect

6)

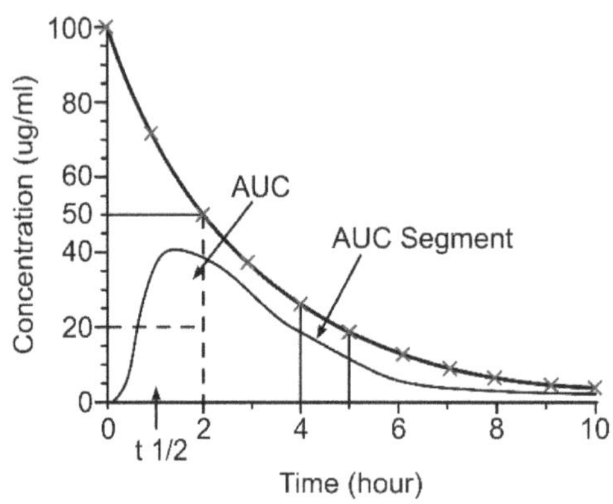

a) Identify the graph shown above and what does it indicate?
b) What is AUC, and AUC segment?
c) What is t1/2?
d) What are the uses of AUC?

7)

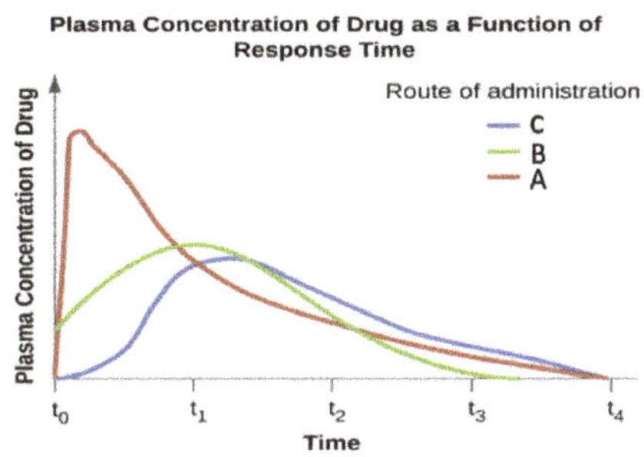

a) Identify the likely routes of administration of drugs based on the responses /effects produced by them
b) What are the limitations of a drug given by route C?

8)

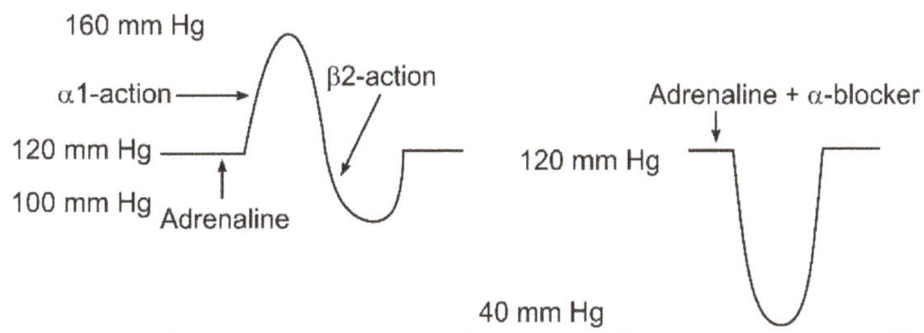

Effect of adrenaline on BP **Vasomotor reversal of Dale**

a) Identify the responses shown by the drugs in the graph
b) Explain the mechanism for the responses

9)

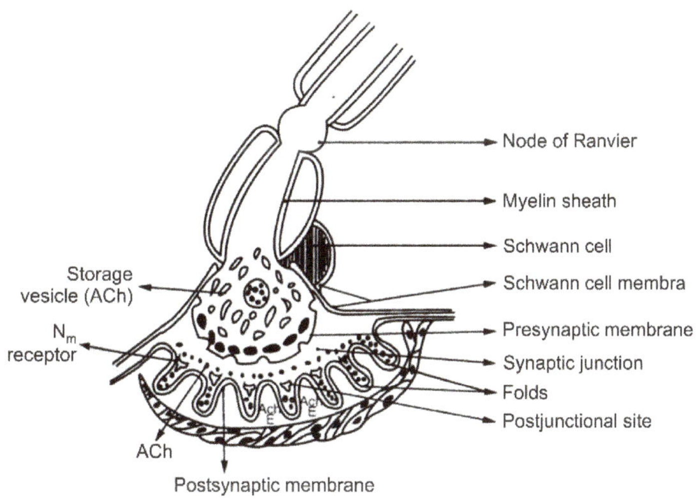

a) Identify the figure shown above
b) Explain the mechanisms of action of two different groups acting at the site

10)

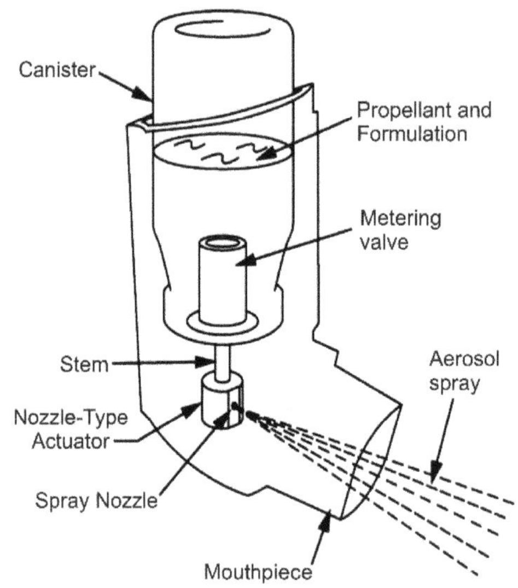

a) Identify the drug delivery system shown above
b) Name the clinical conditions where it can be used
c) Name the drugs that could be delivered through the system

11)

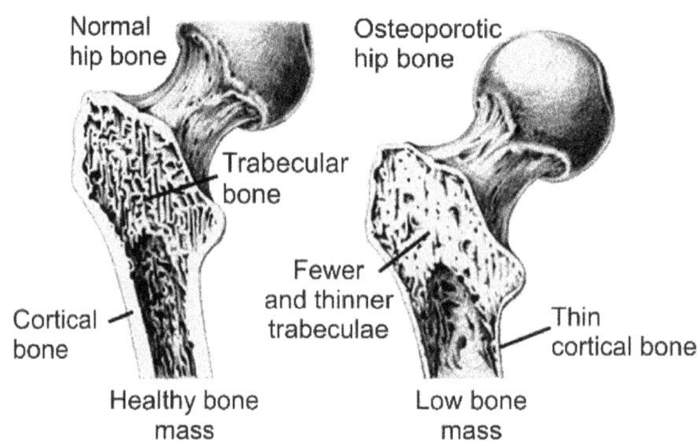

a) Mention the features shown in the bones as presented above
b) Name the drugs used to treat the condition

12)

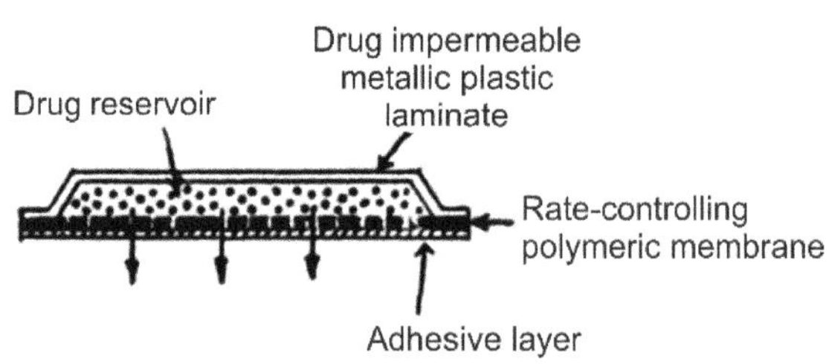

a) Identify the drug delivery system shown in the picture
b) Name the drugs and clinical conditions in which it could be used
c) What are the advantages of this type of drug delivery system

13)

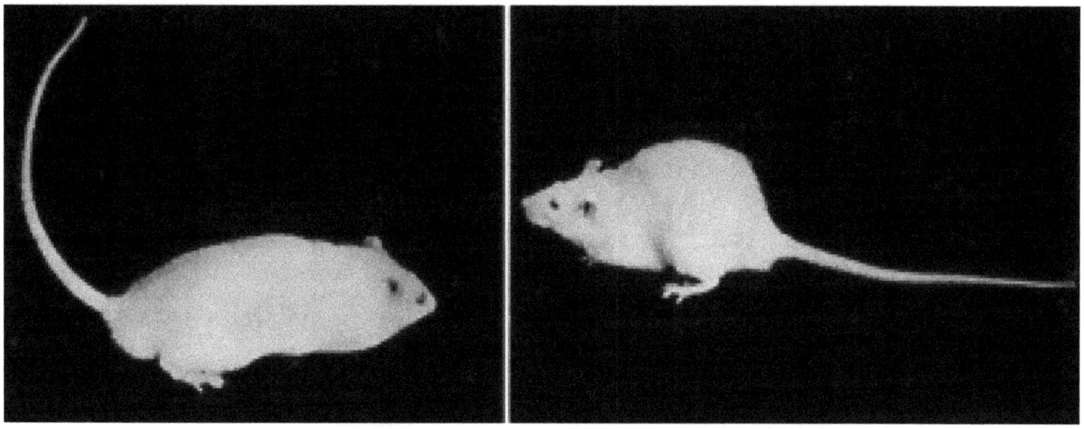

a) Identify the drug responses seen in the mice tail shown in the picture
b) How do you explain the mechanism of action for the same?

14)

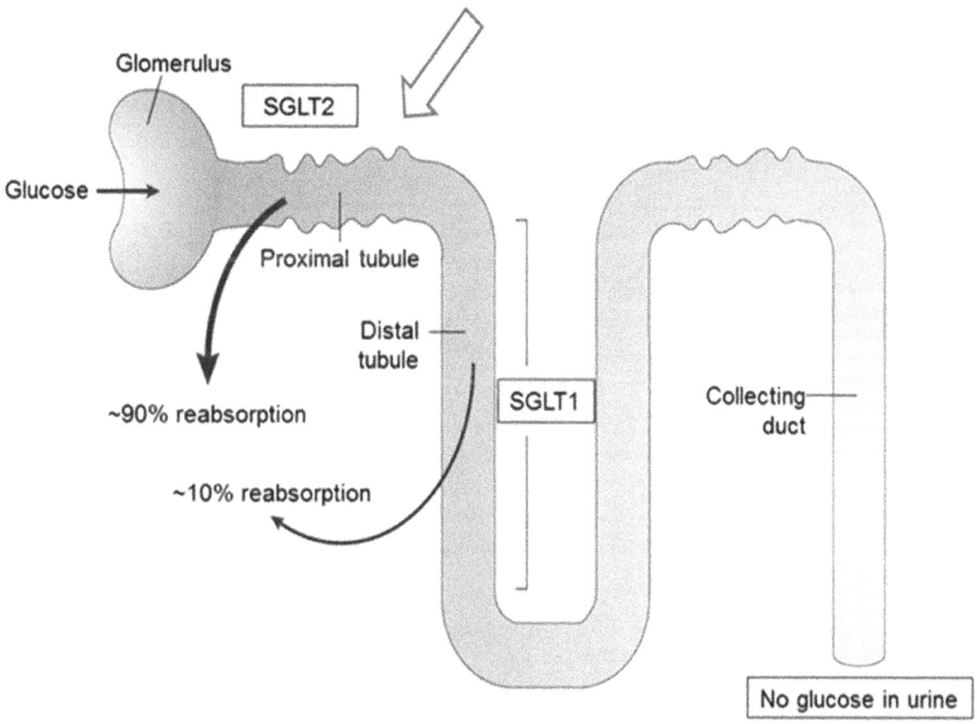

c) Mention the drugs that act at the site (SGLT-2)
d) Name the clinical conditions where they can be used

15)

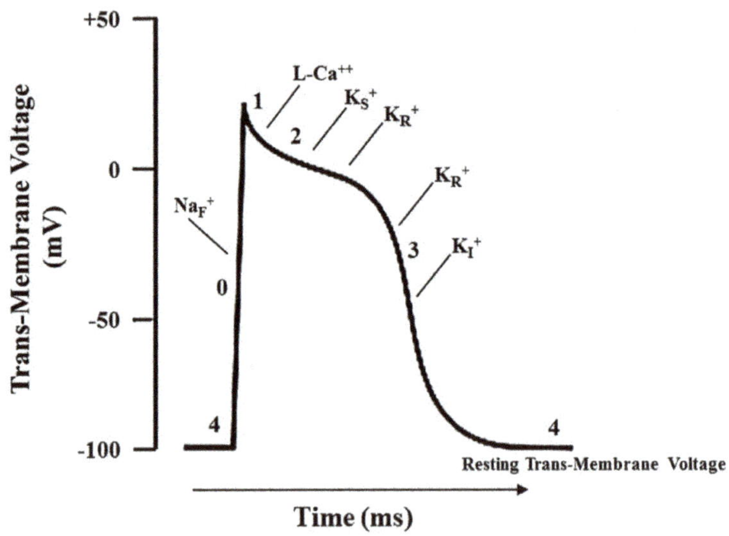

a) Identify the graph shown above
b) What 1,2,3 and 4 stand for in the graph ?
c) Name two drugs which act at site/location 1

16)

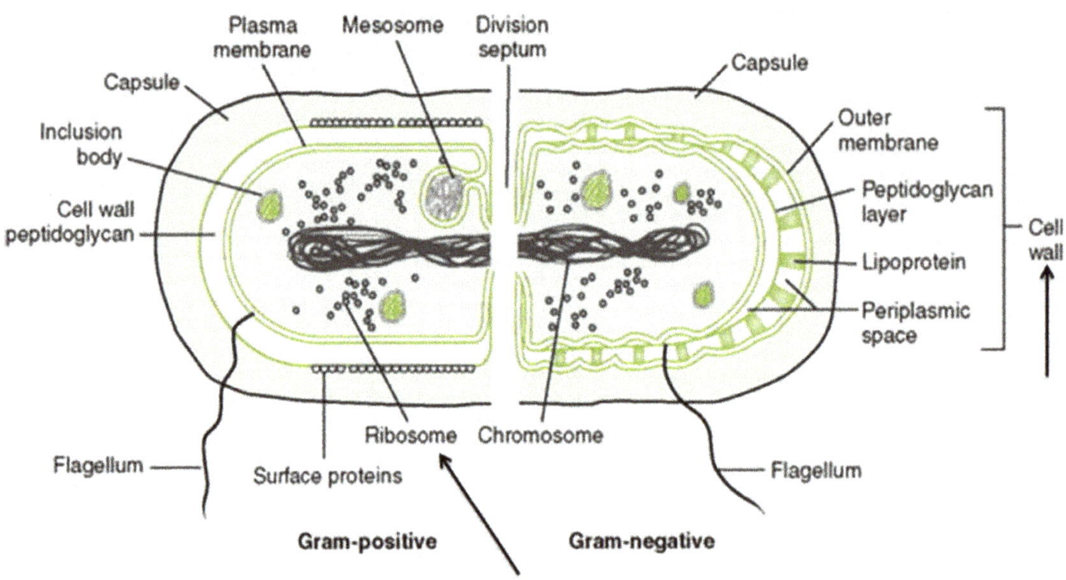

a) Identify the structure of the microorganism shown in the diagram shown above
b) What drugs act at the site specified in the diagram (cell wall, nucleus, ribosomes,)

17)

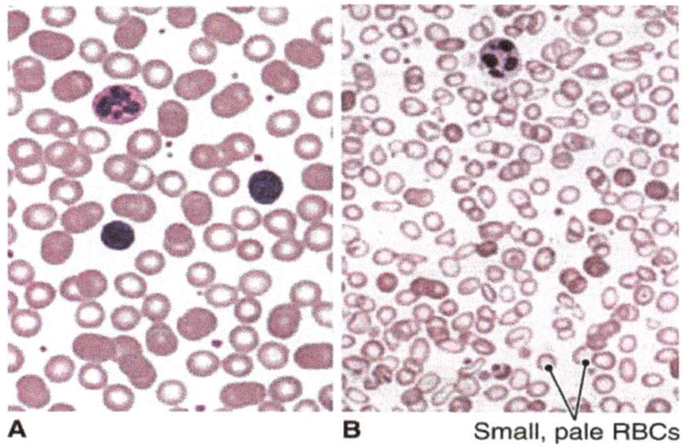

a) Identify the clinical condition based on the peripheral blood smear shown above

b) Name the drugs to treat the condition

18)

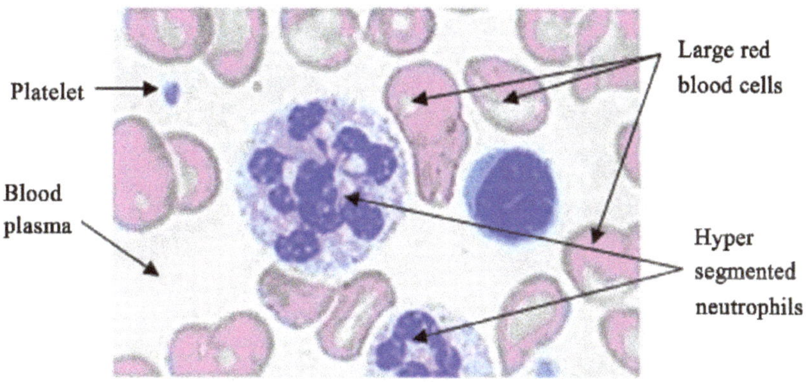

a) Identify the clinical condition based on the peripheral blood smear shown above

b) Name the drugs to treat the condition

19)

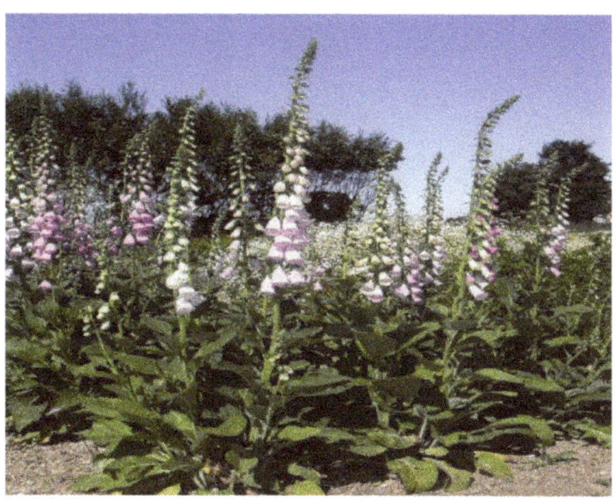

a) Identify the plant shown in the diagram which is a rich source of a potent cardiotonic drug

b) Mention the cardiac action of the drug derived from it

20)

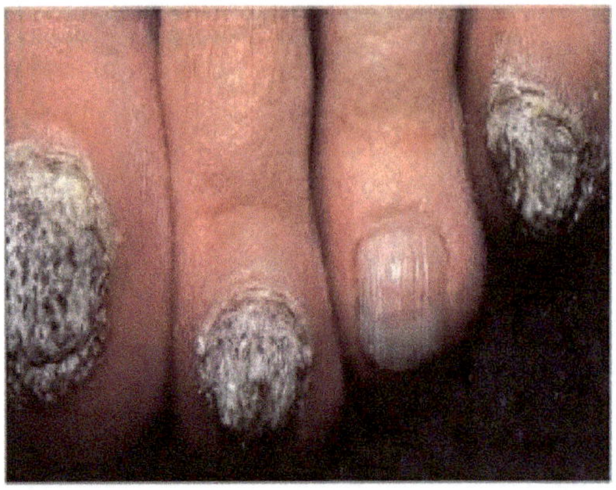

a) Identify the clinical condition based on the presentation as shown above
b) Mention the drugs to treat the condition

21)

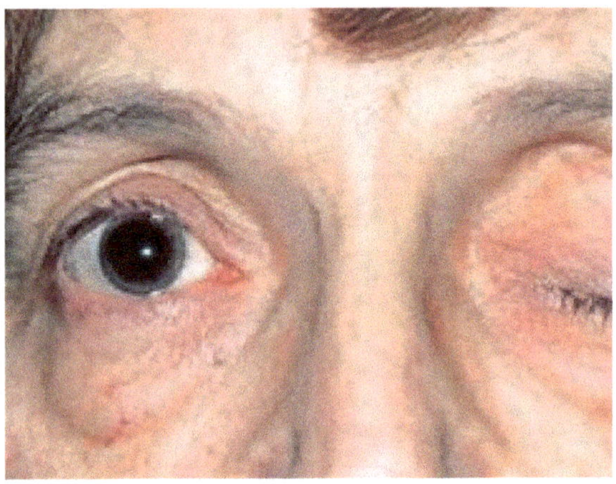

a) Identify the clinical condition of a patient as shown in the above diagram
b) Name the drugs used to treat the condition

22)

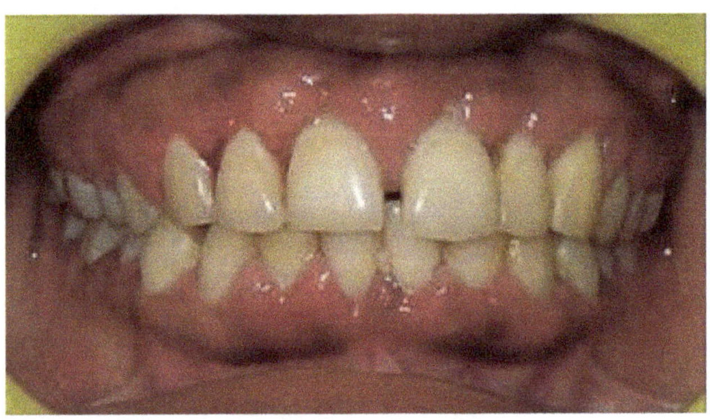

a) Identify the changes seen in the gums of a patient as shown above
b) What drugs could have produced the affect?

23)

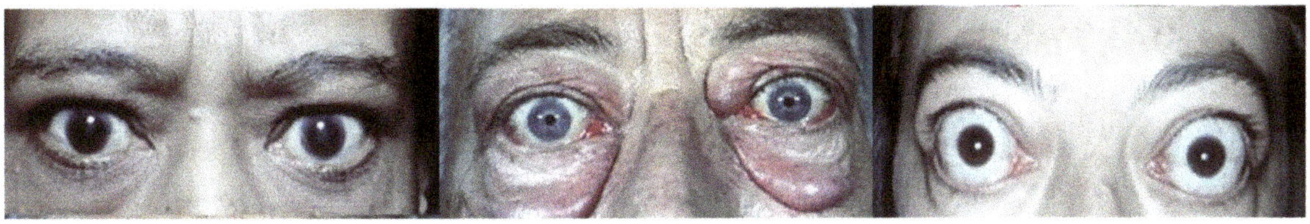

a) Identify the facial features of a patient as shown in the diagram and name the clinical condition
b) Name two drugs to treat the condition

24)

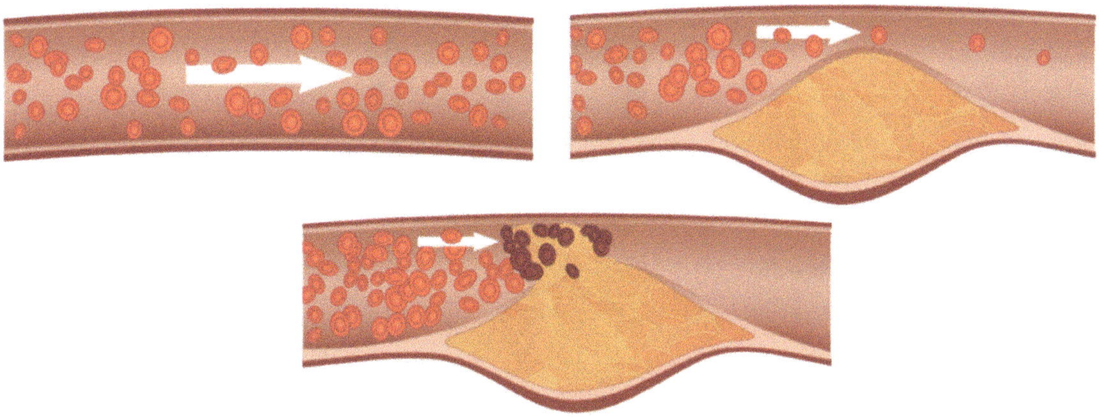

a) Identify the changes seen in the intimal layers of an artery
b) What clinical conditions could be associated with the changes?
c) What drugs could be given to prevent the changes?

25)

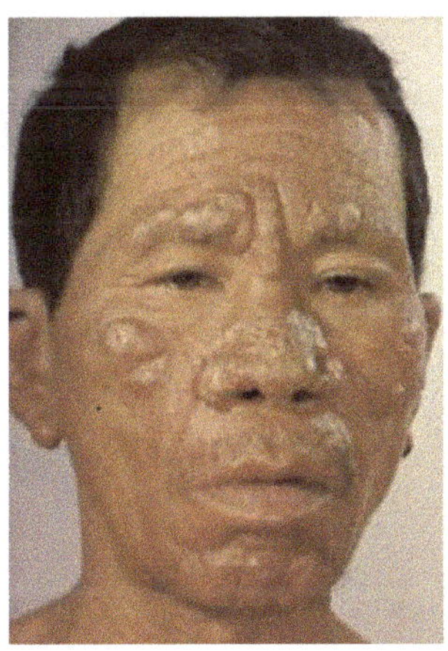

a) Identify the clinical condition of a patient based on the facial features as shown above
b) Name the drugs used in the combination therapy to treat the condition

26)

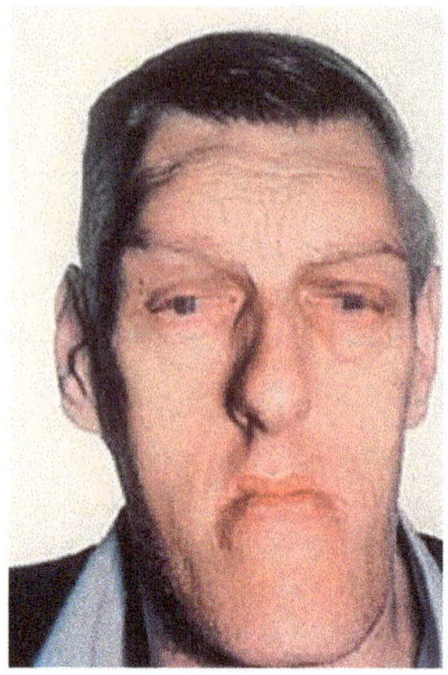

a) Identify the clinical condition of a patient based on the facial features as shown above
b) Name the drugs used to treat the condition

27)

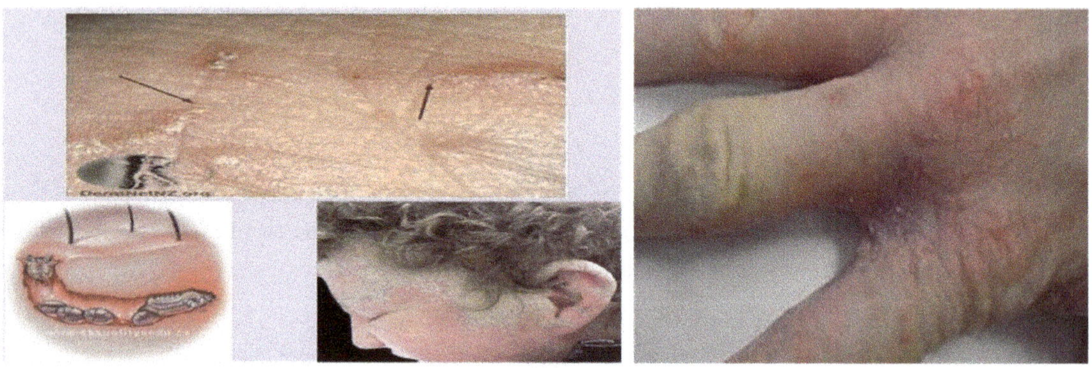

a) Identify the clinical condition of a patient based on the features seen in the skin and web spaces
b) Name two effective drugs to treat the condition

www.ingramcontent.com/pod-product-compliance
Ingram Content Group UK Ltd.
Pitfield, Milton Keynes, MK11 3LW, UK
UKHW061537190726
13845UKWH00006B/136

9 789348 734907